SIGHT AND INSIGHT IN GENESIS

Hebrew Bible Monographs, 56

SIGHT AND INSIGHT IN GENESIS

A SEMANTIC STUDY

Talia Sutskover

SHEFFIELD PHOENIX PRESS

2013

Published by Sheffield Phoenix Press
Department of Biblical Studies, University of Sheffield
45 Victoria Street
Sheffield S3 7QB

www.sheffieldphoenix.com

A CIP catalogue record for this book
is available from the British Library

Typeset by Forthcoming Publications
Printed by Lightning Source

ISBN 978-1-907534-94-2
ISSN 1747-9630

CONTENTS

Preface vii
Acknowledgments xi
Abbreviations xiii

Chapter 1
INTRODUCTION 1
1.1. Some Points Concerning Methodology and Concepts 4
1.2. The Structure of the Sight Field 11
1.3. Literary Aspects of the Semantic Field 19
1.4. Plot and Key-points 33
1.5. The Quantitative Aspect: The Frequency of ראה and Other Sight-Related Lexemes in Genesis 41

Chapter 2
THE CONSTITUENTS OF THE SIGHT FIELD: A DISCUSSION OF MEANINGS AND POSITIONS IN THE FIELD 43
2.1. The Nucleus of the Sight Field 44
2.2. The Centre of the Sight Field 48
2.3. Lexemes of the First Circle: Lexemes Linked Semantically to the Centre 51
2.4. Symbols in the Sight Field 67
2.5. Lexemes Which Participate Both in the Sight Field and in the Field of Cognitive Perception 70
2.6. Lexemes from Nearby Fields 74
2.7. Peripheral Lexemes 78
2.8. Place Names, Personal Names, Words Denoting Time and the Heavenly Bodies 82
2.9. Conclusion 91

Chapter 3
THE DEPLOYMENT OF THE SF IN THE INDIVIDUAL NARRATIVES 92
3.1. The Primeval History 92
3.2. The Abraham Narrative 100
3.3. The Jacob Narrative 116

3.4. The Joseph Narrative 121
3.5. Conclusion 132

Chapter 4
THE THEME OF SIGHT UNIFIES THE SECTIONS OF GENESIS 134
4.1. Diachronic Aspects of Genesis: The Division of the Book into its Parts 134
4.2. Synchronous Aspects in the Book of Genesis: Discerning Coherence 137
4.3. Levels of Sight 143
4.4. The Primeval History 145
4.5. The Abraham Narrative 150
4.6. The Jacob Narrative 157
4.7. 'Seeing the Face': A Unifying Phrase in the Jacob and Joseph Narratives 165
4.8. The Joseph Narrative 170

Chapter 5
CONCLUSIONS: DIVINE SIGHT GIVES WAY TO HUMAN SIGHT IN GENESIS 178

Bibliography 184
Index of References 195
Index of Authors 204

PREFACE

The main aim of this volume, which evolved from my PhD thesis at Tel Aviv University, is to show the dominance of the semantic field of Sight and Insight in Genesis, and how it contributes to the understanding of a principal theme in the book.

Eager to find a thesis topic, I decided to peruse the Hebrew Bible from the beginning. Although I thought I was familiar with the Genesis stories, that reading disclosed that terms relating to the performance of seeing occur frequently, and are often significant in the development of events. For instance: Adam and Eve eat from the forbidden tree of knowledge, after which they open their eyes to realize they are naked. The deluge ends with the rainbow, a visual sign, and as the narrator states, it is to be seen by human beings and by God as a reminder of the deluge. The sinners of Sodom and Gomorrah are punished by blindness; in that same story Lot's wife was punished for looking back. Canaan is not just the Land of Promise, but the Land that God wants to show Abraham. The story of the Akedah contains a lot of seeing, and the place of the revelation is named 'God sees' (ה' יראה), and there are many more. I knew all these added up to a semantic field of sight that is prominent, even dominant, in Genesis.

My analysis started then with the collection of words related to sight. Hence, after an introduction (Chapter 1) that includes a discussion of taxonomy (semantic fields, cohesion, coherence etc.), Chapter 2 is linguistic in character. In it there is a semantic discussion of the words relating to the semantic Field of Sight in Genesis, including its extension into the Field of Cognitive Perception.

When I began discussing my findings with colleagues and friends I was questioned as to their significance. Since sight is such an important and basic human sense, is it not obvious that words of sight will reoccur in any story, in all stories? Intuitively, I knew that sight and insight are not trivial and marginal but rather central to understanding the theme of Genesis. This, however, had to be proved and substantiated. I had to ask myself what textual phenomenon or phenomena impelled me to focus on lexemes of sight.

I tried to find the answer through statistical calculations. Indeed, my findings showed that the verb 'to see' in relation to the sum of all verbs in this book is higher than it is in any other book in the Bible, and also in relation to the number of verbs that appears in each book. However, since I am dealing with the phenomenon of the semantic field I had to check a field of words and not just one verb, even though it is the core of the field of Sight. But which words should be statistically analyzed, which should be chosen to represent the Field of Sight in the entire Hebrew Bible? Should synonymous verbs of sight be chosen: ראה, הביט, and השקיף? But cannot a prophet like Ezekiel enter the semantic Field of Sight by using a unique and different verb of sight, such as חזה, which does not appear at all in Genesis? Or maybe I should choose the synonymous verbs of sight ראה, השקיף and חזה, and add the nouns 'eye', 'light', and 'darkness', all connected to sight? But, then again, is it not possible that the Field of Sight is dominant in a text even though it only utilizes a small or a different selection of these words? It took time to admit that the right approach to the phenomenon of sight in Genesis is not a statistical one. After all, the narrator is a storyteller, not a mathematician. So I had to continue searching for an alternative theory that would explain my hunch regarding the importance of sight related terms in Genesis, or rather the reason why such basic verbs and nouns stand out in this particular biblical text unit.

Looking at the scholarly literature, there was Greimas with his *Structural Semantics* (1983), which includes a discussion of isotopy in texts, but I felt his terminology was too complex to describe this most straightforward textual phenomenon. There were also psycho-linguistic theories that involve computer analysis, such as Stubbs' theory (2001) about processing, but Stubbs was too theoretical and not sufficiently practical. Fortunately there was Buber, whose 'Abraham the Seer' gave me the necessary encouragement to continue my work. In his article he discusses the occurrences of the verb 'to see' in the Abraham narratives, in relation to the developing relationship between Abraham and God. Buber follows this verb from key position to key position in Abraham's life, and uncovers its thematic impact on the understanding of the narrative. I was very glad to discover Buber was with me in realizing the significance of Sight in this part of Genesis, but still I needed to justify the connection I was making between the level of words (the semantic field) and the theme. Buber had done this only in the Abraham narrative and without offering a theoretical background.

At this point, Ruqaiya Hasan's writings suited the way I wanted to describe my findings. Hasan, in *Linguistics, Language and Verbal Art* (1989) and in her work with Halliday, *Language, Context, and Text: Aspects of Language in a Social-semiotic Perspective* (1989), starts to make the connection between the level of words and levels of meaning in literature. She analyzes recurrent semantic patterns in English literature texts, and discusses the ways these patterns contribute to the understanding of the theme. Hasan's theory was exactly what was needed to bridge the gap between the phenomenon of the semantic field that on one hand concerns the level of words, but on the other hand relates to the more abstract and deep level of meaning—the theme.

Accordingly, this volume is divided into a linguistic discussion (Chapter 2), and a more literary one (Chapters 3, 4, and 5). Although there is a general introduction to the book, there are additional forwarding remarks in Chapter 3, immediately before the literary section. Chapter 3 deals with deployment of the Field of Sight in individual narratives in the four main sections of Genesis. In this Chapter I examine the occurrence of terms from the Field of Sight in specific narratives, focusing on the deployment of the Field of Sight at key points of the plots, also discussing the special rhetoric devices that accompany Sight terms and attract our attention. Chapter 4 describes how the Field of Sight is deployed in the larger units of Genesis. Here is where I clarify the way the Field of Sight contributes to the understanding of the overall theme of Genesis. Taken as a whole, this work involves a discussion regarding the level of the words (Chapter 2), and subsequently climbs up for a better view of the macro structure of the text and its overall meaning (Chapters 3, 4, and 5). Readers who want to examine linguistic aspects of the semantic field in Genesis will read Chapter 2. Readers more interested in the literary aspects of the deployment of Sight and Insight in Genesis may prefer to skip that chapter.

Chapter 5 concludes that through the semantic field of seeing in Genesis I have come to realize that many of the stories reveal a developing theme concerning divine and human sight. Genesis begins with a God interested in seeing, who is directly involved in human life but will move backstage as the narratives unfold. God does not reveal himself explicitly in the last unit of the book—the Joseph narrative. On the human level there is general development from a sensual-visual seeing, through abstract sight, to a high level of sight that is actually cognitive acknowledgment of God, or rather blind faith in him. Motifs that were analyzed as local or characteristic of certain narratives in Genesis, are now gathered and included under the theme of Sight and Insight. Such motifs include, for instance, the dream motif in the Joseph narrative, the beauty of the matriarchs, and so forth.

Section 4.6 is based on my earlier essay, 'Lexical Fields and Coherence in the Jacob Narrative', which was published in A. Brenner and F. Polak (eds.), *Performing Memory in Biblical Narrative and Beyond* (Amsterdam Studies and Religion; Sheffield: Sheffield Phoenix Press, 2009), pp. 126-39. In this section I develop and expand the discussion in my PhD concerning the Jacob narrative. In the earlier essay and in the present volume I allude to the physical phenomenon of colours (especially red and white) as connected to the Sight Field.

Section 4.8 is based on my 'The Semantic Fields of Seeing and Oral Communication in the Joseph Narrative', which was published in *JNSL* 33 (2007), pp. 33-50. Here I depart from the findings of my PhD thesis, in that not only is the Sight Field dominant in the Joseph narrative, but rather the semantic fields of Sight and Oral Communication intertwine and compose the central theme of that unit. Hence, although I find that the Sight Field is dominant throughout Genesis, additional semantic fields contribute to the construction of the themes in specific narratives, as pointed out in Chapter 1.

ACKNOWLEDGMENTS

First of all, my deep gratitude to Frank Polak, a phenomenal biblical scholar and teacher, for teaching me the patience required to develop an idea from its early stages until its final appearance on paper, and then allowing it to further develop, substantiate and mature. I am indebted to Frank for his boundless willingness to listen and discuss the ideas in this book.

I also thank Athalya Brenner for reading the manuscript and giving me important advice derived from her immense experience as a biblical scholar and as an author and editor of pivotal works in that field.

Additionally, I am indebted to Meira Polliack for her open support of the idea that the semantic field of Sight may actually be significant in Genesis. This has meant a lot to me

I am deeply thankful for the Bernhard and Rachel Speijer post-doctoral award, the Robert Bosch scholarship, the Tel Aviv University Faculty of Humanities and the Rosenberg School of Jewish Studies there for providing generous grants, all of which allowed me to pursue this research. I thank the board of *JNSL* for permitting me to use large parts of my article 'The Semantic Fields of Seeing and Oral Communication in the Joseph Narrative', published in issue no. 33 (2007), pp. 33-50. Many thanks to Sheffield Phoenix Press, Athalya Brenner, and Frank Polak for allowing me to use large parts of my essay, 'Lexical Fields and Coherence in the Jacob Narrative', published in A. Brenner and F. Polak (eds.), *Performing Memory in Biblical Narrative and Beyond* (Amsterdam Studies and Religion; Sheffield: Sheffield Phoenix Press, 2009), pp. 126-39. Many thanks to Henry Near who contributed immensely to the translation and the creation of the first draft of this manuscript. My thanks also go to David Wesley who edited articles connected to this book.

My thanks go out to my parents, Yael and Jonathan, who walked on their tip-toes every time I came to their house to work on the book. I also thank them for their great love and encouragement as well. Furthermore, on the home front, many thanks to my parents-in-law, Frieda and Ehud, for taking care of the children whenever I needed to continue to work.

Lastly, I wish to thank my husband, Ilan Sutskover, for his endless support throughout all the stages of writing this book, and for his unwavering faith that it would be completed, submitted, and published.

Abbreviations

AB	Anchor Bible
AHw	W. von Soden, *Akkadisches Handwörterbuch* (Wiesbaden: Harrassowitz, 1959–81)
AUSS	*Andrews University Seminary Studies*
BDB	Francis Brown, S.R. Driver and Charles A. Briggs, *A Hebrew and English Lexicon of the Old Testament* (Oxford: Clarendon Press, 1907)
BH	Biblical Hebrew
CAD	Ignace J. Gelb *et al.* (eds.), *The Assyrian Dictionary of the Oriental Institute of the University of Chicago* (Chicago: Oriental Institute, 1956–2007)
CPF	Cognitive Perception Field
CTJ	*Calvin Theological Journal*
DCH	D.J.A. Clines (ed.), *Dictionary of Classical Hebrew* (8 vols.; Sheffield: Sheffield Academic Press/Sheffield Phoenix Press, 1993–2011)
HALOT	L. Koehler and W. Baumgartner, *The Hebrew and Aramaic Lexicon of the Old Testament* (trans. M.E.J. Richardson; rev. W. Baumgartner and J.J. Stamm; Leiden: E.J. Brill, 1994–99)
ICC	International Critical Commentary
JANES	*Journal of Ancient Near Eastern Studies*
JCS	*Journal of Cuneiform Studies*
JNES	*Journal of Near Eastern Studies*
JNSL	*Journal of Northwest Semitic Studies*
JSOT	*Journal for the Study of the Old Testament*
JSOTSup	Journal for the Study of the Old Testament Supplement Series
JSS	*Journal of Semitic Studies*
LXX	Septuagint
MH	Mishnaic Hebrew
NIB	New International Version (UK)
NIDOTTE	W. A. VanGemeren (ed.), *New International Dictionary of Old Testament Theology and Exegesis* (5 vols.; Grand Rapids: Zondervan, 1997)
RSV	Revised Standard Version
SF	Sight Field
TDOT	G.J. Botterweck and H. Ringgren (eds.), *Theological Dictionary of the Old Testament* (15 vols.; Grand Rapids: Eerdmans, 1974–)
TynBul	*Tyndale Bulletin*
VT	*Vetus Testamentum*
VTSup	Supplements to Vetus Testamentum

Chapter 1

INTRODUCTION

Words of sight, seeing, and other lexemes designating human experience can be organized into semantic fields. The term 'semantic field' in the present work follows Lyons's definition, according to which the field is composed of lexemes between which there are defined semantic relations, whether on the paradigmatic or the syntagmatic axes (see further on §1.1.1). Close sound relations between lexemes can stress semantic relations which prevail between lexemes and draw attention to them. In Genesis, lexemes of sight and seeing, which are related by semantic and sound relations, consistently occur at key points, for example, at beginning of episodes, marking the main problem, at climaxes, and in endings. Therefore, from the point of view of the macro-structure of Genesis these lexemes connect between the level of words and plot structure. To cite several of the many examples in which Sight[1] lexemes occur at key points: the beginning of Genesis 6 in which the sons of God see human women, and take them as wives (Gen. 6.2); the opening of the story of the angels visiting Abraham (18.1, 2), and its closure (18.16); the opening of the story of Sodom and Gomorrah (19.1), and its closure (19.28); the opening of the story of Hagar and Ishmael (21.9); the opening of the story of Dinah's rape (34.1-2).

For the centrality of Sight in the broad sense we do not have to go further than the beginning of Genesis. Already in the creation story of Genesis the formula 'And God *saw* that X was good' is repeated at the end of almost all of the creation stages (Gen. 1.4, 10, 12, 18, 21, 25, 31). The first creation was the *light* (1.3-4), which belongs to the semantic field of Sight, since it is a necessary condition for the act of visual perception. Also, one of the significant incidents in the story of the Garden of Eden tells about the *opening of the eyes* of Adam and Eve; 3.7 says 'Then *the eyes* (עיני) of both

1. Following Ungerer, Schmid and Bednarek, who typographically indicate frames by small capitals in brackets, I will indicate semantic fields by using an initial capital letter; see Friedrich Ungerer and Hans-Jörg Schmid, *An Introduction to Cognitive Linguistics* (London: Longman, 2006); M.A. Bednarek, 'Frames Revisited: The Coherence-Inducing Function of Frames', *Journal of Pragmatics* 37 (2005), pp. 685-705 (689).

were opened, and *they knew* (וידעו) that they were *naked* (עירמם)'.[2] This verse alone contains three lexemes connected in various ways to the SF (= Sight Field). Since the field of Cognitive Perception is close to the SF, and sometimes verbs of Sight denote understanding, the verb 'knew' in this verse is also referred to as a SF term (see §1.1.2).

The unique status of lexemes for sight and seeing in the structure of Genesis is often highlighted by paronomasia and other sound plays, such as: 'And the man and his wife were both naked (עֲרוּמִּים), and were not ashamed. Now the serpent was more subtle (ערום) than any other wild creature…' (2.25–3.1); 'And he was afraid (ויירא), and said, "How awesome (נורא) is this place…"' (28.17); 'When Jacob learned (וירא) that there was grain in Egypt, he said to his sons, "Why do you look at one another (תתראו)"' (42.1). Genesis 2.25–3.1 illustrates the use of the homonyms ערום, ערומים, and the rest of the instances a recurrence of the sounds of resh and aleph.

Such occurrences of sight-related lexemes add up to a textual pattern. Their placing at key points and the semantic value and sound-plays that accompany them, assist in establishing a dual role: they serve as meaningful signs in their immediate textual unit, but they also contribute to the deeper meaning of the text, that is, its theme. My point of departure here is a modification of Hasan's work. Hasan[3] recognizes three levels of meaning at which a text can be understood: (1) a basic level that enables a reader to paraphrase a text; (2) a symbolic level, which is based on the notion that some words in a text, if they recur in some foregrounded patterns, can be understood both literally and metaphorically;[4] (3) The theme of the text is considered the deepest level of meaning, and is constituted by making a higher generalization of the word patterns which form the second level of meaning.

Hasan's main interest is finding links between linguistic patterns, the thematic meaning of the text, and its extra-textual significance. This is what I try to do in this work. I will take the semantic field of Sight, trace specific patterns and establish their dual role as carriers of immediate contextual meaning, and as 'structural blocks' for the development of the overall theme of Genesis. I shall show that lexemes of the dominant semantic field of Sight function as mediators between the word level and the abstract theme level.

2. All citations in this book are taken from the RSV, unless otherwise indicated.

3. Ruqaiya Hasan, *Linguistics, Language, and Verbal Art* (Oxford: Oxford University Press, 1989), pp. 94-99.

4. Hasan denotes this level 'the symbolic articulation'. By using this term Hasan does not refer to a metaphoric meaning other than the basic referential meaning, but to a concurrent second function of the word, representing an insight connected to the general interpretation of the text.

It must be admitted that not every occurrence of Sight-related words is thematically meaningful; nevertheless, even if some lexical Sight items appear at less significant positions, they still contribute to the general cohesion and coherence of their text units.[5]

The structure of this book follows the dual role attributed to the Sight lexemes in Genesis. The book consists of two main parts: the first part is of a linguistic character and the second has more of a literary-thematic nature. Chapter 2 deals individually with each of the lexemes included in the SF, discussing their semantic description, and answering such questions as why they are included in the field, and how they are related to the core of the field, which is the verb ראה (see). After the introduction and Chapter 2, the second part of the book, as of Chapter 3 on, is concerned with the application of the theory of semantic fields to a literary text, focusing on the combination of lexemes from the SF at key points in the individual stories, and their contribution to the design of the overall theme of Genesis.

The analysis of the SF in Chapters 3 and 4 will follow the widely accepted division of Genesis into four main units: the Primeval History (Gen. 1–11); the Abraham Cycle (12–25.18); the Jacob Narrative (25.19–36); and the Joseph Narrative (37–50).

A specific factor that always demands consideration is the nature of the object in sight: is the object seen as a concrete object in the world; is it an abstract object; is it a person or is it God himself being seen? Following Sight lexemes at key points in the Genesis units reveals a gradual development in the Sight theme. This development is manifest in two spheres: *the divine sphere and the human sphere*. Four major levels of sight may be defined, based on a close relationship between the SF and the field of Cognitive Perception, with the notion that the same verbs denoting the concrete act of sight often also indicate cognitive perception. The four developmental levels are (see a more extensive discussion at §4.3):[6]

1. Low-level sight, which includes visual perception of concrete objects (e.g. Gen. 8.5).
2. Intermediate-level sight, an act of visual perception involving cognitive insight, or when terms of seeing carry the meaning of cognitive insight (Gen. 30.1). In this example Rachel's eyes see her condition, and at the same time the verb 'saw' refers to her understanding of her difficult state.

5. The terms cohesion and coherence are discussed in §1.3.1.

6. When analyzing the field of Vision in *The French Lieutenant's Woman*, Faber and Wallhead also suggest a scale of levels of sight by which the characters are measured. For example, Mrs Poulteney is put at the bottom of the scale which they term as 'VISION/INTELLECT', whereas Sarah is located at its top (Pamela Faber and Celia Wallhead, 'The Lexical Field of Visual Perception in *The French Lieutenant's Woman* by John Fowles', *Language and Literature* 4 [1995], pp. 127-44 [132]).

3. High-level sight, sight that involves the perception of God in a concrete-visual manner, but at the same time the character expresses recognition that an event involving the seeing of God has taken place (Gen. 28.16-17).
4. Highest-level sight, includes the perception of God and insight as to his providence in an abstract manner, that has nothing to do with the concrete sense of sight. Highest-level seeing is the belief in God without him actually revealing himself directly or indirectly to the character's eyes (Gen. 50.20). In Genesis such an intellectual perception of God may be expressed not by lexemes from the SF, but by an explicit statement that the character recognizes the presence of God in the world and that he/she believes in him without question.

Throughout the literary analysis of Genesis, in search for Sight patterns, I analyze the relationship between divine and human sight, and show the development detected within these spheres as well.

1.1. *Some Points Concerning Methodology and Concepts*

1.1.1. *A Working Definition of the Concept 'Semantic Field'*

It was not easy to find a working definition of the term 'semantic field', first of all since there is a large variety of terms corresponding this term, which were put to use since Trier's (1934) terminology of '*Wortfeld*' (lexical field) and '*Sinnfeld*' (conceptual field) and Ipsen's (1924) and Porzig's (1934) term '*Bedeutungsfeld*' (semantic field) were coined.[7]

Other terms that have been put to use especially since the 1970s are frames (Fillmore), schemas, categories, scenes, and prototypes.[8]

7. Jost Trier, 'Das sprachliche Feld: eine Auseinandersetzung', *Neue Jahrbücher für Wissenschaft und Jugenbildung* 10 (1934), pp. 428-49. Trier explains the general notion of the linguistic field, discussing the theories of Porzig, Ipsen, and others. Also see Trier, 'Sprachliche Felder', in Jost Trier, A. van der Lee and O. Rechmann, *Aufsätze und Vorträge zur Wortfeldtheorie* (The Hague: Mouton, 1973), pp. 93-109 (95-97); G. Ipsen, 'Der alte Orient und die Indogermanen', in J. Friedrich (ed.), *Stand und Aufgaben der Sprachwissenschaft: Festschrift für Streitberg* (Heidelberg: C. Winter, 1924), pp. 200-37 (225); W. Porzig, 'Wesenhafte Bedeutungsbeziehungen', *Beiträge zur deutchen Sprache und Literature* 58 (1934), pp. 70-97 (85, 89).

8. A comprehensive survey of scholarship concerning these terms can be found in Brigitte Nerlich and David D. Clarke, 'Semantic Fields and Frames: Historical Explorations of the Interface between Language, Action, and Cognition', *Journal of Pragmatics* 32 (2000), pp. 125-50. According to the historical survey of Nerlich and Clarke on these terms, Trier and Weisgerber represent 'harder' forms of the semantic field theory—harder than Ipsen's 'softer' idea of a group of words which together form a unit of meaning. Trier and his followers needed meaning to be studied more structurally. Ipsen pointed out that semantic fields are rarely closed entities. The prototype theory is

Since I am applying the theory to the biblical text, in trying to understand the theme and meaning of its units, I need to posit a clear definition that can be used. Hence the definition that lies as a basis for my work is Lyons's, which synthesizes Trier's and Porzig's notions. In trying to clarify the terms, Lyons explains what a conceptual field is. He speaks of the concept of colour:

> The substance of colour is...a conceptual area (Sinnbezirk); it becomes a conceptual field (Sinnfeld) by virtue of its structural organization, or articulation, by particular language-systems.[9]

Then he continues to elucidate this 'structural organization':

> The set of lexemes in any one language-system which cover the conceptual area and by means of the relations of sense which hold between them, give structure to it is a lexical field.

Lyons continues his discussion by stressing the importance of Porzig's notion of 'syntagmatic relations'. By syntagmatic relations Porzig generally referred to the relationships holding within syntagms typically composed of a noun and a verb or a noun and an adjective, such as 'dog' and 'bark' and 'hair' and 'blond'.[10] In Lyons's view, Trier's paradigmatic relations and Porzig's syntagmatic relations must be incorporated to create a satisfactory theory of lexical structure. In his general evaluation of the theory of semantic fields he finally specifies his notion of a semantic field:

> Lexemes and other units that are semantically related, whether paradigmatically or syntagmatically, within a given language-system can be said to belong to, or to be members of, the same (semantic) field.[11]

According to Lyons, the main sense relations of the paradigmatic axis are: synonymy, antonymy, and hyponymy. In addition, I take into account other

described as a bridge between older pre-structuralist field theories and modern field theories of fields and frames. During the 1970s the idea of frames had very much been in the air, finding its basis on social interaction and human experience, not always deriving from literary corpora. Fillmore's frame theory studies the relations between a verb and the syntagmatic components to which it can be related. Schank and Abelson used the terms 'role' and 'script', such as the restaurant script (Roger C. Schank and Robert P. Abelson, *Scripts, Plans, Goals, and Understanding* [Hillsdale, NJ: Erlbaum, 1977]. Bednarek provides a table with the definitions of the term 'frame' and the related terms: scene, script, schema and scenario (Bednarek, 'Frames Revisited', pp. 686-87).

9. J. Lyons, *Semantics* (Cambridge: Cambridge University Press, 1977), pp. 253-54; Porzig, 'Wesenhafte Bedeutungsbeziehungen', pp. 70-97 (85, 89).

10. Lyons, *Semantics*, p. 261.

11. Lyons, *Semantics*, p. 268. The brackets appear in the original text. Lyons continues there: 'A lexical field is therefore a paradigmatically and syntagmatically structured subset of the vocabulary'.

common semantic relations such as instrumentality and conditional relations. I also apply Lakoff's theory of schematic relations (see below).[12] Sweetser's notion of the connection between concrete vision and abstract insight, as will be discussed below, gives me the freedom to include lexemes from the field of Cognitive Perception.[13] Metaphorical extensions such as meronymy may also serve as a criterion for including a lexeme in the field.[14] This is the case for the lexemes 'face' and 'eye', which are connected by meronymy, since the eye is part of the face and can in some contexts represent it, as for example in Isa. 5.21 (see the Hebrew text).

As to additional sense relations, Lakoff, in his book concerning the cognitive phenomenon of categorization, states that in some cases image schemas lead to the inclusion of a word in a certain category. For example, the Japanese classifier *hon* applies to long thin objects such as sticks, pencils, and ropes. But *hon* can be extended to less representative cases such as hits in baseball. The reason for this is that when a baseball is hit, it forms a trajectory, that is, it traces a long thin path along which a solid object travels with force. The image in which the ball travels is a *hon* image—long and thin.[15] In accordance with Lakoff's theory of the image schema, I apply the abstract schema—'the perception of images by the mind'—to sense-visual perception. Due to this abstract schema, the SF is extended to include the verb 'to dream' and the noun 'dream', as shall be discussed further on.

In the SF there is a group of words which belong to it because their semantic definition consists of the schema 'objects which fulfill their function by being seen', for example, the mark of Cain, or the rainbow.

All in all, the definition of the term 'semantic field' applied here is based on the more classical notion of Lyons's lexical field, adding concepts introduced by Lakoff and Johnson into cognitive linguistics, and other sense relations.[16]

12. G. Lakoff, *Women, Fire and Dangerous Things: What Categories Reveal about the Mind* (Chicago: University of Chicago Press, 1987), pp. 104-105, and see the discussion further on.

13. Eva Sweetser, *From Etymology to Pragmatics: Metaphorical and Cultural Aspects of Semantic Structure* (Cambridge: Cambridge University Press, 1990).

14. On the term 'meronymy', see M.A.K. Halliday and R. Hasan, *Language, Context, and Text: Aspects of Language in a Social-Semiotic Perspective* (Oxford: Oxford University Press, 1989), p. 81. Murphy divides the notion of meronymy into part–whole relations, referred to as meronymy, and its converse, whole–part relations, referred to as holonymy (M. Lynne Murphy, *Semantic Relations and the Lexicon* [Cambridge: Cambridge University Press, 2003], pp. 230-35).

15. Lakoff, *Women, Fire and Dangerous Things*, pp. 104-105.

16. These modifications suit my method well, without needing to turn to Fillmore's frame semantics, which call for a syntactic analysis of the category of Sight, an analysis which is unnecessary and uncalled for in the present research. In this work I take Trier's

Moreover, since I am analyzing the semantic field in a text of literary art, and not just the abstract structure of the field in language, the context may offer lexemes with sound resemblance to obvious members of the field. Thus lexemes with sound resemblance to constituents of the field are included. In most cases these kinds of sound resemblances have been discussed by ancient and modern exegetes. One such case is the sound resemblance between the place name Moriah (Gen. 22.2) and the root ראה (see), which has been acknowledged by ancient translations such as Symmachus, who offers τῆς ὀπτασὶας and *visionis* of the Vulgate.

Bednarek, in her discussion on frames, admits that quite often a feature in the frame can be a sub-frame in itself.[17] The same can be said about lexemes of the semantic field. For example, the lexeme 'to cover' (כסה) is analyzed by Balentine as an individual semantic field, but here it is considered as a constituent in the SF.[18]

However, it needs to be pointed out that Ullmann, Lyons and Lakoff, analyze lexical fields or categories in a search for word meanings or in trying to understand the structure of a certain field. They are not interested in the connection between the semantic field, text coherence and plot, which is the interest of the present work.

Several lexical fields in the Hebrew Bible have been discussed and analyzed by biblical scholars: Donald analyses the semantic field of Folly in Proverbs, Job, Psalms, and Ecclesiastes;[19] Sawyer discusses the field of

notion and Lyons's method and contextualize them with the notion of frame semantics in that the *context* and the *situation* of the word are part of its meaning. In this work I chose to work with the term 'semantic field', which is older than the concept of 'frame', since, put in Bednarek's words, 'there is no unified frame theory with specific terms and definitions' (Bednarek, 'Frames Revisited', pp. 686-87). Although definitions of the term 'semantic field' also vary from scholar to scholar the notion of semantic relations usually sees links between the lexemes, and enables a fairly clear-cut working definition. While concepts such as 'frame', 'scene' and 'script' can be considered as developments of the old concepts, the concept of semantic fields has never stopped being used, side-by-side with these parallel concepts. See Richard E. Grandy, 'In Defense of Semantic Fields', in E. LePore (ed.), *New Directions in Semantics* (London: Academic Press, 1987), pp. 259-80; Tamar Sovran, *Semantic Fields: A Linguistic-Philosophical Study of Meaning Relations* (Jerusalem: The Hebrew University Magnes Press, 2000 [Hebrew]); Grzegorz A. Kleparski and Angelina Rusinek, 'The Tradition of Field Theory and the Study of Lexical Semantic Change', *Zeszytynaukowe Uniwersytetu Rzeszowskiego* 47 (2007), pp. 188-205.

17. Bednarek, 'Frames Revisited', p. 691.

18. Samuel E. Balentine, *The Hidden God: The Hiding of the Face of God in the Old Testament* (Oxford: Oxford University Press, 1983).

19. T. Donald, 'The Semantic Field of "Folly" in Proverbs, Job, Psalms, and Ecclesiastes', *VT* 13 (1963), pp. 285-92.

Salvation in the Bible;[20] McAlpine, the field of Sleep—divine and human;[21] Brenner speaks of the field of Colours in the Hebrew Bible and in Late Hebrew, and of the field of Humour in the Hebrew Bible. She also discusses the classification and gendering of terms of love, desire and sexual activity in the Hebrew Bible.[22] Kaddari writes of lexemes of Obligation in the Dead Sea Scrolls.[23] With a focus that is mainly linguistic, the significance of these works lies in the applying of a linguistic method to the biblical text. Beuken has introduced a literary use in the opening of Job,[24] and Polak discusses the contribution of the semantic field to narrative cohesion.[25] Malul discusses the semantic overlap between the fields of Knowledge, Control and Sex in the Hebrew Bible, and Avrahami discusses the categories of the senses, depicting the differences between the traditional Aristotelian model of the five-senses, and the perception of the senses in the Hebrew Bible.[26] Van Wolde analyzes the 'cognitive domains' of biblical terms such as טמא (contaminate).[27] Many of these scholars have arrived at cultural generalizations concerning the authors and origin of the texts.

Kaddari concludes that the role of the semantic field is to organize human experience; regarding the entire system of language, he says the following: 'Language is not just a mirror image of the world outside of it, but it designs

20. J.F.A. Sawyer, *Semantics in Biblical Research: New Methods of Defining Hebrew Words for Salvation* (London: SCM Press, 1972).

21. Thomas McAlpine, *Sleep, Divine and Human in the Old Testament* (JSOTSup, 38; Sheffield: JSOT Press, 1987).

22. Athalya Brenner, *Colour Terms in the Old Testament* (JSOTSup, 21; Sheffield: JSOT Press, 1982); 'On the Semantic Field of Humour, Laughter and the Comic in the Old Testament', in Y.T. Radday and A. Brenner (eds.), *On Humour and the Comic in the Hebrew Bible* (Sheffield: Almond Press, 1990), pp. 39-58; and *The Intercourse of Knowledge: On Gendering Desire and 'Sexuality' in the Hebrew Bible* (Leiden: Brill, 1997).

23. M.Z. Kaddari, *Semantic Fields in the Language of the Dead Sea Scrolls* (Jerusalem: Kiryath Sepher, 1968 [Hebrew]).

24. Willem A.M. Beuken, 'Job's Imprecation as the Cradle of a New Religious Discourse: The Perplexing Impact of the Semantic Correspondences between Job 3, Job 4–5 and Job 6–7', in Willem A.M. Beuken (ed.), *The Book of Job* (Leuven: Leuven University Press, 1994), pp. 41-78.

25. Frank Polak, *Biblical Narrative: Aspects of Art and Design* (Jerusalem: Mosad Bialik, 1999 [Hebrew]), pp. 90-106.

26. Meir Malul, *Knowledge, Control and Sex: Studies in Biblical Thought, Culture and Worldview* (Tel-Aviv: Archaeological Center Publication, 2002); Yael Avrahami, *The Senses of Scripture: Sensory Perception in the Hebrew Bible* (LHBOTS 545; New York: T. & T. Clark, 2012).

27. E.J. van Wolde, *Reframing Biblical Studies: When Language and Text Meet Culture, Cognition, and Context* (Winona Lake, IN: Eisenbrauns, 2009), pp. 206-353.

this world, and it is used as an outline for the spiritual activities of its user'.[28] From the large variety of words belonging to the field of Obligation, he also learns how great an interest the society of the Judean Desert had in that subject.[29] According to Sovran, the synchronic study of different semantic fields in Hebrew and in other languages teaches about preferences and needs, whether implicit or explicit, of the users of the different languages.[30] Moreover, she calls attention to the importance of semantic fields for understanding the processes of perception: 'The semantic field functions as a powerful means, which can expose hidden linguistic intuitions and systems of language and perception'.[31] One of Berlin and Kay's conclusions in their study on colour terms is that the vocabularies in which only a small number of colour terms appeared were typical of speakers of relatively undeveloped technological cultures, whereas vocabularies that contained a large number of lexical terms were typical of speakers of developed technological cultures.[32] So, although we all see the same shades of colours, we express them according to the terms our culture imposes on us. Donald agrees that the field theory can contribute to the understanding of the 'history of ideas and civilization'.[33] Brenner, in her work concerning the field of Humour in the Bible, also stresses the extra-linguistic effects of the semantic field.[34]

These works supply a point of departure for my work. To the best of my knowledge, no systematic analysis of the semantic field of Sight in Genesis has so far been done. Moreover, previous works on semantic fields focus mainly on semantic relations, whereas my method takes the description forward in systematically linking sound plays and paronomasia to the analysis of the semantic field. This would mean that my mapping of the field would both follow previous works and differ from them. Once the structure of the field is established, I take another step forward with the application of additional linguistic and literary textual features, such as plot structure, and the concepts of coherence and cohesion. Ultimately the goal is to have a better understanding of a central theme of Genesis, and like other scholars I am looking for the added bonus of learning through words/fields about human world view, culture and experience.

28. Kaddari, *Semantic Fields*, p. 13.

29. Menahem Z. Kaddari, 'Semantic Fields in the Language of the Dead Sea Scrolls' (Hebrew), *Leshonenu* 29 (1965), pp. 226-37 (236).

30. Tamar Sovran, 'Exploring the Semantic Field of the Positive' (Hebrew), in Shimon Sharvit (ed.), *Studies in Ancient and Modern Hebrew: In Honour of M.Z. Kaddari* (Ramath-Gan: Bar-Ilan University, 1999), pp. 375-81 (381).

31. Sovran, *Semantic Fields*, p. 11.

32. Brent Berlin and Paul Kay, *Basic Color Terms: Their Universality and Evolution* (Berkeley, CA: University of California Press, 1969), p. 104.

33. Donald, 'The Semantic Field of "Folly"', p. 285.

34. Brenner, 'On the Semantic Field of Humour', p. 44.

The semantic field of Sight has been detected in a non-biblical text, in John Fowles's novel *The French Lieutenant's Woman*. In their analysis of this novel, Faber and Wallhead discuss the significance of tracing a foregrounded lexical field in a text, and their words are of great importance to the understanding of the present work, which focuses on the SF underlying Genesis as a whole:

> We propose that semantic field theory can also be applied in literary analysis. A novel is a microcosm constructed by its author out of lexical items which he or she fits together to create the illusion of 'reality', or self-conscious fiction. In the same way that we, as discriminating perceivers, highlight certain parts of our conceptual system by lexicalizing them, an author when writing a novel also deliberately highlights those areas of the lexicon which are most significant within the context of the fictional world being created.
>
> It would thus seem logical that the analysis of the use of particular segments of lexical fields and their metaphorical extension selected or highlighted within the work of a writer should provide valuable information about how and why that writer has constructed this particular fictional universe.[35]

The reason they give for their decision to focus on the field of Visual Perception is that 'there is obvious foregrounding of terms of visual perception'.[36] They suggest that the field serves five functions, of which I will mention two. The first function is that the Vision field is an instrument to define the Victorian age as an age of appearances. The second function is the exploitation of the metaphor proposed by Lakoff and Johnson—'Seeing is Understanding'—in the characterization.

These two functions of the Vision field found in *The French Lieutenant's Woman* are relevant to the present work in that Faber and Wallhead too have pointed at a higher and more abstract generalization which is constructed from the lexemes of the SF. This abstract generalization is what I call, following Hasan, the theme of the narrative. If the dominant semantic field of most of the stories of Genesis is concerned with human and divine sight and the relations between them, it can tell us something about the social and cultural values of the people behind the texts. It is therefore interesting to try to construct an accurate picture of the way this theme develops through the units of Genesis as a whole.

1.1.2. *Sight Includes Visual Perception as Well as Cognitive Perception*

The term 'Sight' signifies a wide range of meaning, including both visual and mental perception. 'To see' means to see visually, but also to perceive mentally. Sweetser, in her work on the terms of the sense of sight, maintains that in Indo-European languages there is a close relationship between the

35. Faber and Wallhead, 'The Lexical Field', p. 128.
36. Faber and Wallhead, 'The Lexical Field', p. 128.

category of sight and the category of cognitive perception.[37] For this reason there are many examples of words that belong to the category of sight in the sensual-visual sense eventually adopting the meaning of cognitive perception; examples are the verb 'to see' and adjectives such as 'brilliant' and 'bright'. This is shown to be true in Biblical Hebrew, and it affects the decision of determining the borders of the SF. To draw a clear line between the SF and the Cognitive Perception field (= CPF) would be artificial. Therefore in building the SF, lexemes with CPF features included in their meaning, such as חפשׂ (to look for), הכיר (to recognize), are also taken into account. Van der Merwe stresses that categories tend to have 'fuzzy borders',[38] whereas according to Sovran, 'Semantic fields are also based on an arbitrary decision of the linguist as to where to end the investigation of their structure'.[39] Hence, here I follow other scholars in allowing myself a relative amount of freedom in deciding upon the borders of my categorization.

1.2. *The Structure of the Sight Field*

This study considers the SF in Genesis, and it may be asked where its borders are to be drawn without entering too far into neighbouring semantic fields.[40] As seen in the quotation given above, Sovran says that in addition to the natural aspect which exists in defining the structure of the field, there is a certain degree of arbitrariness in drawing its border, a procedure which at times involves decisions and limitations determined by the scholar.[41] In her article on the principles of categorization, Rosch discusses the boundaries of categories, and distinguishes between cases in which there is no disagreement about whether a word belongs to a category, as against borderline cases. She prefaces the discussion with an observation also made by the philosopher Wittgenstein, that categories do not necessarily have clear boundaries; nevertheless, they can be intuitively perceived.[42]

37. Sweetser, *From Etymology to Pragmatics*.

38. C.H.J. van der Merwe, 'Lexical Meaning in Biblical Hebrew and Cognitive Semantics: A Case Study', *Biblica* 87 (2006), pp. 85-95 (88). See also W. Croft and D.A. Cruse, *Cognitive Linguistics* (Cambridge: Cambridge University Press, 2004), pp. 89-91.

39. Sovran, *Semantic Fields*, p. 24 (my translation).

40. For an analysis of the sense of sight and the other senses as attested in the Old Testament, see Avrahami, *The Senses of Scripture*. According to Avrahami's findings the Old Testament acknowledges more than the five senses known to modern Western thought. To the five senses she adds the senses of movement, talking, and perhaps eating (Avrahami, *The Senses of Scripture*, pp. 1-17, 109-12).

41. Sovran, *Semantic Fields*, pp. 24-25.

42. Eleanor Rosch, 'Principles of Categorization', in E. Rosch and B.B. Lloyd (eds.), *Cognition and Categorization* (Hillsdale, NJ: Erlbaum, 1978), pp. 27-48 (35-36); L. Wittgenstein, *Philosophical Investigations* (trans. G.E.M. Anscombe; Oxford: Basil Blackwell, 1958), pp. 31e-34e.

In Balentine's discussion of the field Hide, and particularly contexts of hiding the face of God, he cannot avoid also discussing lexemes from neighbouring fields. Balentine creates a division of lexemes into two different fields: the field Hide, and the field Cover. Thus, in addition to the central collocation in the field Hide—hide (סתר) + face (פנים)—he discusses the lexemes כסה, עלף, and כפר, all of which mean 'cover' and belong, according to his standpoint, to the field of Cover, Veil.[43] Commenting on the borders of a field and the unavoidable necessity of dealing with lexemes from neighbouring fields, he says:

> Semantic fields, as well as the categories which may be isolated within them remain, for the most part, inexact. In this respect the semantic field of "hide" words is quite normal. Because of this it is often the case that collocations which appear to be semantically distinctive are in fact paralleled by similar collocations in related areas. Hence it is necessary in this section to test the particularity of the collocation סתר + פנים *against a broader range of similar expressions which occur in 'hide'-related fields.*[44]

1.2.1. *The Nucleus*

Despite Rosch's acknowledgment that the borders of a semantic category are somewhat foggy, she believes, as has been noted, that some items clearly belong to a particular category, and that there are other controversial items—the border-line cases. Rosch calls the clear, without-doubt, instance of a certain word belonging to a category a 'prototype'. The SF serves as a linguistic and cognitive category, and Rosch's remarks about a component which represents the category may be applied to the verb ראה (see): 'categories tend to become defined in terms of prototypes of prototypical instances that contain the attributes most representative of items inside and least representative of items outside the category'.[45] Although Rosch is cautious about trying to identify a particular lexeme as a prototype in a particular category, in this case the verb ראה is a prototypical term in that it is the most obvious and characteristic instance in the SF.[46] Since the

43. Balentine, *The Hidden God*, pp. 14-15.

44. Balentine, *The Hidden God*, p. 14 (my emphasis).

45. Rosch, 'Principles of Categorization', p. 30.

46. Rosch claims that participants usually know what is a prototypical term in a semantic category, even in cases of categories with very fuzzy borders. A prototype will be a term which best represents most of the features included in the category. It also contains semantic features that are very different from contrastive categories. Rosch discusses studies that measure the time it takes participants to answer whether a word belongs to a certain category or not. It turns out that the fastest terms to be responded are the prototypes in their categories. However, she warns about the use of the term 'prototype': 'To speak of a prototype at all is simply a convenient grammatical fiction; what really is referred to are judgments of degree of prototypicality' (Rosch, 'Principles of Categorization', pp. 36-38, 40).

semantic definition of the SF concerns the act of seeing, the verb ראה serves as its nucleus. The noun מַרְאֶה (sight), which derives from the same root, is not as suitable as the verb ראה for constituting the representative nucleus of the category; this is because the noun does not contain the most suitable semantic features.

In the centre, and in all the categories of which the field is built, there is always a group of lexemes, and, in addition, a negative group in whose semantic definition the component '+ negative' appears. In other words, together with the verb ראה there are lexemes or syntagms whose meaning is the negation of sight: לא ראה (did not see), which does not constitute a separate class; the lexeme סנורים, which in the context of Gen. 19.11 means strike of blindness; and the phrase כהות עיניים (27.1), which refers to weakness of sight, to the point of blindness.

1.2.2. *The Centre*
The strongest semantic link to this nucleus is that of synonyms. Other verbs of sight have a synonymous connection to the verb ראה and all these verbs together form the centre of the SF. The verbs found in Genesis which form the nucleus and centre of the SF are ראה, נבט, צפה, שׁעה, שׁאה, שׁקף.[47]

Lexemes are linked semantically to the centre in the following manner. I shall now present a short survey of the structure of the semantic field. A detailed account of the links and the lexemes will be given in Chapter 2.

1.2.3. *Lexemes of the First Circle*
1.2.3.1. As has been noted, lexemes are linked to the centre as a result of various semantic connections. In the first group lexemes are linked to the centre because their semantic definition includes the schema 'an image of a thing which is perceived by the mind':[48] מַרְאֶה (sight, appearance, vision); מחזה (vision), חלם (to dream), חלום (dream), מַרְאָה (vision, as means of revelation),[49] דמות (shape, likeness), צלם (likeness), תֹּאַר (appearance, form).[50]

1.2.3.2. The instrument for seeing: עין (eye). This category also includes various phrases which consist of the lexeme עין, such as מצא חן בעיני (found favour with...), and נשא עיניים (lifted the eyes). The construct ארבות השמים, which is taken as a metaphor for eyes (§2.3.2.2), is also a constituent in this category.

47. On the nuances which nevertheless exist between these verbs of sight, see §2.2.
48. On the term 'schema', see G. Lakoff, *Women, Fire and Dangerous Things*, p. 104 (see also §1.1.1).
49. So BDB, p. 909.
50. All references associated with these lexemes in Genesis are treated in Chapter 2.

1.2.3.3. The necessary condition of seeing and a sufficient condition of not seeing: אור (light), חשך, חשכה, עלטה (darkness).

1.2.3.4. Lexemes whose semantic definition includes the schema: 'creating a condition for seeing', and its opposite 'creating a condition for not seeing'. Examples for the first: גלה (to uncover), ערוה (nakedness), ערום (to be naked, exposed, bare), מחשׂף (peeling, stripping). Examples of the negative side: חבא (to hide), כסה (to cover), כסות עינים (covering the eyes), מכסה (a covering), סתר (to hide, conceal), עלף (to cover; faint). The lexeme צעיף (wrap, veil) constitutes a sub-class in this category, since it is a means for creating conditions of not seeing.

1.2.3.5. Lexemes whose semantic definition in the given contexts contains the schema 'objects that function by being observed': אות קין (Cain's mark), קשׁת (rainbow), אות הברית (the sign of the covenant), פצלה (stripped sections of the sticks).

1.2.4. *Symbols in the Sight Field*
The lexeme נחשׁ (snake) is a term in the SF symbolizing both craftiness and, outside Genesis, death and healing. The lexeme עין in the sense of a spring of water, and מעין (spring of water), symbolize in Genesis, it is suggested, the divine presence.

1.2.5. *Lexemes of the Second Circle*
1.2.5.1. *Lexemes which Belong Both to the Sight Field and the Cognitive Perception Field.* This category includes lexemes which consist of semantic components both from the SF and from the CPF, such as: בקשׁ (to discover, find, search for), חפשׂ (to search), מצא (to reach, find), נכר (in the hiphil, to recognize).

There are three other subsidiary groups in this category. One includes lexemes of clothes and supplementary accessories which serve to identify their wearer or owner.[51] These cases involve concrete vision as well as perception. Examples of such are: Joseph's long-sleeved robe (כתנת פסים), and Judah's חותם (seal), פתיל (cord) and מטה (staff). Also included are בגד (garment, covering) and שׁני (crimson thread).

1.2.5.2. *Lexemes from the Neighbouring Fields of Cognitive Perception, Education, and Emotion.* This category mostly included lexemes from the CPF. In the case of the SF, the meanings of the verb ראה (to see), which is

51. Matthews states that clothing serves as a means of visual communication (Victor H. Matthews, 'The Anthropology of Clothing in the Joseph Narrative', *JSOT* 65 [1995], pp. 25-36 [25-26]).

located in the centre of the field, dominate two neighbouring fields: that of Sight and that of Cognitive Perception. As noted above (§1.1.2), Sweetser's study has shown that there is a natural process whereby the verb 'to see' acquires the meaning of understanding. It is important to point out that the meaning of concrete visual sight is the primary meaning of the SF, whereas the abstract meaning of cognitively perceiving is secondary, from the point of view of the diachronic development of the meanings in verbs of sight. On the synchronous level it is impossible to ignore the aspect of cognitive perception which exists in the SF, and, as a result, of a number of additional lexemes which reflect this aspect in their meaning. As a result of the synonymous relations between the verb ידע (to know) and the secondary meaning of the verb ראה, the first is included in the SF. As we shall see below, following Talmon, there are examples of exchanges between the meanings of the verbs ראה and ידע.[52] The verb חשׁב (to assume, impute, reckon) from the CPF is also part of the complex structure of the SF; this is because of its semantic propinquity to the verb ידע. There is an interesting link between the roots ידע and חשׁב, which is found, for instance in Ps. 144.3; and apart from this, the verb ראה appears in collocation with the verb חשׁב in Gen. 38.15.

Other lexemes such as זכר (to remember, name, mention), שׁכח (to forget), and פקד (to make careful inspection) also belong to fields neighbouring the SF, but the semantic component of 'cognitive perception' which they possess links them, too, to the SF.

The root ירא (fear) belongs to the field of Emotions, and the root ירה (to direct, teach) to the field of Education, which are both close to the SF. These roots also share a strong phonetic resemblance to the core root of the SF—ראה (see). Thus they are included in it because of semantic and sound propinquity.

1.2.6. *Peripheral Lexemes*

Some lexemes are peripheral to the SF, since they are linked to words from the field, which are not central in it. In a sense, they are indirectly connected to the field, that is, by the mediation of another lexeme from the field.

1.2.6.1. The lexeme ראשׁ (head) is peripheral in the SF, since it is metonymically linked with the lexeme עין (eye), from the first circle of the SF.

1.2.6.2. The lexeme פנים (face, front, surface) and the preposition פני are also considered as peripheral, but only in contexts where they appear in collocation with a verb of sight.

52. Shemaryahu Talmon, 'Synonymous Readings in the Textual Traditions of the Old Testament', *Scripta Hierosolymitana* 8 (1961), pp. 335-83 (340-42).

1.2.6.3. The lexemes אֵשׁ (fire) and לַפִּיד (torch) belong to the periphery of the SF because their basic semantic definition contains the semantic component 'light', which is a lexeme in the SF.

1.2.6.4. Another group of lexemes is addressed as peripheral, because it consists of lexemes linked through the schema 'states of consciousness which can be determined mainly by the closing or opening of the eyes of their experiencer': יקץ (to awake), ישׁן (to sleep or fall asleep), לון (to spend the night), תרדמה (deep sleep), שׁכר (be drunk). Indeed, these are cognitive states, and they primarily belong to the CPF. However, since the eyes, the instrument of sight, play a crucial role in their semantic definition, they constitute this peripheral sub-category in the SF.

1.2.6.5. In addition, I address colour terms as peripheral to the SF, since colour is the phenomenon whereby, so Brenner notes, 'energy distribution reaches the eye of the observer, is then transmitted through the observer's vision and interpreted and turned into a sensation'.[53] The involvement of the eyes is what makes the phenomenon of colour peripheral to the SF. I shall not elaborate on the Colour field since this has already been done by Brenner, and it is only peripheral to the SF.

1.2.6.6. Lastly, the term *hinneh* is also peripheral in the SF, since it sometimes presents the vision which is being seen.

1.2.7. *Names of People and Places, Words of Time and Celestial Lights*
1.2.7.1. Names of individuals and of places that include lexemes from the SF are considered as lexemes of the field. For example, the name ראובן (Reuben) includes the verb ראה (to see), and so does the name ה' יראה (God sees), which Abraham gives the mountain of the Akedah.

1.2.7.2. Another group consists of words concerning time whose semantic definition includes a connection to light or darkness: בקר (morning), יום (day), לילה (night), שׁחר (morning, the first light of the morning).

1.2.7.3. In the SF I have included the lexemes referring to the celestial objects, such as 'sun', 'moon', and 'stars', since it is explicitly said that these objects indicate the time of day, and their semantic definition includes the crucial component 'light', which is a term of the first circle.

53. Brenner, *Colour Terms in the Old Testament*, p. 3.

1.2.8. *Tables of the Categories of the Semantic Field of Sight*

Table 1. *The Nucleus of the Sight Field*

Seeing	*The negation of seeing: not-seeing*
ראה	סנורים עינים כהות

Table 2. *The Centre of the Sight Field*

נבט צפה שׁאה שׁעה שׁקף

Table 3: *Lexemes of the First Circle of the Sight Field*

<table>
<tr><td rowspan="2">The schema: ‘the image of the object which is perceived by the mind’</td><td rowspan="2">The means of seeing (+ collocations consisting of this lexeme)</td><td rowspan="2">Necessary conditions for seeing and a sufficient condition for not-seeing</td><td colspan="2">The schema: ‘creating conditions for seeing’ and its opposite: ‘creation of conditions for not-seeing’</td><td rowspan="2">The schema: ‘objects which fulfil their function by being seen’</td><td rowspan="2">Symbols in the Sight Field</td></tr>
<tr><td>(+)</td><td>(-)</td></tr>
<tr><td>מַרְאֶה
מחזה
חלם
חלום
מַרְאָה
דמות
צלם
תֹּאַר</td><td>עין
ארבות־
השמים

מצא־
חן־בעיני
נשׂא־עינים
…</td><td>אור
חשך
חשכה
עלטה</td><td>גלה
זרח
ערוה
עָרוֹם
מחשׂף
חבא
כסה</td><td>כסות־
עינים
מכסה
סתר
עלף
צעיף</td><td>אות
קשׁת
מול
פצלה</td><td>נחשׁ
עין
מעין</td></tr>
</table>

Table 4. *Lexemes of the Second Circle of the Sight Field*

<table>
<tr><td>Lexemes which participate both in the Sight Field and in the Field of Cognitive Perception</td><td colspan="3">Lexemes from nearby fields</td></tr>
<tr><td></td><td>Lexemes from the field of Cognitive Perception alone</td><td>Lexemes from the field of Emotion</td><td>Lexemes from the field Education</td></tr>
<tr><td>בקשׁ
חפשׂ
מצא
נכר</td><td>אמן
בין
זכר
חשׁב</td><td rowspan="3">ירא</td><td rowspan="3">ירה</td></tr>
<tr><td>Clothes and other supplementary appurtenances which serve to identify their owners:</td><td>ידע</td></tr>
<tr><td>בגד
כתנת פסים
שׁני, מטה, פתילים, חותם</td><td>דעת
עָרום
פקד
שׁכח</td></tr>
</table>

Table 5. *Peripheral Lexemes*

<table>
<tr><td>Lexemes connected by metonymy to one of the lexemes in closer circles, and other remote relations</td><td>Lexemes which include the semantic component 'light'</td><td>Lexemes which include the schema: 'states of consciousness which can be determined mainly by the closing or opening of the eyes of their experiencer'</td><td rowspan="2">Colour terms</td><td rowspan="2">The presentative particle הנה in specific contexts</td></tr>
<tr><td>ראשׁ
פנים
פני</td><td>אשׁ
לפיד
תנור</td><td>יקץ
ישׁן
שׁנה
לין
מלון
שׁכר
תרדמה</td></tr>
</table>

Table 6. *Place Names, Personal Names, Words Denoting Time and the Heavenly Bodies*

Place names and personal names	*Words denoting time*	*Heavenly bodies*
אור כשדים	בקר	מאור
אל ראי	יום	המאור הגדול
אלון מורה	ליל	שמש
אלוני ממרא	שחר	ירח
ארץ המוריה		המאור הקטן
באר לחי ראי		כוכב
שור		
ה' יראה		
זרח		
לוט		
ממרא		
מצפה		
עין משפט		
עינים		
ער		
ערי		
פניאל/פנואל		
ראובן		

1.3. *Literary Aspects of the Semantic Field*

The previous pages dealt with the SF as evinced in the range of lexemes in the book of Genesis. I discussed the linguistic aspects of this work, that is, matters such as the definition of the semantic field, the lexemes of which it is composed, and the semantic links which form the basis of their mutual connection in the creation of the field. We noted that the SF is constructed of a centre, composed of verbs of sight, and of a circle of lexemes linked to the centre by various semantic connections such as 'instrumentality', and 'necessary conditions for seeing', as well as a second circle of lexemes, and peripheral lexemes. An additional category is that of place names, personal names, words denoting time, and the heavenly bodies, all of which include Sight words. This linguistic investigation serves as the basis of a literary investigation. It will be recalled that at the beginning of this work I described the phenomenon of the exceptional prominence of the SF in Genesis, thanks to its frequent appearance at key junctures in the different narratives, which is often highlighted by paronomasia and other sound plays. So, the literary discussion is conducted at several levels. First of all I shall clarify the connection between the lexemes of the SF found in the narratives, and the terms cohesion, coherence, plot, and theme. Then I shall consider the evidence systematically, in order to show that there is a consistent and comprehensive phenomenon of the appearance of the SF especially at the beginning of episodes, at their end, and at climactic points.

1.3.1. *Cohesion, Coherence and Semantic Fields*

Although there are differences in opinion as to the exact definition of cohesion and coherence, cohesion is often considered as the quality which creates the primary basis of textual connectedness by explicit textual signals, whereas coherence considers connectedness to be of a cognitive nature.[54] According to Berlin, cohesion refers to the ways lexical elements in the text 'are linguistically connected within a sequence. That is, how one sentence is linked to the next and how the elements in one part of the text are connected to those in others.'[55] Coherence, on the other hand, is a matter of semantic and pragmatic relations in the text[56] and can be a product of a number of factors, some of which are outside the text itself, such as, the knowledge of the subject, the logical connection between the text's parts, and the plot. Spooren and Sanders speak of cognitive relations between clauses, such as, contrast, claim-argument, and evaluation.[57] Longacre considers the plot as a device contributing to the coherence of the text. He sees the plot as part of the underlying structure of the text, and as standing against the phenomenon of cohesion, which belongs to the surface structure.[58] Cun argues that 'coherence is attained when connectors or lexical devices represented by words or phrases make the paragraph consistent in subject and meaning'.[59] Widdowson adduces an example of a well-connected text with cohesive

54. Ted Sanders and Henk Pander Maat, 'Cohesion and Coherence: Linguistic Approaches', in K. Brown *et al.* (eds.), *Encyclopedia of Language and Linguistics* (Elsevier: London, 2006), pp. 591-95 (591). Bednarek opens her discussion concerning frames and coherence with the remark, that like the frame concept, 'coherence is a rather fuzzy notion in linguistics and there is as yet no generally accepted definition or theory of coherence' (Bednarek, 'Frames revisited', p. 692). For a list of references regarding the concepts of cohesion and coherence; see Wolfram Bublitz, Uta Lenk and Eija Ventola (eds.), *Coherence in Spoken and Written Discourse: How to Create It and How to Describe It* (Pragmatics and Beyond, 63; Amsterdam: John Benjamins, 1999), pp. 267-95.

55. Adele Berlin, 'Lexical Cohesion and Biblical Interpretation', *Hebrew Studies* 30 (1989), pp. 29-40 (29-30). See also Rachel Giora, 'Notes Towards a Theory of Text Coherence', *Poetics Today* 6 (1985), pp. 699-715. Kress speaks of cohesion as created by the 'formal elements and principles which make a collection of sentences into a text' (Gunther Kress, 'Cohesion', in Paul Cobley [ed.], *The Routledge Companion to Semiotics and Linguistics* [London: Routledge, 2001], pp. 173-74).

56. Tanya Reinhart, 'Conditions for Text Coherence', *Poetics Today* 1 (1980), pp. 161-80 (163).

57. W. Spooren and T. Sanders, 'The Acquisition Order of Coherence Relations: On Cognitive Complexity in Discourse', *Journal of Pragmatics* 40 (2008), pp. 2003-26 (2004).

58. Robert E. Longacre, *The Grammar of Discourse* (New York: Plenum Press, 1996), p. 33.

59. Antonia Cun, 'Coherence in Discourse', *The Scientific Journal of Humanistic Studies* 1 (2009), pp. 62-67 (62).

device, but which is still not coherent. The reason for this, he says, is the lack of a frame of reference, or a contextual connection.[60] Habermas and Bluck speak of referential, spatial, temporal, causal, and thematic coherence, and the extent to which a story conforms to relevant cultural models.[61]

Halliday and Hasan, in their seminal book *Cohesion in English* (1976),[62] explain cohesion as a phenomenon whereby one linguistic element can be deciphered correctly only with the help of another linguistic element. These relations between linguistic elements lead the reader to see the text as a complete unit. Thus, the term 'they' assumes something other than itself in a text, and relates to some referent mentioned before or after it. In the Hebrew Bible for instance, Gen. 1.5 reads: 'and the darkness he called Night'. In this clause the verb קרא (to call), includes the pronoun for the third person singular, and refers to God, who appears immediately before it: 'God called the light Day' (Gen. 1.5). In Gen. 30.37 we find 'Then Jacob took fresh rods of poplar and almond and plane', and immediately thereafter, in the same verse, 'and peeled white streaks in them', the prepositional phrase 'in them' (בהן) relates to the referents mentioned before it. Cohesion is usually considered to be a characteristic which is created by explicit lexical means: that is to say, by verbal and grammatical repetitions.[63]

In a later book, *Language, Context and Text* (1989), Hasan refines her view on the means of cohesion. She maintains that it is pairs of words with a semantic link between them that create cohesion between the clauses in a text. The link between two such words is called a 'cohesive tie', a term which had been already used in Hasan and Halliday's previous book, but is here developed further.

There may exist several types of cohesive ties between words. One of them is co-reference; in this case, two words relate to the same referent in the text. Such, for instance, are the connections between a noun and a pronoun referring to it which is repeated in a subsequent clause.[64] For example, in Gen. 7.16, the personal pronoun 'you' is used, 'Go forth from the ark, you and your wife, and your sons and your sons' wives with you',

60. H.G. Widdowson, *Discourse Analysis* (Oxford: Oxford University Press, 2007), pp. 41-51.

61. T. Habermas and S. Bluck, 'Getting a Life: The Emergence of the Life Story in Adolescence', *Psychological Bulletin* 126 (2000), pp. 748-69. See Ageliki Nicolopoulou, 'The Elementary Forms of Narrative Coherence in Young Children's Storytelling', *Narrative Inquiry* 18 (2008), pp. 299-325 (304).

62. M.A.K. Halliday and R. Hasan, *Cohesion in English* (London: Longman, 1976).

63. M. Canale, 'From Communicative Competence to Communicative Language Pedagogy', in J.C. Richards and R.W. Schmidt (eds.), *Language and Communication* (London: Longman, 1983), pp. 2-26.

64. Halliday and Hasan, *Language, Context, and Text*, pp. 73-74.

and Noah is mentioned in the previous verse. Both 'Noah' and 'you' refer to the same referent, and the link between them is co-referential.

Another type of connection is referred to as 'co-extension'. In this case the elements between which the connection is created belong to the same general category of meaning. This is the case, for instance, when one of two clauses contains the word 'gold' and the other 'silver'. These clauses are connected, on the basis that the terms gold and silver belong to the same group of meaning—the group of precious metals. This link is very similar to the use of a semantic field in a text. We might equally say that gold and silver belong to the same semantic field.

Hasan speaks of several types of possible semantic links which may unite elements belonging to the same group of meaning. Semantic relations such as synonymy, antonymy, hyponymy, hyperonymy, and meronymy may connect between elements belonging to the same group. In her view, silver and gold are linked by antonymic relations. Hasan refers to meronymy as part–whole relations. For instance, when the word 'root' appears in one clause, and the word 'leaf' in another, since the reader knows that these are the parts of the tree, a relationship of cohesion between the clauses is established (based on meronymy).

In addition, repetitions of the same lexical element also create meaning relations included in ties of co-extension. Here, however, as Hasan explains, there is no real relation of meaning, since the same word is repeated. Repetition of the same lexical element creates a simple link, because the same meaning is repeated again and again in the text. She states that a particular word may appear in various declensions, and in this case, too, a link of meaning between its occurrences is created.[65]

Meaning relations between words within an existing text can be broadened out when they include more than two constituents. Hasan calls the occurrence of many elements linked by different relations of meaning 'cohesive chains'. When the same element is repeated either lexically or by means of some alternative, such as a personal pronoun, an identity chain—for example, 'girl' and 'she'—is created. Many chains, however, contain lexical elements which are similar rather than identical: this is a similarity chain, such as 'go', 'walk', 'went'. In the terminology used in this book, the latter chain is a group of words which belong to the field of Walking. Similarly, the simple repetition of the same root (if we speak of Hebrew forms) also serves as a reason to include the lexemes in a semantic field.

Hasan shows that the more interaction there is between the various chains which constitute the text, the more coherent the text will be considered. The interaction takes place in the framework of the syntactical status of the

65. Halliday and Hasan, *Language, Context, and Text*, p. 81.

words in the clause. For instance, Hasan discusses a nursery tale in which the following chains appear: (a) girl, girl, girl, girl (repetition of the same word in four different clauses); (b) teddy bear, teddy bear…; (c) washed, combed, washed, brushed. Chain 'a' interacts with chain 'c', which interacts with chain 'b' in such sentences as 'The girl washed the teddy bear', 'The girl combed the teddy bear', etc. The more contact there is between the chains, the more coherent the text will be seen to be.[66] Hasan adduces an example from another text which includes two chains alongside another five, but the two have no points of contact with the other five. This text was far less coherent than the former example, and the presence of cohesive chains is the reason for this.

As to the relationship between cohesion and coherence, Halliday explains that 'An important contribution to coherence comes from COHESION: the set of linguistic resources that every language has…for linking one part of the text to another.'[67] In other words, cohesion is a means of attaining coherence. Hallilday and Hasan add, further, that coherence contains a set of expectations created during the reading of the text with regard to its continuance.[68] Olshtein and Celce-Murcia speak of coherence as the correspondence between the understanding of the world by the reader, from his own experience, and the system of ideas and statements which can be understood from the text.[69]

Biblical scholars have put to use the notion of coherence in different ways. Leder, for example, discusses the coherence of Exodus from the point of view of its plot. He finds that Exodus 1–2 present a narrative problem, which is the enslavement of Israel and the enforced building of the store cities, followed by three major conflicts, taking the reader to the resolution of the narrative. The resolution, which is the construction of the tabernacle, after overcoming the conflicts, solves the narrative problem presented at the initial chapters.[70] Long discusses literary and theological coherence in the narratives concerning the reign of Saul; Kim speaks of conceptual coherence between the collections in the book of Proverbs; Kessler searches for coherence in Jeremiah; Hunter in Lamentations, and there are others.[71]

66. Halliday and Hasan, *Language, Context, and Text*, pp. 91-93.

67. Halliday and Hasan, *Language, Context, and Text*, p. 48.

68. Halliday and Hasan, *Language, Context, and Text*, p. 72.

69. E. Olshtein and M. Celce-Murcia, 'Discourse Analysis and Language Teaching', in D. Schiffrin, D. Tannen and H.E. Hamilton (eds.), *The Handbook of Discourse Analysis* (Malden, MA: Blackwell, 2001), pp. 707-24 (717-18).

70. Arie C. Leder, 'The Coherence of Exodus: Narrative Unity and Meaning', *CTJ* 36 (2001), pp. 251-69.

71. V. Philips Long, *The Reign and Rejection of King Saul: A Case for Literary and Theological Coherence* (Atlanta: Scholars Press, 1989); Seenam Kim, *The Coherence of*

1.3.2. *The Semantic Field as Intermediary between Lexical Cohesion and Theme by Means of the Plot*

Apart from the general argument that coherence is about overt textual signals, whereas coherence has to do with logic connections in the text, there is another difference between these two textual characteristics, one which lies not only in the means used for their creation but also in the type of textual unity to which they lead. In other words, the means of attaining cohesion are morphological, and the meaning which they contribute to a text is different from that contributed by the means of coherence. Reinhart and Giora adduce instances in which it is possible to find cohesion without coherence: there may be a situation in which the text is cohesive, but not conceptually and logically coherent.[72] It follows from this that means of cohesion contribute to the immediate contextual link between clauses, but do not necessarily contribute to the deeper meaning relations which must exist in a well-constructed text. Thus, the means of cohesion contribute to the construction of the meaning which exists between clauses, whereas the term 'coherence' is connected to meaning at a deeper level, that which concerns the more extensive units of the text. But how are the level of words and the deep level of meaning to be bridged? The key to understand this is to bear in mind that meaning is coded as wording. Hasan, as noted in the beginning of this introduction, proposes three levels of deriving meaning from a text, just as the semiotic system of language is divided into three—phonology, lexico-grammar, and semantics—and the main units with which they deal are sounds, wording, and meaning, respectively. Similarly, meaning is derived from a text on three levels: the lowest is the level of the connection between words, which Hasan names 'verbalization'; the highest level is the 'theme'; and the intermediate level 'symbolic articulation'.[73]

According to Hasan, the lowest stratum of understanding meaning takes place at the time of the first encounter with it. The reader must be familiar with the language in which the text is written, including the entire linguistic resource of the community. At this level of understanding subjects such as the tenses of the verbs and the relationships between the tenses are dealt

the Collections in the Book of Proverbs (Eugene, OR: Pickwick Publications, 2007); Martin Kessler (ed.), *Reading the Book of Jeremiah: A Search for Coherence* (Winona Lake, IN: Eisenbrauns, 2004); Jannie Hunter, *Faces of a Lamenting City: The Development and Coherence of the Book of Lamentations* (Frankfurt am Main: Peter Lang, 1996); Mieke Bal, *Death and Dissymmetry: The Politics of Coherence in the Book of Judges* (Chicago: University of Chicago Press, 1988); Thomas B. Dozeman, Thomas Römer and Konrad Schmid (eds.), *Pentateuch, Hexateuch, or Enneateuch: Identifying Literary Works in Genesis through Kings* (Atlanta: Society of Biblical Literature, 2011).

72. Reinhart, 'Conditions for Text Coherence'; Giora, 'Notes Towards a Theory of Text Coherence'.

73. Hasan, *Linguistics, Language, and Verbal Art*, pp. 94-101.

with. But this level is not sufficient for a complete understanding of the text. At this level one understands the individual clauses of which the text is composed and the relations between them. Such understanding enables the reader to paraphrase the text which he/she has read. But there is also a higher level of understanding.

Hasan calls the highest level of meaning 'the theme'. She illustrates understanding of the theme through Robert Frost's poem 'The road not taken'. We may say that this poem is about a man who has decided to take a particular road, hoping to return and try another one; in the course of his life, however, it becomes clear to him that he cannot retrace his steps. Yet it is also possible to describe the meaning of the poem in words that are not necessarily taken from the poem itself: for instance, one may say that the poem describes the limitations and immutability of human choice. Both of these formulations will be correct, and both of them lead to the highest level of abstraction which can be derived from a literary creation—the level of the theme. In Hasan's words:

> The stratum of theme is the deepest level of meaning of verbal art; it is what a text is about when dissociated from the particularities of that text. In its nature, the theme of verbal art is very close to a generalization, which can be viewed as a hypothesis about some aspect of the life of social man.[74]

These two levels of meaning, the highest and the lowest, are linked by the intermediate stratum, which Hasan calls 'symbolic articulation'. Hasan draws an analogy between this level and the lexico-grammatical level of the three strata of linguistic study, in that the symbolic level, like the lexico-grammatical level, contains the system of symbols which create the meanings of the highest stratum—the theme.

In order to understand the level of symbolic articulation it has to be recognized that actions, processes and states described in a text have a dual status: they can be interpreted literally, but sometimes they also have another meaning, and serve as signs or symbols which may indicate a more general abstract meaning in the text. Hasan illustrates this with Angus Wilson's short story 'The Widower'.[75] Here, the widower who is the hero of the story carries out several actions: he cuts wood, goes into the house, boils water and makes himself tea. Hasan interprets this as a catalogue of ineffectual movements in relation to the cosmic movement of time. Moreover, the impression that these actions, which fill up the widower's time, are so predictable serves as reinforcement of our understanding of his character as a man who acts as an automaton. But the series of predictable actions could be interpreted differently; for instance, they could create the opposite

74. Hasan, *Linguistics, Language, and Verbal Art*, p. 98.

75. Hasan brings this story as an appendix in her book: *Linguistics, Language, and Verbal Art*, pp. 107-15.

feeling, as the security in the inevitability of the workings of the world. Hasan maintains that it is the micro-patterns—the use of certain words, the delicate phrases which appear throughout the story and which are emphasized by de-automatization—which prompt us to interpret the story in this way. In a great many of the phrases in the story there are words which belong both to the world of machines and to the human world. Therefore, the level of symbolic articulation is 'wherever the linguistic meanings become signs with deeper meaning'.[76] In Hasan's article 'Rime and Reason',[77] the categories of the code of the language (i.e. words, phrases) are used to symbolize a set of situations, events, or processes, just as they are used in language in general. But, in literary art these situations and events, in their turn, are used to symbolize a certain theme. A literary text has to have a code which is instantial to it, 'for the reason that certain discrete situations which per se do not have a given symbolic value, are assigned such a value by being placed in a certain arrangement'.[78] Hasan stresses that the consistency of foregrounding and the thematically motivated use of language patterns ensure a reader's sensitivity even to apparently ordinary phenomena in language which might otherwise go unnoticed. The dominant semantic field discovered in a text is considered here as a foregrounding pattern whose function is to drive the reader's attention to the central theme. According to my thesis, this is done through the occurrence of the relevant semantic field at key points of the plot.

Since the semantic field is composed of repetition of words between which there are semantic links, it may be said that it is another of the cohesive phenomena which serve to increase coherence—as Hasan and Halliday have demonstrated—by means of cohesive chains.

One of the principal aims of this study, however, is to consider whether the lexemes which constitute the SF also help to design a theme in the text; and, if so, how they do it. I suggest that the connecting link between the lexemes from the semantic field and a main theme of the story is the plot. Indeed, the most prominent phenomenon connected to the words of the field is their appearance at turning-points in many and different plots. In other words, the lexemes of the SF have an additional function to those of words from other fields which may occur in the text: the function of sustaining the theme by appearing at key-points in the plot.[79]

76. Hasan, *Linguistics, Language, and Verbal Art*, p. 98

77. Ruqaiya Hasan, 'Rime and Reason in Literature', in Seymour Chatman (ed.), *Literacy Style: A Symposium* (New York: Oxford University Press, 1971), pp. 299-326 (309).

78. Hasan, 'Rime and Reason', p. 311.

79. To strengthen this inference I quote Hasan, who claims that cohesive chains (see §1.3) belong to the sphere of microstructures of the text, and are expressed in the plot:

Lexemes from the semantic field, as distinct from other means of cohesion, do not necessarily appear in consecutive or adjacent verses. As I shall show in the analysis of individual chapters in Genesis, they appear at turning-points in the plot. They can be omitted from whole sections of the plot, and still contribute to the overall rationale of the whole episode, provided that they are prominent in a particular section of the plot. Of course, lexemes from the field may also be distributed throughout the episode, appearing in almost each and every verse. Eventually, the plots of individual narratives are jointly observed to form the macro-plot in Genesis.

Chapter 4 deals with the coherence of Genesis as a whole, and discusses the theme related to the SF in Genesis in greater depth. In this chapter I discuss the various levels of sight as they are expressed on the divine and the human level: in other words, low vision, which is concrete and sensory; intermediate sight, which is combined with understanding; elevated sight, linked with seeing God in concrete visual fashion; and the highest level of sight, which is expressed by the belief in God without his being revealed.

1.3.3. *Can Any Semantic Field Be Theme-Related?*

Since seeing is an everyday act, some readers of this work may argue that it is trivial to the structure of any story in which human beings are the central characters. Here I once again follow Hasan's footsteps. According to Hasan, special attention should be paid to simple language uses. She shows how verb tenses and prepositions may point to a main theme of a narrative, and states that:

> It is not the patterns per se that are artistic; it is the mode of their utilization that creates an important parameter of artfulness in verbal art.[80]

This is true of semantic fields found in a text as well. It is really the specific pattern of their appearance that elevates these lexical items, relative to the other lexical items which together constitute a text. In Genesis a textual pattern emerges in which sight lexemes occur at key positions, and this makes them worthwhile for studying as part of the theme of the book in spite of their frequency and assumed triviality.

Hasan, who analyzes Angus Wilson's story 'Necessity's Child', comes to the conclusion that a word such as 'talk' is one of the words which sustain the main theme of the story. Hasan believes that in this story words connected with the thought and speech of the characters reveal the central theme of the plot. As a result, she emphasizes words connected with understanding

'These micro features of the text support the macro patterns of the plot' (Hasan, *Linguistics, Language, and Verbal Art*, p. 89). These macro-patterns lead to the understanding of the theme.

80. Hasan, *Linguistics, Language, and Verbal Art*, p. 96.

and speech, some of which are very frequently found in many stories, such as 'talk', 'muse', 'gossip', 'conversation'. In the story which she analyzes words connected with talking and thinking are significant, since thought and the way people describe their thoughts are a central issue for the understanding of its characters and theme.[81] The example presented in this study augments that of Hasan, according to which a central theme of the story may be borne by a relatively frequent word.

Although rarity of lexical items is not considered a criterion in the method I propose here, some of the words connected to the SF are uncommon and rare. There is a large variety of lexemes from the SF in Genesis, some of which are not to be instantly expected in a narrative, such as: ויכרם (he recognized them, Gen. 42.7), ויתנכר (he acted as stranger to them, Gen. 42.7), צעיף (veil, 38.14), אות־הברית (the sign of the covenant, 9.12). This rarity has drawn my attention to the dominance of the SF in the Genesis narratives.

1.3.4. *The Presence of Other Semantic Fields in the Same Narrative*

Another matter which should be addressed is the question of the presence of other dominant semantic fields in the narratives of Genesis apart from the SF. If we claim that the SF is foregrounded in Genesis, how is it that when analyzing the Joseph Narrative the fields of Sight and Oral Communication are combined to emphasize the theme of this specific section of Genesis? The answer to this problem can be compared to the lens when filming a motion picture. Before the camera has zoomed in on an object which is far away we can only notice general characters in that frame. This can be compared to the SF in Genesis. However, once the lens has zoomed in closer to the objects in that frame, we start noticing the details. When 'getting closer' and reading into the various stories in the Joseph Narrative, we may discover that the SF is not foregrounded by itself and it is intertwined with the field of Oral Communication. When 'zooming in on' Genesis 38 we discover that the focus is on cognitive perception, which is one specific aspect in the SF. As in cinematography, focus depends on the 'distance' at which the narrator and the readers wish to stand and describe or understand the story. So, the book of Genesis is constituted of close and distant 'camera frames'. Hence, when grasping the text of Genesis as a whole, the SF does stand out. Nevertheless, it is also possible that in that same zoom additional semantic fields will be shown to be dominant as well. This work focuses on the textual patterns stressing the SF. Further investigations may show the foregrounding of additional semantic fields.

81. Hasan, *Linguistics, Language, and Verbal Art*, pp. 86-87.

1.3.5. *The Semantic Field and the Leading Word*

Scholarship concerning the leading word is relevant to the understanding of the function of the semantic field, since both phenomena involve the repetition of a particular root, a repetition which contributes to the understanding of the structure and meaning of the narrative. Martin Buber, in a lecture given in 1927, coined the term 'Leitwort', afterwards referred to as 'leading word',[82] and defined it as follows:

> A word or word root that is meaningfully repeated within a text or sequence of texts or complex of texts; those who attend to these repetitions will find a meaning of the text revealed or clarified, or at any rate made more emphatic.[83]

Hence, Buber himself emphasizes that the word does not have to be repeated in exactly the same form; its root could reappear in various conjugations. From the examples he adduces it is apparent that sometimes he applies an even more liberal approach and addresses words only close in meaning to the leading word which he had identified. For instance, in the story of Korah's rebellion in Numbers 16–17, Buber maintains that one of the principal leading words is עדה (congregation), whereas the root קהל (to assemble), whose meaning is close to that of the first, is introduced into the story in order to reinforce the leading word.[84] So, in fact, Buber at times analyzes semantic categories and not just leading words.

Similar to the function of the semantic field as shown in this essay, according to Buber, the prime purpose of the leading word is to attract the reader's attention and consideration, and thereby to reveal central meanings in the text. At one point Buber calls the meaning found in the text 'the secret meaning'.[85] In his analyses he classifies various words as primary or secondary leading words; in one short story he may identify several leading words. For example, in the story of the Tower and City of Babel (Gen. 11.1-9) Buber discerns seven leading words: כל־הארץ (the whole earth), שׂפה (language), הבה (let us), עיר ומגדל (city and tower), בנה (to build), שׁם (name), and פוץ (to scatter). According to Buber, similarity of sound between the verses in which the leading word recurs causes the reader to pay attention to the phenomenon of the leading word.

82. See, e.g., Yairah Amit, 'The Multi-Purpose "Leading Word" and the Problems of its Usage', *Prooftexts* 9 (1989), pp. 99-114.

83. Martin Buber, 'Leitwort Style in Pentateuch Narrative', in Martin Buber and F. Rosenzweig (eds.), *Scripture and Translation* (trans. L. Rosenwald and E. Fox; Bloomington: Indiana University Press, 1994), pp. 114-28 (114).

84. Buber, 'Leitwort Style in Pentateuch Narrative', pp. 117-19.

85. Buber, 'Leitwort Style in Pentateuch Narrative', p. 120.

As for the ways to recognize a leading word in a text, according to Amit it will be accompanied by estrangement. Estrangement (or foregrounding) is the alteration of the routine meaning of a linguistic expression.[86] The purpose of foregrounding is to draw attention to something exceptional, something which has changed, and this may guide the reader to the connection between the texts in which the leading words are involved.[87] Polak explains further that foregrounding of a leading word is created primarily by means of special stylistic effects. It may be by doubling a word, and other semantic patterns such as contradiction and equivalence. He also remarks that sound resemblance between words may strengthen an associative link between them.[88] The same phenomenon—foregrounding—has the effect of bringing to the reader's attention the repetition of words from the semantic field.

Frisch has discussed the phenomenon of the leading word in various episodes in the Pentateuch and Prophets. He discusses the verbs ראה (see) and שׁמע (hear) as leading words in Genesis 21, and in the narrative of the Akedah in Genesis 22. It appears that although Frisch discusses the leading root ראה he cannot avoid broadening the scope of his discussion to include other lexemes, which are connected with it through the semantic field. In his work Frisch maintains that there is a theme connecting Genesis 21 with Genesis 22 which leads to 'a parallel between individuals and between their histories'.[89] Thus, Frisch uses the principle advanced in the present study, according to which lexemes from the SF in Genesis sustain the unifying theme of the book.

In another of Frisch's studies he expands his discussion of leading words, and considers the question of how they are reflected in translations into English. Frisch analyzes the occurrences of the root שׁוב (return) in Deut. 30.1-10. He finds that the verb is 'thoroughly dispersed throughout the whole of the literary unit, and it epitomizes its subject'. Frisch speaks of the

86. See Hasan and Mukarovsky on foregrounding (§1.4 nn. 111, 112). Prince, in his dictionary has the entry 'defamiliarization', explaining that this is the making of the familiar strange by impeding automatic habitual ways of perceiving (Gerald Prince, *A Dictionary of Narratology* [Lincoln: University of Nebraska Press, 1987], p. 18).

87. Amit, 'The Multi-Purpose "Leading Word"', p. 101.

88. Before Buber, Walzel pointed out the phenomenon of the repetition of a word, a root, or a group of words, and called it a 'leading motif'. Walzel made a distinction between a phonetic and a symbolic function. He, too, noted the connection between repetition of words and the meanings created in the text as a result of this repetition (O. Walzel, *Das Wortkunstwerk* [Darmstadt: Wissenschaftliche Buchgesellschaft, 1968 (1st edn 1926)], pp. 157-58, 178-81, mentioned in Polak, *Biblical Narrative*, p. 91).

89. Amos Frisch, Amos, 'שׁמע and ראה as a Pair of *Leitwörter*' (Hebrew), *Proceedings of the Twelfth World Congress of Jewish Studies: Jerusalem, July 29–August 5 1997* (Jerusalem: World Union of Jewish Studies, 1999), pp. 89-98 (93, 97).

formation of a framework describing the acts of Israel, and within it another framework which relates to the acts of God. In other words, this verb contributes to the cohesion and to the logical coherence of the text.[90]

Berlin speaks of the creation of lexical coherence in texts by means of repeated words, even if they do not refer to the same referent.[91] To a great extent, this recalls the phenomenon of the leading word. Berlin adduces the example of the word מספר ('to count' or 'to say') in Ps. 147.4-5, which functions as a means of coherence despite its ambiguity: once it alludes to the counting of the stars, and once its meaning is 'to tell', or 'to say'. Berlin begins by saying that her aim is not only to describe the means of cohesion in this text; in the last resort, it is important to find an interpretation which results from this cohesion. In other words, she identifies prominent lexemes, which bear the theme of the unit analyzed.

The connection between the leading word and the structure of the text unit has also been explored. Rosenzweig's discussion makes it possible to connect the leading word with the structure of the story, hence the key to understanding the link between the semantic field and the plot can be found by the mediation of his studies. Rosenzweig uses slightly different terminology for the phenomenon of the leading word from that of Buber, referring to it as a 'Stichwort'.[92] In his essay, he emphasizes that it is impossible to separate the form of the story from its content. Sometimes, he says, there are complete formulaic verses, not just single words, which are repeated in the biblical text, and which link different stories. He maintains that unlike Homer's phrases, whose purpose is 'pictorial', these phrases drive the story onwards: 'they are not the colours of things but the joints of the story'. The form and the content adhere to each other, and it is impossible to separate them: 'Form—real form, not "poetic form", and substance—true substance, not apparent, indicable "content"—are indivisible'.[93] When discussing the form of biblical narrative Rosenzweig maintains that it is like—'a dialogic element framing the narrative about an alteration of question and answer,

90. Amos Frisch, 'The Conveyance of the *Leitwort* in English Translations of the Bible (KJV, JPS, RSV, JB, NAB, NEB, NJPS, NRSV)' (Hebrew), *Studies in Bible and Exegesis* 6 (2002), pp. 235-51.

91. Berlin, 'Lexical Cohesion', p. 33.

92. Amit translates this as 'key word' (Amit, 'The Multi-Purpose "Leading Word"'). Also see Talia Stadler-Sutskover, 'The Leading Word and its Roles in Judges 19–21', in Johann Cook (ed.), *Bible and Computer: The Stellenbosch AIBI-6 Conference. Proceedings of the Association Internationale Bible et Informatique 'From Alpha to Byte' University of Stellenbosch 17–21 July, 2000* (Leiden: Brill, 2002), pp. 295-307 (296-97). For a discussion of this terminology, see Franz Rosenzweig, 'The Secret of Biblical Narrative Form', in Buber and Rosenzweig (eds.), *Scripture and Translation*, pp. 129-42 (133 n. 8).

93. Rosenzweig, 'The Secret of Biblical Narrative Form', pp. 139-40.

speech and counterspeech, proposition and qualification'.[94] These phrasings and others show that Rosenzweig draws connections between the occurrence of the leading word, narrative structure, and key points, and that it can be found not only in prose, but also in poetry, prophecy, and even in biblical law, since in these genres, too, some events or passages are more significant than others. By contrast, Buber does not explicitly discuss the structural element of a narrative—its plot. In the examples relating to Abraham, however, he considers the important stages in Abraham's history.[95] His discussion does not include explicit reference to the development of the plot, but it does emphasize the contribution of the leading word to the understanding of the theme of the story. Moving into more recent scholarship concerning the leading word, according to Polak's definition, the leading word can be recognized by two criteria: that the word recurs frequently, and that it makes a substantial contribution to the understanding of the structure or meaning of a textual unit.[96] The most helpful point to my analysis is that Polak, following Rosenzweig, links the phenomenon of the leading word to plot structure, a notion which also lies underneath the present discussion which assumes a connection between the semantic field and the plot. Polak also points out, as stated above, the existence of stylistic/rhetorical structures which draw the reader's attention to the leading word, structures which help to emphasize the word in relation to its surroundings.

I extend the discussion of these matters to the sphere of semantic fields, and refine it. On the one hand, I attempt to track the repeated appearance of lexemes from the SF at key points in the plot of the individual story. If words from the SF do in fact appear frequently and consistently at certain strategic points, we may say that the phenomenon of the dominant semantic field has a fundamental connection to the plot. The basic connection with the plot lays the foundation for the claim that the words of the field contribute to the design of a central theme of the book. In her discussion of the theme, Hasan speaks of the principle of consistency, according to which significant events appear again and again at the same points in the plot (for example, at the end of sub-plots).[97] On the other hand, in addition to considering the plot I carefully consider whether lexemes from the SF are accompanied by stylistic/rhetorical phenomena which stress their occurrences as compared with lexemes from other fields.

94. Rosenzweig, 'The Secret of Biblical Narrative Form', p. 141.

95. M. Buber, 'Abraham the Seer (Genesis 12–25)', in N.N. Glatzer (ed.), *On the Bible: Eighteen Studies by Martin Buber* (trans. S. Meyer; New York: Schocken Books, 1968 [first published in 1939]), pp. 22-43.

96. Polak, *Biblical Narrative*, p. 93.

97. Hasan, *Linguistics, Language, and Verbal Art*, p. 95.

1.4. *Plot and Key-points*

Since I maintain that lexemes from the SF stand out against other lexemes which constitute the stories of Genesis, mainly because they appear at key-points in the plot, I shall now consider the term 'plot'. The plot of a narrative can be addressed from two points of view: *fable* (*fabula*) or *sujet*. Chatman defines the fable thus: 'Basic story stuff, the sum total of events to be related in a narrative'.[98] This is the abstract framework of events as they take place in the story itself, but without presenting the characters or describing the circumstances in detail.[99] Chatman calls the *sujet* 'plot', and describes it as the events put into discourse, or the events put in a modus of presentation.[100] In Genesis there are various types of narratives. Many of these are structured as pediments, or pyramids;[101] others are genealogical lists or dialogues. Both in the common type of plot and in lists and dialogues there are key-points, which are more significant than others. I suggest that lexemes from the SF are frequently to be found at these prominent plot positions.

Plots which are constructed as pediments are usually divided into five main stages: exposition, complication, turning-point, unravelling and ending.[102]

1. *Exposition*. The exposition is the part of the plot in which the narrator presents the characters, their characteristics, information concerning time and place, and other data important for the development of the story. Amit speaks of the static or customary nature of the data described in the exposition.[103]

98. S. Chatman, *Story and Discourse: Narrative Structure in Fiction and Film* (Ithaca, NY: Cornell University Press, 1978), p. 19. This terminology has been coined by Russian Formalists such as Boris Tomashevski ('Thematics', in L.T. Lemon and M.J. Reis [ed. and trans.], *Russian Formalist Criticism: Four Essays* [Lexington: University of Nebraska Press, 1965 (first published 1925)], pp. 61-98). For a discussion concerning these terms, see S. Onega and J.A. Garcia Landa, *Narratology: An Introduction* (London: Longman, 1996), pp. 1-41.

99. Polak, *Biblical Narrative*, p. 6.

100. Chatman, *Story and Discourse*, p. 43.

101. On Freytag's 'pyramid' or 'triangle', see Gustav Freytag, *Freytag's Technique of the Drama* (trans. Elias J. MacEwan; New York: Johnson Reprint Corp, 1968). Also see Prince, *A Dictionary of Narratology*, pp. 36-38.

102. For a discussion on these plot stages, see Freytag (previous note), Polak, *Biblical Narrative*, pp. 115-20, and Yairah Amit, *Reading Biblical Stories* (Jerusalem: Ministry of Defence, 2000 [Hebrew]), pp. 55-56.

103. Amit, *Reading Biblical Stories*, p. 43. Also see M. Sternberg, 'What Is Exposition? An Essay in Temporal Delimitation', in J. Halperin (ed.), *The Theory of the Novel, New Essays* (New York: Oxford University Press, 1974), pp. 25-70.

2. *Complication.* Aristotle's definition of 'complication' is: 'By "tying" I mean the part reaching from the beginning (of the story) to the scene which is the last before the shift to good or bad fortune'.[104] Polak defines the complication as the stage in the plot which describes how the balance is disturbed by distress, ambition, or injury by a rival. The Israeli narratologist Joseph Ewen, in his dictionary of literary terms, adds the important detail that sometimes the complication takes place in several stages.[105]
3. *Turning-point.* Aristotle's definition of the turning-point is: '"Peripety" is the shift of the action towards the opposite pole'.[106] Bal states that it is the moment at which the situation changes, when a line is broken.[107]
4. *Unravelling (or denouement).* Aristotle says very little about the unravelling: 'that from the beginning of the shift to the end (of the play)'.[108] The turning-point is a specific moment or event, and the events which follow it, whose function is to untie the knot, constitute the stage of the unravelling.
5. *Ending (or quiescence).* Sometimes the narrative ends in a state of quiescence, but sometimes there is a further complication. In some narratives the complication is constructed as a series of delays which grow towards the climax.[109] Sometimes biblical narratives come to an end with an explanation (Midrash) of a name and the observation that a new customary situation has been established.[110]

Longacre divides the plot rather differently. First, he divides the plot into the central and secondary stream of events. The exposition is one type of secondary information. Longacre maintains that every discourse aspires to advance. A well-constructed discourse advances to a particular point. This advance flows through a climactic development (or developments), which he calls a 'peak', though I shall continue to use the accepted term, 'turning-point'. According to Longacre, every plot has a peak, and some

104. Aristotle, *Poet.* 55b.26-27.

105. J. Ewen, *Milon LeMunachei HaSiporet* (Jerusalem: Academon, 1978 [Hebrew]), p. 84.

106. Aristotle, *Poet.* 52a.22. Polak explains the turning-point as the stage in the story at which the wheel turns around (Polak, *Biblical Narrative*, p. 117).

107. Mieke Bal, *Narratology: Introduction to the Theory of Narrative* (Toronto: University of Toronto Press, 1997), p. 102.

108. Aristotle, *Poet.* 55b.28-29.

109. Polak, *Biblical Narrative*, p. 117. As an example of a complication constructed as a series of delays, Polak adduces the story of Samson and Delilah in Judg. 16.6-21.

110. Amit, *Reading Biblical Stories*, pp. 55-56.

parts (pre-peak) precede it, while others (post-peak) follow it, and it contains an incident which triggers off the events. The plot is composed of a series of episodes leading to the peak, which can be identified by means of the characteristics found in the surface structure. When the peak approaches there is a stylistic change of some kind in relation to the style of the rest of the plot. For example, there may be a longer and more detailed dialogue than those in the other parts of the plot, particular types of verb may be used, and so forth.[111] I shall make use of this change principle in my analysis of the different narratives in Genesis. According to Hasan, certain events in a plot stand out more than others, and she refers to this textual phenomenon as 'foregrounding', which is the same as estrangement mentioned before. In her view, this emphasis on certain events is accomplished by the use of linguistic norms opposed to those customary in the text.[112] This is close to Longacre's idea of peaking. Hasan, following Mukarovsky, stresses that different events cannot achieve special importance in the framework of the text if the reader does not recognize first its automatic patterns.[113] The emphasis on particular events encourages the reader to pay special attention to the events on whose background the important events stand out. Thus, the meaning of the plot is not only built on the prominent, important events, but also on the contrast between foreground and background.[114]

As has been said, not all texts are built as pediment plots. Some of the narratives are very short: for example, journey narratives tell of characters' movements from place to place, and are no more than an account of the execution of certain actions (Gen. 12.8). There are also lists (Gen. 5, 36) and blessings (Gen. 49). Nonetheless, even in texts of this type there are key-points, such as the beginning and the end; and in a list one item may be particularly significant—for instance, the first or the last item. In these genres, too, it is possible to distinguish background details such as the time or the place of the list or blessing.

111. Robert E. Longacre, 'Interpreting Biblical Stories', in T. van Dijk (ed.), *Discourse and Literature: New Approaches to the Analysis of Literary Genres* (Philadelphia: John Benjamins, 1985), pp. 169-85; and *Joseph: A Story of Divine Providence: A Text Theoretical and Textlinguistic Analysis of Genesis 37 and 39–48* (Winona Lake, IN: Eisenbrauns, 1989), p. 18.

112. Hasan, *Linguistics, Language, and Verbal Art*, p.94.

113. Mukarovsky coined the term 'automatization', which is the contrast of 'de-automatization', or 'foregrounding' (J.R. Mukarovsky, 'Standard Language and Poetic Language', in P.L. Garvin [ed.], *A Prague School Reader on Esthetics: Literary Structure, and Style* [Washington, DC: Georgetown University Press, 1964], pp. 17-30).

114. Hasan, *Linguistics, Language, and Verbal Art*, p. 95.

I shall now give examples of the appearance of lexemes from the SF at key positions in the episodes in Genesis. A large compilation of examples will show that the principle of consistency is fulfilled, and that the SF has a strong connection with the sub-plots in Genesis, and, in the final analysis, with its unifying theme.

1.4.1. *Sight Field Lexemes in Background Details*

Background details of the plot usually stand beside the main sequence of events, that is to say, the main plot line. Background details may be embodied in the names of the characters, place names, the time at which the plot takes place, or various circumstances which are important for the future development of the plot. They generally, though not always, appear in the exposition.[115] In the following I adduce examples of various types of background details from Genesis in which lexemes from the SF appear.

1.4.1.2. *Sight Field Lexemes Indicating the Time of the Occurrence.* Comments on the time of day may contribute to the understanding of the plot.[116] Indications of time may also belong to the SF, if they contain a lexeme from the field. Lexemes such as 'morning', 'evening' and 'night', which indicate various levels of light, are linked to the SF, since they have implications for the characters' conditions of sight.

Thus, for instance, in the story of Laban's deception of Jacob in Genesis 29, when Laban gives Jacob Leah instead of Rachel, it is said that Laban takes Leah and delivers her to Jacob *in the evening* (בערב, 29.23). Only *in the morning* (בבקר, 29.25) does Jacob realize that it is Leah who is by his side. Thus, morning and evening are significant because of their implications for the conditions of sight and the degree of consciousness of the characters. It is not surprising that Lot's daughters ply him with drink and lie with him specifically *at night* (19.33-35); for, in addition to his being befuddled by the wine, the objective conditions of sight hinder his vision of his daughters. Sometimes, when it is said that a particular action takes place in the morning, this constitutes a hint that the character commits his act in the best possible conditions of vision and consciousness; for example, 'So Abraham rose early *in the morning*' (Gen. 21.14; 22.3).

115. According to Bar-Efrat, the storyteller may display expositional details in the course of the story. Thus, for instance, in the story of Abraham's servant looking for a wife for Isaac (Gen. 24.15-16), it is only when the servant notices her that we are introduced to her (Shimon Bar-Efrat, *Narrative Art in the Bible* [trans. Dorothea Shefer-Vanson in conjunction with the author; Sheffield: Almond, 1989], p. 117; see also Sternberg, 'What Is Exposition?').

116. Polak, *Biblical Narrative*, pp. 242-43.

1.4.1.1. *Sight Field Lexemes Indicating the Place of the Occurrence.* Words from the SF sometimes constitute a component in place names which are mentioned as background details to what is happening in the plot. Thus, for example, after Sarah has dealt harshly with Hagar, she flees to a spring (עין) of water located on the way to Shur (בדרך שור, 16.7). The words עין (spring/eye) and שור (Shur/to see) are constituents in the SF. Tamar disguises herself and waits for Judah as a harlot at the entrance to Enaim (פתח עינים, 38.14), and he comes to her in this place. עינים can be translated literally as 'eyes'. Abraham is enjoined to go to the land of Moriah (מריה, 22.2) and to sacrifice his son there.[117]

Place names do not always appear in the exposition or the opening of the plot. Though appearing at the end of the story, and not in the opening as should be expected from background information, explanations of place names are still tagged as background details. In these cases the central character names the place explicitly at the end of the main chain of events. This is the case regarding place-names in 22.14 ה' יראה ('Yhwh will provide', RSV, literally: 'Yhwh will see'), 16.14 באר לחי ראי (Beer Lahai Roi), and 32.30 פנואל (Penuel).

1.4.1.2. *Sight Field Lexemes in the Names of the Characters.* Words from the dominant semantic field may appear in the names of the characters in the plot. In Genesis, for instance, the name Reuben (ראובן) is connected with sight. This connection is mentioned explicitly in Gen. 29.32: 'And Leah conceived and bore a son, and she called his name Reuben (ראובן); for she said, "Because Yhwh has *looked* (ראה) upon my affliction; surely now my husband will love me"'. The personal name of Lot (לוט), who is the central character in Genesis 19, is connected to the SF since it means hiding or covering. Although the repetition of the root מלט in 19.18-22 is considered to be a pun on the name לוט,[118] the name may also be interpreted as linked to the SF, indicating concealment.

1.4.2. *Characteristic or Action of a Central Character—at the Opening or Close to a Fateful Event*

Traits of character or physical attributes are among the background details of the plot. They are static details, which do not form part of the plot's chain of events. But there is often a reason for mentioning these characteristics, because the plot is somehow bound up with them. In Genesis the beauty of

117. See the discussion about Moriah and its connection to the SF in §2.8.1.5.

118. Garsiel suggests that Gen. 14.12-13 may contain a word-play on the name Lot, and that Lot is thereby close to the word פליט ('survivor'; see Moshe Garsiel, *Biblical Names: A Literary Study of Midrashic Derivations and Puns* [trans. Phyllis Hackett; Ramath Gan: Bar-Ilan University Press, 1995], pp. 238-39).

three of the matriarchs—Sarah, Rebekah, and Rachel—is mentioned, and this beauty is also linked to the overarching theme of sight (see Chapter 5). Here, however, I shall mention other instances in which a background detail describing an attribute of a character is essential to the future development of events. These matters stand out in the plot for two reasons: because background details on which the plot depends are repeatedly mentioned; or because these details are placed either at the beginning of the story, or as an introduction placed very close to a fateful event, a violent happening or a revelation—which triggers this event.

In Genesis 27 Jacob succeeds in his scheme to steal the blessing only because Isaac's 'eyes were dim', as we are told in the exposition (27.1). There is a similar instance in Gen. 48.10: 'The *eyes* of Israel were *dim* with age, so that *he could not see*'. In this passage Jacob blesses both of Joseph's children—Ephraim and Manasseh. As he makes the blessing he stretches out his hands and places his right hand on the head of Ephraim, the younger son, and his left hand on the head of Manasseh, the first-born. Yet, according to the words of Joseph in v. 18, it appears that when he asked his father to put his right hand, and not his left, on the first-born Jacob acted against his wishes. It would be possible to relate this act to his feeble sight, but it becomes clear that the deed was done with completely clear vision: the story is phrased in language connected, though only indirectly, to the SF—'And Joseph said to his father, "Not so, my father; for this one is the first-born; put your right hand upon his *head* (ראשו)". But his father refused, and said, "*I know* (ידעתי), my son, *I know* (ידעתי); he also shall become a people, and he also shall be great…' (Gen. 48.18-19).

The story of the Garden of Eden provides another example. In it, we are told of a very important trait of one of the chief characters—the serpent. Here one of the features of its character is described in the exposition (Gen. 3.1): 'The serpent was more *subtle* (ערום) than any other wild creature'. This characteristic of the serpent is critical to the development of the plot; because of his 'subtlety' he succeeds in tempting the woman to eat of the forbidden fruit, and for this he is punished.

A character's critical action is described in terms of vision in the exposition, in Gen. 34.1-2: 'Now Dinah the daughter of Leah, whom she had borne to Jacob, went out to visit (לראות) the women of the land and when Shechem the son of Hamor the Hivite, the prince of the land, *saw* (ראה) her…' Whether Dinah's visit (literally: sight) was good or bad is a matter of interpretation, but its position at the strategic point of the beginning of the story draws special attention to these SF lexemes. Had Dinah not gone to see or visit the daughters of the land, Shechem would not have *seen* her and raped her. These acts expressed in SF lexemes and done by the central figures in the story serve as a 'trigger' for the sequence of events which follows them, and are rather like the mention of the subtlety of the snake.

Genesis 18.1 opens with a divine revelation: 'And Yhwh *appeared* (וַיֵּרָא) to him by *the oaks of Mamre* (באלני ממרא)'. The visit of the three men described after this must be read in the light of this introductory statement. Sight is mentioned again in the following verse: 'He *lifted up his eyes and looked* (וישׂא עיניו וירא), and behold, three men stood in front of him. When he *saw* (וירא) them…' (Gen. 18.2).

Genesis 30 opens with the mention of Rachel seeing: 'When Rachel *saw* (ותרא) that she bore Jacob no children, she envied her sister' (30.1). The story of the expulsion of Hagar also opens with the verb 'to see': 'But Sarah *saw* (וַתֵּרֶא) the son of Hagar the Egyptian, whom she had borne to Abraham, playing…' (21.9). A short episode involving the change of Jacob's name to Israel opens with a Sight-related word: 'God *appeared* (וַיֵּרָא) to Jacob again, when he came from Paddanaram' (35.9).

1.4.3. *Sight Field Lexemes at the Turning-Point or Near It*

The appearance of lexemes from a certain field at the turning-point, or close to it, is a significant feature for the disclosure of a dominant semantic field. In Genesis there are several narratives at whose climax there appears an explicit reference to the seeing or understanding of one of the main characters. Alternatively, there may appear a negative reference to Sight: the character does not see, or something is not understood. These narratives can be referred to as 'Narratives of Insight'.[119] Not all the examples here fall into this category, but the ones that do have special importance—each in their own section. Thus, for instance, the turning-point of the Garden of Eden narrative occurs after Adam and Eve have eaten of the fruit of the tree of knowledge. After this action comes a dramatic change: 'And the *eyes* of both of them were *opened* (ותפקחנה עיני שׁניהם), and they *knew* (וידעו) that they were naked (ערמם)' (Gen. 3.7). This Sight statement is central to the story, and makes it an Insight Narrative.

In the description of Lot's hospitality with which the Sodom and Gomorrah narrative opens in Genesis 19, the men of Sodom ask Lot to deliver his guests to them so that they may *know* them (ונדעה אתם, 19.5). Lot refuses, but offers his virgin daughters as a substitute (19.6-8). The verbal aggression of the men of Sodom grows worse, and quickly turns to physical violence as they come near to break the door (19.9). Then the turning-point occurs: the angels take Lot into his house, and strike the men

119. This is somewhat close to the *Bildungsroman* (an educational novel), but refers to short and isolated narratives such as those of Genesis. These Insight Narratives focus on the understanding of specific and limited pieces of information not known to the character prior to the main turn of events (see Jerome Hamilton Buckley, *Season of Youth: The Bildungsroman from Dickens to Golding* [Cambridge, MA: Harvard University Press, 1974]).

of Sodom with *blindness* (סנורים, 19.11, see §2.1.2.1). In this story the turning point describes a state opposite to that of seeing, in which the character does not see, or does not come to a state of understanding—it can be referred to as a 'Narrative of Blindness'.

The story of Lot's lying with his daughters appears immediately after the destruction of Sodom and Gomorrah. This, too, I suggest, is a Blindness Narrative, because when his daughters lie with him in turn, one night after the other, the text repeats: 'he *did not know* (ולא־ידע) when she lay down or when she arose' (19.33, 35). Lot does not gain any sight or insights in this story. He is not conscious of what is happening to him, because he is drunk; it is even hinted that what he really sees is blurred, because of the emphasis on the events taking place at night time.[120]

The story of the uncovering of Noah in Gen. 9.18-29 tells of Ham's *seeing* his father naked (9.22). The events described before this also seem to be an important element in the story, and they, too are described in terms of Sight: 'And he drank of the wine, and became *drunk* (וישכר); and lay *uncovered* (ויתגל) in his tent' (9.21). As opposed to Lot, who does not understand what has happened to him during his drunkenness, Noah wakes up from his wine and understands what Ham has done to him (9.24). This also can be considered as an Insight Narrative.

The climax of the story of Joseph is connected to Sight, even though it contains no lexemes from this field. The climactic scene is Joseph's recognition by his brothers, which is introduced by the words: 'So no one stayed with him, when Joseph *made himself known* (בהתודע) to his brothers' (45.1). The turning point is composed of Joseph's weeping and introducing himself to his brothers face to face. The latter is described in the words: 'I am Joseph' (45.3). After a monologue he again makes himself known, and this time uses explicit SF lexemes: 'And now *your eyes see*, and the *eyes* of my brother Benjamin *see*' (45.12).

1.4.4. *Sight Field Lexemes at the Unravelling and Ending*

Sometimes SF lexemes appear at the unravelling or the ending of a story. Thus, for instance, words connected with the SF can be traced at the unravelling of the story of Lot's drunkenness: 'When Noah *awoke* (וייקץ) from his wine, and *knew* (וידע) what his youngest son had done to him…' (9.24). Genesis 40 ends with a further complication rather than with quiescence, and is told in words connected with the SF: 'Yet the chief butler did not *remember* Joseph, but *forgot* him' (40.23). In 33.10, Jacob sums up his meeting with his brother Esau using SF lexemes: 'accept my present from

120. For a discussion on the meaning of the narrative of Lot and his daughters, see Talia Sutskover, 'Lot and his Daughters (Gen 19:30-38): Further Literary and Stylistic Examinations', *JHS* 11 (2011), pp. 2-11.

my hand; for truly to *see* your *face* is like *seeing* the *face* of God, with such favor you received me'. In the story of the Creation, at the end of most days the conclusion 'And God *saw* that it was good' is repeated; and at the end of the creation comes the concluding phrase: 'And God *saw* (וַיַּרְא)everything that he had made, and *behold* (והנה), it was very good' (Gen. 1.31).

1.4.5. *Turning-points in a List*
Sometimes a name connected with Sight appears in a genealogical list. It may be the first name (Reuben, 29.32) or the last (Reumah, 22.24). In cases in which there are no names connected with Sight, a detail from the background may be connected to Sight, for example, the place where the family listed lives. This is the case in Ishmael's genealogy, which is said to be dwelling 'from Havilah to *Shur*' (25.18). The place name Shur is a constituent in the SF.

These examples show that lexemes from the SF frequently appear at various strategic points in the plot: at the beginning, at the conclusion, and at the turning-point. In addition, SF lexemes are also significant as background details. Thus, at this stage the principle of 'consistency' is already fulfilled by the appearance of SF lexemes in the framework of the plot. I shall now adduce statistical data about the occurrences of the verb 'see' (ראה) in Genesis.

1.5. *The Quantitative Aspect: The Frequency of* ראה *and Other-Sight Related Lexemes in Genesis*

Although the number of lexemes of sight in Genesis does not constitute a criterion for the existence of a unifying semantic field in the text, I nonetheless consider it appropriate to present a number of figures concerning the nucleus of the field—the verb ראה (to see)—as against other books of the Bible. The amount, in percentages, was established by dividing the number of appearances of the verb by the overall number of verbs in the book. The number of appearances of nouns was also divided by the total number of nouns in the book. These results were multiplied by a hundred. The different frequencies of the words of the semantic field in Genesis were compared with the other pentateuchal and historical books: Exodus, Leviticus, Numbers, and Deuteronomy—as well as Joshua, Judges, Samuel, Kings, Ezra, Nehemiah, and Chronicles. The data were collected by means of the Accordance and Bible Windows search engines.

The verb ראה appears in Genesis 142 times. This constitutes 2.809% of all the verbs in the book, which number 5056. This is a higher frequency than in any of the other books which were examined. Its frequency is also greater than that of any other verb of sight, and this confirms that it is the nucleus of the field. Brenner, too, maintains that one of the characteristics of a term which is at the centre of a field, or in its main layer, is that it appears more frequently than other words in the field.[121] If we evaluate the data in Genesis by ranking scales, it will be seen that Genesis is in the 96th percentile: in other words, the average number of appearances of ראה in Genesis is significantly higher than the average number of its appearances in all the books examined. Other verbs of sight appear less frequently both in Genesis and in the other books examined. For instance, נבט and שקף each appear only three times in Genesis, and only in 1 Samuel does the root נבט appear once more than in Genesis. These frequencies are low, however, and we must exercise caution in drawing far-reaching conclusions from them.

The noun מַרְאֶה (sight, appearance) appears twelve times in Genesis: 0.168% of the 7152 nouns in the book. Only in Leviticus is there a greater proportion. Yet most of the instances in that book are concentrated in one chapter, ch. 13, which deals with the laws of skin disease, and its diagnosis by the priest. Thus, this concentration of the word is no indication of its overall meaning in Leviticus.

Other words in the field may also belong to other fields; thus, it is not to be expected that all the words in the field will appear most frequently in Genesis. For instance, the lexeme עין (eye) has 1.119% appearances relative to the other nouns in the book, but there are other books in which it appears more. The appearances of this lexeme must be considered in detail: its different meanings should be distinguished, as should the question of when it appears as part of the phrases מצא חן בעיני (found favour in the eyes of), היה רע בעיני (was evil in the eyes of), and so on. Despite these reservations, there are many instances of this lexeme in Genesis.

The lexeme אור (light) appears more frequently in Genesis than in the other books: six instances, which constitute 0.084% of the nouns in this book. The lexeme חשך (darkness) appears in Genesis four times—0.056%—of all the nouns. This frequency is relatively high, though its two appearances in 2 Samuel—0.057%—are close to it. In these cases, too, caution must be observed when dealing with lexemes that appear infrequently.

Although the fact that lexemes of Sight appear frequently in our text is of some importance, I do not believe that a detailed examination of the data, and the conclusion that they are found most frequently in Genesis, are the reasons for its clear prominence. As has been remarked above, it is the consistent appearance of the lexemes at key points in the different plots, and the various rhetorical devices accompanying them, which emphasize the appearances of lexemes from the SF.

121. Brenner, 'On the Semantic Field of Humour', p. 51

Chapter 2

THE CONSTITUENTS OF THE SIGHT FIELD: A DISCUSSION OF MEANINGS AND POSITIONS IN THE FIELD

This section presents a list of the lexemes making up the SF, organized in categories according to the semantic guidelines that have been set forth in the Introduction (§§1.1, 1.2). In the centre stand verbs of sight, with synonymous semantic relations linking them together. Lexemes that are linked to the centre by various semantic relations form the first circle of the field. The second circle of lexemes is formed by items which belong to close semantic fields, and then stand peripheral lexemes, which are connected to the SF by the mediation of another lexeme, which belongs to the first circle. Lastly, there is a special category of personal names, names of places, and words denoting time, all of which contain lexemes from the SF. I wish to point out that since de Blois and Mueller in their *Semantic Dictionary of Biblical Hebrew* have a comprehensive view of semantic domains in the Hebrew Bible in general, they accordingly arrange semantic domains differently than suggested in this work, which focuses on Genesis alone. For example, according to de Blois and Mueller, the domain Hide is a subcategory in the categories of Position and Location, whereas here it is rather connected with the process of sight.[1] In addition, as can be seen in dictionaries of Biblical Hebrew, many of the lexemes possess rich and diverse semantic definitions, but here I only mention those points that are relevant to the discussion of the function of specific lexemes in the SF. I have generally made use of BDB, *HALOT*, *TDOT*, *Otzar Leshon haMikra*, *DCH*, and *A Dictionary of Biblical Hebrew* by Kaddari[2] for semantic definitions of the lexemes, but have mentioned explicit references to these dictionaries and other references as well when it was necessary for specific discussions.

1. Reinier de Blois, with the assistance of Enio R. Mueller, *Semantic Dictionary of Biblical Hebrew* (United Bible Societies, 2000–2009), <http://www.sdbh.org/home-en.html>.

2. Menahem Zevi Kaddari, *A Dictionary of Biblical Hebrew* (Ramath Gan: Bar Ilan University Press, 2006 [Hebrew]).

2.1. *The Nucleus of the Sight Field*

The nucleus (§1.2.1) of the SF is the verb ראה (to see) and lexemes which mean 'not seeing'. In the following paragraphs I will address each of the lexemes individually.

2.1.1. ראה *(to See)*

According to *HALOT*, the primary meaning of the verb ראה in the qal conjugation is 'to see with one's eyes'.[3] As indicated by *Webster's Dictionary*, the primary meaning of 'to see' is 'to get knowledge or an impression of through the eyes and the sense of sight; perceive visually, look at; view'.[4] The second meaning, according to Webster, is 'to get a clear mental impression of; grasp by thinking; understand'. In other words, its primary meaning is perceiving by means of the eyes, while the secondary meaning is perceiving by the mind, understanding in general. As stated in *HALOT*, the second meaning of the verb ראה is 'to see, parallel with ידע to understand'.[5] BDB gives the meaning 'see = perceive' as the fifth category in the entry (the first meaning is identical to that given in *HALOT*).[6]

The verb ראה functions as the nucleus of the SF, since in most instances it embodies the basic meaning of the SF, the act of perceiving by means of the eyes. Its other meaning, 'grasp by thinking', is secondary, in the sense that Sweetser refers to as 'a metaphorically motivated secondary sense'.[7] As I have maintained in the Introduction (§1.2.1), the verb ראה is prototypical in this category, since it possesses the semantic features most representative of items inside the field and least representative of items outside it.[8]

The verb ראה of the SF is the lexeme which occurs in Genesis more frequently than any other lexeme in the field, with 142 appearances (considering

3. When I speak here of secondary or primary meanings, I follow the order of meanings as found in the dictionaries cited. I may also refer to them as first, second, third, etc. The principle of organizing these meanings is stated by Baumgartner: 'The safe principle of modern semantics is to look first for the original meaning of a word (in many cases more concrete and restricted than the secondaries) and from this to derive the word's more abstract and even more spiritual meanings. As a rule today one endeavours to draw a genetical sequence of the meanings a word is apt to assume. That principle has, as far as possible, been followed in this dictionary' (*HALOT*, I, p. lxx). Also see n. 7 below.

4. David B. Guralnik and Joseph H. Friend (eds.), *Webster's New World Dictionary of the American Language: Encyclopedia Edition* (Cleveland: World Publishing, 1964), p. 1319.

5. *HALOT*, p. 1157.

6. BDB, p. 907.

7. According to Sweetser, a metaphorically motivated secondary sense is acquired when the speakers become unconscious of the metaphor (Sweetser, *From Etymology to Pragmatics*, pp. 5-8).

8. See Rosch, 'Principles of Categorization', p. 30.

that the total number of uses of verbs in Genesis is 5056). Similarly, the verb סתר (to hide), which is central to the field of Hide, appears more frequently than any other of the lexemes which make up this field.[9] Prototypical terms often appear more frequently than non-prototypical terms in a particular field.

In addition to its two main meanings, the verb ראה has the following meanings: in Gen. 22.8 it means 'to choose, select something for oneself'[10]: 'God will *provide* [RSV, according to most dictionaries "choose"] himself (יראה לו) the lamb for a burnt offering'; and, similarly, in Gen. 41.33: 'Now therefore let Pharaoh *select* (ירא) a man discreet and wise'.

Sometimes this verb appears with the shade of meaning 'to inspect', as in the story of the Tower of Babel in Gen. 11.5: 'And Yhwh came down *to see* (לראת) the city and the tower'. In Gen. 39.23 ראה has the meaning 'to look after':[11] 'the keeper of the prison *paid no heed* (ראה, or: did not look after, did not worry about) to anything that was in Joseph's care'.

Comparison with other Semitic languages shows that the root ראה also exists although as *r'y* and bears the same meaning in Arabic, Geez and Aramaic (*HALOT*). In Akkadian both the verb *amāru(m)* and *dagālu(m)* mean 'to see'.[12]

Other verbs of sight (see §2.2) are linked synonymously to ראה, and all the verbs of sight together constitute the centre of the field. Even though they are linked synonymously, the meaning of the following verbs of sight is not completely identical with that of the verb ראה, and they frequently bear shades of meaning of their own.[13]

2.1.2. *The Negation of Seeing: Not-Seeing*

There are several ways of expressing not-seeing, apart from contexts in which the negation particle לא ('no') stands beside the verb of ראה. In Genesis neither the adjective עִוֵּר (blind, e.g. Exod. 4.11) nor the noun עִוָּרוֹן (blindness, e.g. Deut. 28.28) is found, but there are other expressions for not-seeing.

9. Balentine, *The Hidden God*, p. 2.
10. *HALOT*, p. 1159.
11. *HALOT*, p. 1158.
12. *CAD*, A/2, p.5; D, p. 21.
13. The verb חזה also belongs to the SF, since it is a synonym of ראה, but it is not found in Genesis. This verb appears mainly in poetry (BDB, p. 302). In the narrative it appears in Exod. 18.21 (meaning 'to select'); 24.11; Num. 24.4, 16 (Balaam's prophecy, a poetic text). In Ezra 4.14 the verb חזה appears in Aramaic, in which language it is the central verb in the field of sight. The verb שׁוּר, one of whose meanings is 'to see', is discussed in the section on names and places, since it appears in Gen. 16.7 as part of the place-name דרך שׁור, 'the way to Shur'.

2.1.2.1. סנורים *(blindness)*.[14] The lexeme סנורים appears in Gen. 19.11, and in one other verse of the Bible: 2 Kgs 6.18 (twice). In Genesis 19, the men of Sodom are stricken with blindness by the angels, and the result, from the point of view of the Sodomites, is that 'they wearied themselves groping for the door' (19.11). In other words, their sight was impaired, and as a result they had difficulty in finding the entrance to Lot's house, which they had previously been about to break into (19.9) with a view to molesting his guests.

The second context in which this lexeme occurs is outside Genesis, at the time of the Aramean threat to Israel in Elisha's days. When the Aramean army reaches Dothan and surrounds the town, an army of horses and fire chariots miraculously surrounds Elisha to help him. Elisha sees this, but his young servant does not see the supporting force. So Elisha asks God to open the young man's eyes: 'So Yhwh *opened the eyes of* the young man, and he *saw*; and behold, the mountain was full of horses and chariots of fire...' (2 Kgs 6.17). When the Aramean army descends to fight against Elisha, he asked God to 'Strike this people, I pray thee, with blindness (בסנורים)', a request which God granted (2 Kgs 6.18 [RSV translation]). After the Aramean army had been stricken with blindness, Elisha leads them to Samaria. It seems, however, that they still did not see, for in v. 20 Elisha asks God to open their eyes, that they may see: 'So Yhwh *opened their eyes*, and *they saw*; and lo, they were in the midst of Samaria'. That is to say, after God struck the Arameans with סנורים they were unable to see.

The dictionaries interpret the word סנורים as 'blindness', 'sudden blindness', 'dazzling, deception'.[15] According to Speiser, the etymological derivation of the word is from a loanword based on the Akkadian form *šunwurum*, which is a form of adjective composed of the root *nwr*, to which is added the prefix *š*, which gives the meaning of stress, strengthening. In Hebrew the letter *š* was transformed to *s*. The meaning in Akkadian would be 'very strong light'.[16] Stol analyzes this noun differently. He points out the possibility of a relationship between this form and the Akkadian form *sinlurmā* (which also occurs as *si-nu-ri*), which means both night blindness and day blindness. Stol claims that the first component of the word is a reference to Sīn, the Babylonian moon god.[17] Both of these etymologies indicate that the men of Sodom were struck with blindness—whether through a flash of very bright light, or through being struck directly by night blindness.

14. M. Stol, 'Blindness and Night-Blindness in Akkadian', *JNES* 45 (1986), pp. 295-99.

15. *DCH*, VI, p. 172; BDB, p. 703; *HALOT*, p. 761.

16. E.A. Speiser, 'The "Elative" in West-Semitic and Akkadian', *JCS* 6 (1952), pp. 81-92. See also E.A. Speiser, *Genesis* (AB, 1; Garden City, NY: Doubleday, 1964), pp. 139-40.

17. Stol, 'Blindness and Night-Blindness in Akkadian', pp. 295-99 (296).

Speiser continues that in the Bible the Hebrew root indicating ordinary blindness is עור which is found in Lev. 22.22, Deut. 28.28, and elsewhere. But in these contexts the most appropriate interpretation is not ordinary blindness, the lack of ability to see, for these are situations which reflect a sudden flash, caused by strong divine light.[18] Ahuvia, on the other hand, believes that the instances of the word סנורים in the Hebrew Bible show that neither the men of Sodom nor the Aramean army were in a state of blindness—namely, a state in which they did not see, for the men of Sodom continue to look for the door, and the Aramean army continues on its way without any of its soldiers realizing that it had been stricken in any way. Ahuvia claims that this lack of awareness is evidence that they have not been struck by blindness caused by a strong flash of light. In his view, their state is the opposite of being open-eyed—the state described in 2 Kings 6; in this situation, something is eradicated from the normal state of sight, but this is not physiological blindness. In his view, the word סנורים is derived from the root סנר, which is related to שׂריון—both mean 'covering'. Moreover, Ahuvia finds no reason for the narrator to use euphemism in biblical contexts, and to say that they were stricken with an excess of light (סנורים) instead of directly using the form עוורון (blindness).[19]

Rabin differs completely from Ahuvia. He contends that the word שריון is borrowed from Hurrian, and that it cannot be compared with סנורים. As for the contention that there is no reason to use euphemism to describe blindness, he cites the Aramaic phrase סגי נהור, whose literal meaning is 'much light', or 'strong light' as a description of blindness. Stol cites evidence from Arabic and from Akkadian texts in which euphemism is used to describe the blind.[20] The reason was, apparently, the desire to fend off the evil eye.[21]

2.1.2.2. עינים כהות *(dim eyes)*. Genesis says of Isaac once only that his eyes were dim: 'When Isaac was old and his *eyes were dim* so that *he could not see* (ותכהין עיניו מראת)' (Gen. 27.1). Speiser and Westermann translate literally, 'his eyes were too dim to see', and add that it means that his sight was so weak that he was unable to see.[22]

18. Speiser, 'The "Elative"', p. 82, and Speiser, *Genesis*, pp. 139-40.

19. Abraham Ahuvia, 'סנורים = the Covering of the Eyes' (Hebrew), *Tarbiẓ* 39 (1970), pp. 90-92.

20. Chaim Rabin, 'Comments on: "סנורים = the Covering of the Eyes"' (Hebrew), *Tarbiẓ* 39 (1970), pp. 214-15.

21. Stol, 'Blindness and Night-Blindness in Akkadian', pp. 295-99.

22. Speiser, *Genesis*, p. 208. Westermann reads 'his eyes were so dim that he could not see' (Claus Westermann, *Genesis 12–36: A Commentary* [trans. J.J Scullion; London: SPCK, 1985], p. 432.)

Outside Genesis this expression appears once, with reference to Eli: 'At that time Eli, whose *eyesight had begun to grow dim* (ועינו החלו כהות), so that *he could not see*' (1 Sam. 3.2). Unlike Eli's eyes, it is said that Moses' eye did not grow dim in his old age (לא־כהתה עינו, Deut. 34.7).

2.2. *The Centre of the Sight Field*

Verbs of sight are linked synonymously to the nucleus of the field; nonetheless, they possess independent shades of meaning. The following verbs of sight will be considered in alphabetical order: נבט, צפה, שאה, שוף, שעה, שקף.

2.2.1. נבט

The root נבט, from which the verb הביט (hiphil) is derived, indicates an act of seeing, and is translated by the BDB as 'look'. According to *HALOT*, the principal meaning of the verb in the hiphil conjugation is 'to look in a particular direction'. The verb appears three times in Genesis: in 15.5, 19.17 and 19.26. In 15.5 it means to look at a particular spot, '*Look* towards heaven' (הבט־נא השמימה), and in 19.17 to look backwards, '*do not look* back (אל־תביט) back', 'But Lot's wife behind him *looked* (ותבט) back' (19.26). According to Morag, the Akkadian verb *nabāṭu*, whose root has the same consonants as in Hebrew, and which means 'to light', is also evidence of the semantic connections between the fields of Light and Shining and those of Germination, Development and Growth.[23]

2.2.2. צפה

This verb appears once in the qal conjugation in Genesis, in 31.49: 'And the pillar *Mizpah* (והמצפה), for he said, "Yhwh *watch* (יצף) between you and me, when we are *absent* (נסתר) one from the other"'. The verb צפה usually means 'to see', to perceive by means of the eyes, but it has its own shade of meaning: to see for a length of time, to keep watch, and even 'lie in wait for' or 'spy keep watch'.[24] The verse cited above emphasizes the contradictory meanings of watching and being hidden (סתר).

2.2.3. שאה

In *HALOT* the root שאה III is listed as the root from which the verb משתאה (hithpael), which appears only in Gen. 24.21, is derived. There, it is claimed that this is a secondary form of the verb שעה, or a textual error for this

23. Shelomo Morag, '"ומתערה כאזרח רענן" (Psalms XXXVI, 35)', in *Studies on Biblical Hebrew* (Jerusalem: Magnes Press, 1995 [first published in 1972, Hebrew]), pp. 194-217 (197); *CAD*, N/1, p. 22.

24. BDB, p. 859; *HALOT*, p. 1044.

verb.[25] The context in which משתאה appears is Abraham's servant's journey to Haran, in order to find a wife for Isaac. All of the signs which the servant asks God to bring about on his way to Haran are fulfilled. The young women go to draw water, as he asked, and when he asks one of them for water from her pitcher, she also offers it to his camels. The events which take place as the servant had requested are, for him, a sign that this women is meant to be the wife of his master's son. The servant's reaction to the fulfilment of the events is phrased in the language of sight: 'The man *gazed* (משתאה) at her in silence to learn whether Yhwh had favoured his journey or not' (Gen. 24.21). The servant examines Rebekah with his eyes, but does not open his mouth.[26] He has to see whether the women will really give water to the camels, as he requested. When the camels have finished drinking he understands that God has made his journey successful, and he quickly heaps jewels upon her. Medieval Jewish commentators, however, interpreted this verb as meaning 'alarm' and 'wonder': 'from משומם, as in an astonished man, silent and full of thoughts' (Rashi), 'as if wondering (משתומם)' (Ibn Ezra), 'wondering and thinking' (Rashbam).

2.2.4. שעה

The verb שעה appears only twice in Genesis, in the qal, each time in the same context: 'And Yhwh *had regard* (וישע) for Abel and his offering, but for Cain and his offering he *had no regard* (לא שעה)' (Gen. 4.4-5). In Akkadian the verb *še'ûm* is composed of the same root, and means 'to seek'.[27]

This verb appears several times in parallelisms in contexts related to sight. Isaiah 17.7 reads: 'In that day men will regard (ישעה) their Maker, and their eyes (ועיניו) will look (תראינה) to the holy one of Israel'. Hence, the meaning of the verb שעה is 'to gaze, look at'.[28] The following verse reads: 'They will not have regard (ולא ישעה) for the altars, the work of their hands, and they will not look (לא יראה) to what their own fingers have made' (Isa. 17.8). Here again, the parallelism confirms the meaning of the verb שעה.[29]

Returning to Gen. 4.4-5, the meaning of שעה is 'to gaze, look at': God turned his gaze onto Abel's sacrifice, and not onto Cain's.[30] There are also

25. *HALOT*, p. 1368. Westermann also believes that *aleph* is written here instead of *ayin* (Westermann, *Genesis 12–36*, p. 381.

26. *HALOT*, p. 1368. Speiser interprets similarly (Speiser, *Genesis*, p. 180).

27. *HALOT*, pp. 1609-10; *CAD*, Š/2, p. 355.

28. *HALOT*, p. 1610.

29. In Isaiah there are some verbs whose formation is close to that of שעה. In Isa. 32.3 the verb תשעינה, is derived from the root שעע, here meaning that the eyes will 'be sealed', or 'pasted over'. In Isa. 41.10, 23 the verb שתע occurs, meaning 'to be afraid' (*HALOT*).

30. C. Westermann, *Genesis 1–11: A Commentary* (trans. J.J Scullion; Minneapolis: Augsburg, 1984), p. 296. Medieval Jewish commentators attempt to solve the theological

contexts in which the gaze is not turned onto, but away from, somebody. Thus in Isa. 22.4 (שעו מני), Job 7.19 (לא־תשעה ממני), and Job 14.6 (שעה מעליו).[31]

This verb is also subject to a shift in meaning from visual perception to cognitive perception. For instance, according to *HALOT*, in Exod. 5.9, this verb means 'to be concerned about, pay attention to', 'and *pay no regard* (ואל־ישעו) to lying words'. This shift in meaning may also be true for the occurrences in Genesis.

2.2.5. שקף

The verb השקיף, which derives from the root שקף, appears three times in Genesis in the hiphil: in Gen. 18.16, 19.28, and 26.8. Various dictionaries connect it with the Arabic noun *saqfun*, meaning 'ceiling', 'roof', or 'sky'[32], and to the Arabic verb *ašrafa*, which means 'overtop, overlook', and derives from *šarufa*, 'to be high'.[33] In Modern Hebrew, as in Biblical Hebrew, the verb שקף appears only in the niphal and hiphil in the meaning of 'to look down from above'. According to the dictionaries, in the Bible it means to look outwards and downwards. In the Bible, the verb appears in the following contexts: in the story of Abraham's hospitality to the angels in Gen. 18.16, 'Then the men set out from there, and *they looked toward* (וישקפו על־פני) Sodom'. From 13.10-13 we know that Lot chose the plain of Jordan, which is geographically low. It seems that Abraham also looked down on the region of Sodom from the direction of Elonei Mamre; similarly in ch. 19.28. In 26.8 Abimelech king of the Philistines *looks* (וישקף) through the window, and sees Isaac 'fondling (RSV, "caressing" according to NIB) Rebekah his wife'. It may be that here, too, the observer was at a greater height than the object observed.

Differences of height between the observer and the object observed are expressed outside Genesis. In 2 Sam. 6.16 Michal, Saul's daughter, looks through the window, and sees (נשקפה בעד החלון ותרא) David 'leaping and dancing'. Taking into account the geographical conditions, it seems probable

problem which arises from the text: How did Cain know that God turned his gaze onto Abel's sacrifice, but did not accept Cain's? Rashi and Ibn Ezra say that fire descended and consumed Abel's sacrifice, and from this it was clear that God accepted it. Skinner's solution is that this is one of the anthropomorphic descriptions of God (J. Skinner, *A Critical and Exegetical Commentary on Genesis* [ICC; Edinburgh: T. & T. Clark, 1930], pp. 104-105).

31. Clines takes שעה to mean 'take your gaze from me' (Job 7.19), and 'look away from' (Job 14.6) (D.J.A. Clines, *Job 1–20* [WBC 17; Dallas, TX: Word Books, 1989], p. 327).

32. E.W. Lane, *An Arabic–English Lexicon* (Beirut: Librairie du Liban, 1968), p. 1383.

33. BDB, p. 1054; *HALOT*, p. 1645; Lane, *An Arabic–English Lexicon*, p. 1536.

that the window through which she looks is higher than the sight she sees. According to 1 Sam. 13.18, the Philistine army turned toward the border that 'looks down upon' (נשקף) the valley of Zeboim. Shortly before this Saul and Jonathan were in Gibeah of Benjamin, a region higher than the valley of Zeboim. These differences of height are presumably the reason for the use of the verb שׁקף of all sight verbs.

In 2 Sam. 24.20, the verbs ...וירא and ...וישקף describe Araunah the Jebusite seeing David. Araunah stands within the threshing-floor, and looks down on David from the raised area. In the same context, in 1 Chron. 21.21 the verbs ...וירא and ...ויבט occur. The context shows that it was not without reason that the verb וישקף was replaced by the verb ויבט, since, according to Chronicles, David was standing at the same height as Ornan; for it is stated there specifically that 'David came to (עד) Ornan'.

2.3. *Lexemes of the First Circle: Lexemes Linked Semantically to the Centre*

Lexemes linked to the centre by various semantic relations belong to the first circle of lexemes. The semantic relations may be of several types, such as a connecting abstract schema, a metaphor, or relations of instrumentality. The first group consists of the following lexemes: מַרְאֶה (sight, appearance, vision); מחזה (vision), חלם (to dream), חלום (dream), מַרְאָה (vision, as means of revelation), which all share the schema 'an image of a thing perceived by the mind'.[34] The lexemes מַרְאֶה and מחזה are connected with an external image which is perceived through the eyes, whereas in the lexemes חלם, חלום, and מַרְאָה the vision is mental, and does not reach the mind through the eyes. The same image perceived by means of the eyes is also the basis of the semantic definition of the lexemes: דמות (shape, likeness), צלם (likeness), and תֹּאַר (appearance, form). They also belong to the first circle.

2.3.1. *The Schema: 'The Image of the Object which is Perceived by the Mind'*

2.3.1.1. מַרְאֶה. The first translation of מַרְאֶה in *HALOT* is 'seeing'. Ben Yehuda defines it as a verbal noun from ראה, meaning 'what the eye sees, the appearance and the form'.[35] The act of sight is included in the semantic definition of this noun, hence it is considered a constituent in the SF. In passages outside Genesis, such as Exod. 3.3, 'and *see* this great *sight*' (ואראה את־המראה), and Song 2.14, 'let me *see your face*' (הראיני את־מראיך), the

34. On the term 'schema', see Lakoff, *Women, Fire and Dangerous Things*, p. 104 (also see §1.1.1).

35. Eliezer Ben Yehuda, *A Complete Dictionary of Ancient and Modern Hebrew* (Ben-Yehuda Hozaa-La'Or: Jerusalem, 1948–59 [Hebrew]), p. 3299.

function of the noun מַרְאֶה as an internal object[36] is especially prominent. Functioning in this way it is semantically redundant to the understanding of the verb of sight.

It is interesting to see the collocations in which מַרְאֶה occurs in Genesis. The lexeme appears eleven times in Genesis, five times in the construct-genitive relations: יפת־מראה (beautiful to behold [RSV], or just beautiful [*HALOT*], 12.11; 29.17; 39.6 [–יפה]; 41.2, 4); twice in the construct-genitive with טבת—טבת מראה (pleasing, beautiful, 24.16; 26.7); and twice within the construct-genitive—רעות מראה (poor in appearance, 41.3, 4). It appears once in the phrase נחמד למראה (pleasant, desirable to the sight, Gen. 2.9), and once with the possessive suffix מראיהן (their appearance, Gen. 41.21). In most of these cases, the definition of the lexeme מראה is 'appearance' (noun).

In the story about her dangerous trip to Egypt Sarah is said to be יפת מראה (Gen. 12.11); Rebekah is טבת מראה (24.16; 26.7), and Rachel יפת תאר ויפת מראה (beautiful and lovely, 29.17). In the story of his temptation by Potiphar's wife Joseph, Rachel's son, is said to be יפה־תאר ויפה מראה (handsome and good looking, 39.6). The cows in Pharaoh's dream are described as יפות מראה (41.2, 4) and רעות מראה (41.3, 4), and in the Garden of Eden God makes 'every tree that is *pleasant to the sight* (נחמד למראה)' grow from the ground (2.9).

2.3.1.2. מחזה. According to biblical dictionaries,[37] the meaning of the noun מחזה is 'vision', perhaps in the ecstatic state. Since we are dealing with a vision, it is seen by someone, and hence it belongs to the category of the schema: 'image of a thing which is perceived by the mind'. This lexeme appears once in Genesis, at 15.1. Apart from this, it appears in three other biblical contexts: Num. 24.4, 16, and Ezek. 13.7. In every other case, other than the instance in Gen. 15.1, the verb חזה appears together with the noun מחזה: 'who *sees* (יחזה) the vision (מחזה) of the Almighty' (Num. 24.4; there is a similar wording in v. 16). Similarly, in Ezek. 13.7: 'Have you *not seen* (...הלוא חזיתם) a delusive vision (מחזה)'. According to the BDB, חזה is generally found in poetical texts.[38]

36. P. Joüon and T. Muraoka, *A Grammar of Biblical Hebrew* (Subsidia Biblica, 27; Rome: Editrice Pontificio Istituto biblico, 2006), p. 450, §125q: 'The internal object is an abstract noun of action, identical with or analogous to the action expressed by the verb'.

37. E.g. BDB, p. 303; *HALOT*, p. 568.

38. Close to the noun מחזה is חזיון, which similarly means 'vision, revelation', but since it is not found in Genesis it is not included in the present description of the SF.

2.3.1.3. חלם. According to Ben Yehuda's dictionary, the meaning of the verb חלם is 'to see a dream in sleep',[39] and חלום (dream) is defined as 'a vision which a person sees while asleep, and which seems to him as if he were seeing it in reality'.[40] Genesis 41.5, for example, provides evidence of the dream's taking place in sleep: 'And he fell asleep and dreamed a second time'. In Akkadian, the form *šuttu*, meaning 'dream', is derived from the same root as the noun *šittu*, 'sleep'.[41] In *HALOT* חלם is translated as 'to dream'.[42] Webster defines 'dream' as '1. a sequence of sensations, images, thoughts, etc. passing through a sleeping person's mind'.[43] Thus, both sight by means of the eyes in a waking state and dreaming are connected with an act of perception of images by the mind. This is the schema which connects dreaming and visual perception (sight), and, therefore, this lexeme belongs to the SF.

The verb חלם appears 14 times in Genesis, in the following places: 28.12; 37.5, 6, 9 (twice), 10; 40.5, 8; 41.1, 5, 11 (twice), 15; 42.9.

2.3.1.4. חלום. The noun חלום (dream) is connected to the SF by the semantic connection of the abstract schema 'an image perceived by the mind, but not through the eyes'; for regular sight, which is done through the eyes, also involves the perception of images by the mind. The status of the verb חלם in relation to the centre is very similar to that of the noun חלום.

The dream is, then, a vision, and in several verses the collocation ראה + בחלום (to see + in a dream) occurs.[44] Thus, for instance, in Gen. 31.10, we find: 'I *lifted up my eyes* (ואשׂא עיני), and *saw in a dream* (וארא בחלום)

39. This is also the definition according to Samuel Ephraim Loewenstamm and J. Blau (eds.), *Otzar Leshon haMikra* (Jerusalem: The Bible Concordance Press, 1957–68), III, p. 159.

40. In *HALOT* the definition 'to dream' of the verb חלם is the second of the two principal definitions of the qal (and also of the hiphil—qal and hiphil are the two main conjugations in which this verb is found in the Bible). The first definition of the qal is 'to become strong', and in the hiphil החלים it is defined as 'to restore to health'. In the BDB the definitions are separated into two homonymous entries: חלם I and חלם II. The parallel term in Arabic, *ḥalama*, denotes both dreaming and arriving at sexual maturity (Lane, *An Arabic–English Lexicon*, p. 632). Fidler points out that it may be that the physiological phenomenon of sexual excitement while dreaming was also known to the ancients; hence the closeness between the two meanings in Arabic (Ruth Fidler, *'Dreams Speak Falsely'? Dream Theophanies in the Bible* [Jerusalem: Magnes Press, 2005 (Hebrew)], p. 24 n. 85, and see references there).

41. *CAD*, Š/3, pp. 140, 405.

42. *HALOT*, p. 320.

43. Webster, *Webster's New World Dictionary*, p. 442.

44. In Akkadian, too, people *see* in their dreams (M. Ottoson, 'חלום', *TDOT*, IV, p. 423).

that the he-goats…' There is another example from the early prophets, and Gen. 41.22: 'I also *saw in my dream* (וארא בחלמי) seven ears…' There is another example from 1 Kgs 3.5: 'In Gibeon Yhwh *appeared* (נראה) to Solomon in *a dream* (בחלום)'. A play on this collocation of 'seeing in a dream' is found in Gen. 37.20. Instead of the usual construction in which the agent himself sees in his own dreams, here Joseph's brothers are the agents, and they want to see what will become of Joseph's dreams: 'Come now, let us kill him and throw him into one of the pits…and *we shall see* (ונראה) what will become of his *dreams* (חלמתיו)'.

The lexeme חלום is found 34 times in Genesis, 29 of them in the Joseph Narrative. In Job it appears in parallelism with חזיון לילה (vision of the night), and also with חזיון (vision) alone: 'He will fly away like a *dream* (כחלום יעוף), and not be found; he will be chased away like a *vision of the night* (כחזיון לילה)' (Job 20.8), 'Then thou dost scare me with *dreams* and terrify me with *visions*' (Job 7.14 [RSV translation]). This parallelism shows the close semantic resemblance between these terms.[45] In Job 33.15, חלום and חזיון are found not in parallelism but as a syntagm: 'In *a dream*, in *a vision of the night* (בחלום חזיון לילה), when deep sleep falls upon men, while they slumber on their beds'.[46]

2.3.1.5. מַרְאָה. The noun מַרְאָה is interpreted as 'a vision', as a special image in that it serves as a means of a revelation of God or his words (see 1 Sam. 3.15).[47] It is connected to the SF since it is a vision, hence, through the schema, 'image of a thing which is perceived by the mind', which is a constituent in its semantic definition. This noun appears in Genesis once only, in the plural: 'And God spoke to Israel in *visions of the night* (במראת לילה), and said…' (46.2). The lexeme appears twelve times in the Hebrew Bible. In Num. 12.6 it appears in parallelism with חלום (dream): 'I Yhwh make myself known to him *in a vision* (במראה), I speak with him *in a dream* (בחלום)'.

2.3.1.6. דמות. This noun is derived from the root דמה, which has the meaning of 'compare, liken' (*HALOT*). *Otzar Leshon haMikra* defines this noun as 'equality, likeness, shape'. It is found in Genesis three times, at 1.26 and 5.1, 3. According to the BDB, in Gen. 1.26 the meanings of דמות (likeness) and צלם (image) are close: 'Then God said, "Let us make man in our *image* (בצלמנו), after our *likeness* (כדמותנו)"'. Along with this definition

45. Fidler, *'Dreams Speak Falsely'? Dream Theophanies in the Bible*, p. 24.

46. See also the discussion of dreams as a poetic phenomenon in the sections dealing with the coherence of the Joseph Narrative (§3.4.1 and §4.8).

47. BDB, p. 909, and Fidler, *'Dreams Speak Falsely'? Dream Theophanies in the Bible*, p. 24.

דמות here means the external form. God intends to create a man whose external form will be like that of himself. In an ancient Aramaic inscription found at Tell Fekheriye דמות means 'statue'.[48]

The principal meaning of this noun, then, is the external form, shape—in other words, again, an image—which is grasped through the eyes and perceived by the mind. It is this abstract semantic schema that connects it to the SF.

2.3.1.7. צלם. In Ben Yehuda's dictionary, the definition of צלם is 'The image of a thing, a person, and the like, its (his) likeness and bodily form'.[49] The Akkadian noun, *ṣalmu*, means a statue, a painting, or a form, and especially a statue of a god or the king; that is to say, a statue with religious significance.[50] A statue with a religious significance can be found in Amos 5.26: 'You shall take up Sakkuth your king, and Kaiwan your star-god, your images (צלמיכם), which you made for yourselves'; and not also Ezek. 7.20: 'and they made their abominable images (צלמי תועבתם) and their detestable things of it'; as well as 1 Sam. 6.11: 'And they put the ark of Yhwh on the cart, and the box with the golden mice and the images (צלמי) of their tumours'. There is a similar root in Arabic, *ṣanama*, which means a carved, cut or incised form.[51] The external form, the image which is perceived by the mind, constitutes the semantic component which connects the lexeme with the SF. The lexeme צלם is found five times in Genesis: at 1.26, 27 (twice); 5.3, and 9.6. In each of these instances, the context is that man was created in the image of God.

2.3.1.8. תֹּאַר. Ben Yehuda's definition of תֹּאַר is 'figure, shape, appearance'.[52] This noun, too, like the previous one, is concerned with external appearance, an image of some sort which is perceived by the mind; it is connected, therefore, with the SF. According to *HALOT* (pp. 1676-77), the collocation יפה תֹּאַר appears three times in Genesis, and means 'beautiful in form'. The lexeme תֹּאַר appears a total of four times in Genesis: 29.17; 39.6; 41.18, 19.

48. A. Abou-Assaf, P. Bordreuil and A.R. Millard, *La statue de Tell Fekheriye et son inscription bilingue assyro-araméenne* (Etudes assyriologiques, 7; Paris: Editions recherches sur la civilisation, 1982), pp. 23-24. The inscription is dated to the mid-ninth century BCE.

49. Ben Yehuda, *A Complete Dictionary*, p. 5498 (my translation from the Hebrew).

50. *CAD*, Ṣ, p. 78.

51. Lane, *An Arabic–English Lexicon*, p. 1735. BDB has *ṣalama* with *laam* instead of *nuun* as the second consonant of the root (I thank Professor Nasser Basal for pointing this out to me).

52. Ben Yehuda, *A Complete Dictionary*, p. 7644.

2.3.2. *The Means of Seeing*

2.3.2.1. עין *(eye)*. The lexeme עין, with its inflections, is connected with the verb ראה because it serves as a means of performing the act of seeing.[53] The eye is the organ which senses rays of light that are transferred to the mind.[54] In Akkadian there is a similar root, *īnu*, with the same meaning.[55] In Akkadian a person who has found favour in somebody's sight is called *ša īnšu maḫru*,[56] the literal meaning of which is: 'which is acceptable to his eye'. Both in Mesopotamia and in Egypt the belief in the evil eye was widespread, and it was based on the assumption that the eye can function as an independent force. Both in Ugaritic and in the Bible, the words 'eye' and 'head' occur as synonyms in parallelism.[57]

As been noted, in the Bible the eye is the instrument of sight, and in many texts it is referred to as being defective: Lev. 21.20 (תבלל בעינו, 'a defect in his eye'—*HALOT*), Deut. 28.65 (כליון עינים, 'failing eyes'). Zechariah 11.17, Gen. 27.1, and Deut. 34.7 all refer to כהות עיניים (dim eyes); Gen. 29.17 mentions Leah's soft eyes (ועיני לאה רכות), plausibly meaning that they were weak.[58] In Gen. 48.10 eyes are described as 'heavy', and so forth.

2.3.2.1.1. *Collocations featuring the Lexeme* עין. Various collocations and phrases are included in the SF because they include the component עין. The following collocations and phrases are found in Genesis:

53. Zadka uses the term 'instrument' in connection with עין, pointing out that the parts of the body serve as instruments of performing various actions: the eye sees and has mercy and desires, the mouth can speak and command, the heart can love, pity and think (Y. Zadka, '"Noah found grace in the eyes of the Lord": A Semantic and Syntactic Analysis' [Hebrew], *Criticism and Interpretation* 24 [1988], pp. 113-40 [118]).

54. Egyptian religion distinguished between light and divinity, and this belief was extended to the human domain since the human eye perceives light. The relationship between man and god was expressed through sight, and blindness symbolized a departure from divinity: just as the eyes of the god were perfect and unflawed, it was expected that human eyes would be perfect (E. Otto, *Gott und Mensch nach den ägyptischen Tempelinschriften der griechisch-romischen Zeit* [Heidelberg: C. Winter, 1964], pp. 101-105).

55. *CAD*, I–J, p. 153.

56. *CAD*, I–J, p. 64.

57. F.J. Stendebach, 'עין', in *TDOT*, XI, pp. 28-44 (30).

58. Commentators are divided on the meaning of the description of Leah's eyes. RSV: 'Leah's eyes were weak'; KJV: 'Leah was tender eyed'. Speiser prefers 'tender' rather than 'weak', explaining that traditional translation has been influenced by popular etymology of the name Leah as weak. What the narrative appears to be saying is that Leah had lovely eyes, says Speiser, but Rachel was an outstanding beauty (Speiser, *Genesis*, p. 225). It seems that Rashbam interprets Leah's eyes as blue, or bright coloured, saying that *rakkōt* means 'beautiful', and that 'black eyes are not as nice as white eyes'. Skinner: 'they lacked the lustrous brilliancy which is counted a feature of female beauty in the East' (Skinner, *Genesis*, p. 383). According to Westermann, the present meaning suggests that *rakkōt* means 'dull, lustreless' (Westermann, *Genesis 12–36*, pp. 462-63).

(1) מצא חן בעיני. This phrase is found in Gen. 6.8; 18.3; 19.19; 30.27; 32.6; 33.8, 10, 15; 34.11; 39.4; 47.25, 29; 50.4. Stendebach translates: 'to find favour in the eyes of'.[59] Harman maintains that it functions as an endorsement or blessing given by God to righteous men, and that it is also used in the context of attempts by people to find favour in the sight of another (33.8, 10).[60] It should be noted that wherever this phrase appears it refers to the relationship between a patron and a subject: the inferior person asks for favour in the eyes of his/her superior.

(2) נתן חן בעיני. This phrase, which means 'to give favour with', is found at Gen. 39.21. Its meaning is close to that of the previous expression מצא חן בעיני. Here, God 'gives Joseph favour' in the sight of the chief jailer: he ensures that Joseph will find favour in his sight.

(3) וישא עיניו וירא. Literally, this long formula of seeing means 'and he lifted his eyes and saw'. However, the lifting of the eyes signifies the beginning of the process of seeing, and the principal weight of the meaning is borne by the verb וירא (and he saw).[61] The formula is found in Genesis at 13.10, 14; 18.2; 22.4, 13; 31.10, 12; 33.1, 5; 37.25; 43.29.

(4) נשא עין. This phrase, 'to raise the eyes', meaning 'to look up, look at', occurs once only in Genesis. When Potiphar's wife looks at Joseph, it is said that: 'his master's wife *cast her eyes upon* (ותשא...את־עיניה) Joseph, and said, "Lie with me"' (Gen. 39.7). It may be that when the narrator did not add the verb ותרא after the phrase 'she raised her eyes' he intended to emphasize that Potiphar's wife was not fully engaged in the cognitive perception of what she has seen; rather, her sight was superficial. The very raising of the eyes at Joseph, done by a married woman, was a forbidden act. Westermann sees here an expression of concrete sight, which symbolizes desire. Both he and Speiser mention Ishtar's desire for Gilgamesh, which is phrased similarly.[62]

(5) בעיני X. Various collocations which include the nominal phrase בעיני (in the eyes of) have the abstract meaning: 'in the opinion of…' (*HALOT*). Rubinstein speaks of clauses in which he who is perceived is syntactically

59. Stendebach, 'עין', p. 37.

60. A.M. Harman, 'עין', in *NIDOTTE*, III, pp. 385-90 (386).

61. Frank Polak, 'Epic Formulae in Biblical Narrative and the Origins of Ancient Hebrew Prose' (Hebrew), *Te'uda 7* (1991), pp. 9-54 (10). For a more detailed analysis, see Polak, 'Linguistic and Stylistic Aspects of Epic Formulae in Ancient Semitic Poetry and Biblical Narrative', in S. Fassberg and A. Hurvitz (eds.), *Biblical Hebrew in Its Northwest Semitic Setting* (Winona Lake, IN: Eisenbrauns, 2006), pp. 285-304.

62. Claus Westermann, *Genesis 37–50: A Commentary* (trans. J.J Scullion; London: SPCK, 1987), p. 65; Speiser, *Genesis*, p. 303. See *The Gilgamesh Epic*, VI.6 (Benjamin R. Foster [trans. and ed.], *The Epic of Gilgamesh: A New Translation, Analogues, Criticism* [New York: W.W. Norton, 2001]).

realized and explicit. In his article, Rubinstein adduces the example דוד חכם בעיני (David is wise in my eyes), which he interprets as: אני חושב דוד חכם (I think: David is wise).[63] The following collocations are found in the Genesis:

(a) קל בעיני. This phrase occurs twice in Genesis, each time in the same context: 'and when she *saw* (ותרא) that she had conceived, she looked with contempt on her mistress (ותקל גברתה בעיניה)' (16.4); and again in 16.5, when Sarah tells Abraham of the incident. The meaning of this phrase in this context is that from the moment Hagar discovers that she is pregnant, she despises her mistress.[64] Dictionaries of Biblical Hebrew translate as 'to be insignificant in the eyes of, meaning to count as nothing', and 'trifling, i.e. of little account'.[65]

(b) טוב בעיני. There are three syntactical variations of the collocation טוב + בעיני, that is, the root טוב (good) followed by the noun עין ('eye', in the sense of 'in the opinion of someone'). The meaning of all of them is similar.

(i) עשׂה הטוב/כטוב בעיני. The phrase 'X did good in the eyes of…' occurs only twice in Genesis, at 16.6 and 19.8.

(ii) וייטב הדבר בעיני. The phrase 'X was good in the eyes of…' is found in Gen. 34.18; 41.37 and 45.16. Malul analyzes the occurrence of this phrase in 2 Sam. 3.36, and claims that since the verb הכירו ('took notice of') in the same verse has the validity of legal recognition, the phrase וייטב בעיניהם ('and it pleased them') also has the meaning of agreement on an official or legal level.[66] It may be assumed that this explanation also holds good for the instances of this expression in Genesis.

(iii) בטוב בעיניך. Abimelech tells Abraham to dwell where it pleases him (Gen. 20.15). בטוב בעיניך means 'where it pleases you', or 'where it is good in your eyes'.

(c) וירע (הדבר) בעיני. This phrase may be translated as 'And it was bad in the sight of', 'evil, wicked behaviour'.[67] It is found in Gen. 21.11, 12; 28.8; 38.7, 10; 48.17.

63. Eliezer Rubinstein, 'The Hidden Perceiver' (Hebrew), *Hebrew Computational Linguistics* 19 (1982), pp. 63-68.

64. Westermann, *Genesis 12–36*, p. 240. Skinner translates 'was despised' (Skinner, *Genesis*, p. 286). According to Rashi, in his commentary on these verses, Hagar did not believe that Sarah was a righteous woman, since she did not become pregnant, whereas she, Hagar, became pregnant after her first sexual encounter.

65. *HALOT*, p. 1103 (קלל); BDB, p. 886. The phrase appears a total of five times in the Bible, two occurrences in the qal in Genesis and three times in the niphal in 1 Sam. 18.23; 2 Sam. 6.22; 2 Kgs 3.18.

66. M. Malul, 'Law in the Narratives: A Study of the Expressions הכירו and וייטב בעיניהם in 2 Sam 3:36', *JNSL* 17 (1991), pp. 23-36.

67. *HALOT*, p. 1251.

(d) חרה בעיניו. This phrase appears in Gen. 31.35 and 45.5. According to *Otzar Leshon haMikra*, like חרה לו it means 'to become or be angry, to regret'.[68] Westermann translates the phrase in 31.35 as 'do not be angry with me', and in 45.5, rather differently, '...reproach yourselves'.[69]

(e) מצחק בעיני. In the story of Sodom and Gomorrah, it is said of Lot, as translated by Westermann: 'but his sons in law thought he was joking (ויהי כמצחק בעיני)' (Gen. 19.14).[70] According to the Ramban, the sons-in-law were laughing at Lot. Rabbi Joseph Bekhor Shor maintains that ויהי כמצחק means that the sons-in-law were treating Lot as a fool, since they did not believe him.

(f) היה בעיניו כ. This phrase occurs twice in Genesis, at 27.12, 'Perhaps my father will feel me, and *I shall seem to* be mocking him (והייתי בעיניו כמתעתע)', and at 29.20, 'So Jacob served seven years for Rachel, and *they seemed to him* but a few days (ויהיו בעיניו כימים אחדים)'.

(6) נדדה הַשֵּׁנָה מן עינים. Literally: 'the escape of sleep from the eyes'. This phrase occurs once in Genesis, at 31.40, meaning that the person is unable to fall asleep.[71] It occurs once more in the Bible, at Est. 6.1.

(7) אל תחס עינכם על. Occurs once in Genesis, at 45.20. Rabbi David Kimhi comments: 'It is usually the custom of the Hebrew tongue to relate this root to the eye, even though pity is not in the eye, but in the heart, since when the eye sees, there will be pity in the heart'. According to *HALOT* תחוס עין על means 'to be troubled about'.[72] In *Otzar Leshon haMikra* the phrase is interpreted: 'Do not be sorry for them'.

(8) שית יד על העינים. 'To place the hands on the eyes of' occurs in Gen. 46.4. On this occurrence Ibn Ezra comments: 'And Joseph will lay his hand on your eyes when you die, for this is the custom of the living towards the dead'.

(9) כסות עינים. This phrase, which *HALOT* translated as 'covering of the eyes',[73] is found at Gen. 20.16. According to Rashi, the money which Abimelech gave to Abraham was intended to restore Sarah's honour. From the next part of the verse, לכל אשר אתך ('in the eyes of all who are with you'), Rashi understands that the money also served to cover the eyes of

68. The expression ...ויחר ל ('and he was angry with...') also occurs in Genesis (for instance: 4.5, 6; 18.30; 34.7), but is not included in the SF, since it does not include the lexeme עין (eye). Nonetheless, the similarity in meaning between the two phrases strengthens the notion that בעיני (in the eyes of) in the above examples does not have a concrete sense, but refers to an individual's opinion.

69. Westermann, *Genesis 12–36*, p. 487; Westermann, *Genesis 37–50*, p. 140.

70. Westermann, *Genesis 12–36*, p. 295.

71. Speiser, *Genesis*, p. 242; Westermann, *Genesis 12–36*, p. 487.

72. *HALOT*, p. 298.

73. *HALOT*, p. 489; BDB, p. 492.

others, and to ensure that they would not slight her. According to Speiser, the covering is meant for the eyes of the others, and is intended to hide her guilt. In his view, Sarah's sin was that she had gone with Abimelech, and Abimelech gave Abraham money in order to absolve both him and Sarah from guilt in the eyes of those who accompanied her and of the public in general.[74]

(10) חכלילי עינים. This phrase is found in Jacob's blessing on Judah in 49.12. According to *HALOT*, the meaning of the lexeme חכלילי is 'sparkling'; accordingly in Gen. 49.12 this phrase means 'with eyes sparkling from wine'. Kapelrud, however, claims that חכלילי עינים means 'dark eyes'.[75] He compares Akkadian, where *ekēlu* means 'to be dark'.[76] Brenner points out the parallelism in this verse, which is expressed in the contrast between 'wine' and 'milk', and claims that it is apparently based on the axis light/ dark, rather than on the chromatic scale.[77] Dullness, or blurred vision resulting from excessive drinking, seem more appropriate to her than a bloodshot (red) condition of the eyes. Clines offers the meanings 'dull', 'sparkling', or 'red'.[78] The overall context of the blessing for Judah is a positive one in whose framework he is promised superiority over his enemies (49.8-9) and long-lasting power (v. 10), and that the period of his sovereignty will be a time of prosperity in the land: there will be an abundance of vines and grapes (v. 11). The verse under consideration here, 49.12, is suggested to mean that the Judaean governor will be 'dark-eyed' because of the abundance of wine, and his teeth white because of the abundance of milk in the land. Thus, the context of this verse, too, is abundance and prosperity in the Land of Canaan.

The word חכלילי is also found in the same syntagm with עינים (eyes) in Prov. 23.29. Here, the context again indicates that the meaning is dimness and darkening of the eyes because of excessive drinking of wine.

2.3.2.2. ארבות השמים. The construct ארבות השמים is found twice in Genesis, only in the context of the Flood narrative, '…on that day all the fountains (מעינת) of the great deep burst forth, and the windows of the heavens (וארבת השמים) were opened' (Gen. 7.11), and at the end of the Flood, 'the fountains (מעינת) of the deep and the windows of the heavens (וארבת השמים) were closed…' (8.2). According to the BDB and *HALOT*, in Eccl. 12.3 the ארבות are a metaphor for eyes, or for the sockets of the eyes: 'In the day

74. Speiser, *Genesis*, pp. 148, 150.
75. Arvid S. Kapelrud, 'Genesis xlix 12', *VT* 4 (1954), pp. 426-28.
76. *CAD*, E, p. 64.
77. Brenner, *Colour Terms in the Old Testament*, pp. 86-87.
78. *DCH*, III, p. 218.

when the keepers of the house tremble, and the strong men are bent, and the grinders cease because they are few, and those that look through the windows (הראת בארבות) are dimmed'. Because of the connection with Ecclesiastes, it might be said that in Genesis, too, this is a metaphor for eyes, as if the heavens are a mythic creature with eyes; but, according to the other occurrences of the word ארבות, it is more probable that the meaning is 'hatches' or 'windows' through which the rain descends.

2.3.3. *Necessary Conditions for Seeing and Not-Seeing*

2.3.3.1. אור.[79] The eyes see on condition that there is light (אור). This idea is well illustrated in the description of the plague of darkness in Egypt: 'And Moses stretched forth his hand toward heaven; and there was a *thick darkness* in all the land of Egypt three days; they *saw not* one another, neither rose any from his place for three days; but all the children of Israel had *light* (אור) in their dwellings' (Exod. 10.22-23).

The lexeme אור is found in Genesis as a noun six times, at 1.3 (twice), 4 (twice), 5, and 18, and as a verb three times: twice in the infinitive construct, Gen. 1.15, 17, and once in the perfect of qal, 44.3. Light is connected with the SF since it is a necessary condition for seeing. Seeing may take place because the light is absorbed by the seen object, or is reflected from it and penetrates the eyes. It is impossible to see anything without the existence of a certain amount of light, however small, in the vicinity.[80] It should be noted that the nouns אור (light) and חשך (darkness) are found in Genesis only in ch. 1, in the context of the creation of the world.[81]

2.3.3.2. חשך. The noun חשך (darkness) is found in Genesis only four times, at 1.2, 4, 5, 18. According to the dictionaries, it means 'darkness', 'obscurity'. Since this noun is the opposite of light, it is one of the conditions for not-seeing.

2.3.3.3. חשכה. This noun is found only in Gen. 15.12. The meaning of חשכה here is darkness, the absence of light. This lexeme is chiefly found in poetical contexts, whereas in Genesis 15 it refers to supernatural darkness (BDB).

79. Various celestial lights are all discussed in the paragraph on lexemes which denote time (§2.8.2).

80. Brenner, *Colour Terms in the Old Testament*, p. 3.

81. According to Zohori, light may carry symbolic meanings such as salvation, success and wellbeing. It can also refer to the Torah (Menahem Zohori, '"Light"—Its Meanings in the Hebrew Bible' [Hebrew], in *Bamiqra Uvolamo: Studies and Essays on Biblical and Oriental Subjects* [Jerusalem: Carmel, 1998], pp. 7-18).

2.3.3.4. עלטה. The lexeme עלטה means darkness, or thick darkness.[82] It is found only in Genesis, in the story of the covenant between the divided parts (Gen. 15.17), like the preceding lexeme. The lexeme עלטה is also found in Ezekiel three times, all in ch. 12 (vv. 6, 7, 12).

2.3.4. *Lexemes Whose Semantic Definition Contains the Schema 'Creation of Conditions for Seeing' and its Opposite 'Creation of Conditions for Not-Seeing'*

As can be seen from the heading, this category consists of lexemes whose semantic definition contains the schema 'creation of conditions for seeing' and its opposite 'creation of conditions for not-seeing'. This action cannot involve causation, since it is impossible to cause a person to see, but it is possible to create the conditions under which he/she is able to see. This group contains verbs and nouns, verbs shall be mentioned first.

2.3.4.1. גלה. This verb is found for the first time, in the hithpael, in the story of Noah's drunkenness, at Gen. 9.21: 'And he drank of the wine, and became drunk, *and lay uncovered* (ויתגל) in his tent'. In this situation the verb ויתגל describes Noah undressing and exposing himself to his sons.[83] In the second instance it is in the niphal, when Jacob builds an altar to God in Bethel, and calls it Elbethel 'because there God had *revealed himself* (נגלו) to him' (35.7). Both Noah and God reveal themselves, and by this they create the conditions for seeing for other characters (for Noah's sons and for Jacob). Hence, the semantic definition of this verb includes the abstract schema 'creation of conditions for seeing', and for this it is included in the SF.

2.3.4.2. זרח. This verb means both 'to rise, shine' or 'to come out, to appear'.[84] It is only found at Gen. 32.31. Morag elaborates on this relationship between the semantic fields of Shining and Growth.[85]

2.3.4.3. ערוה. The root of the noun ערוה is ערה, which means 'to expose' or 'to uncover';[86] it includes the schema: 'to create conditions for seeing'. The lexeme ערוה appears five times in Genesis, at 9.22, 23 (twice); 42.9, 12 (ערות הארץ). Its meaning is 'nakedness, genital area of a man or of a

82. BDB, p. 759; *HALOT*, p. 832.

83. *HALOT*, p. 192. See the discussion in §4.4 regarding the possible interpretations of what has occurred between Noah and his son.

84. *HALOT*, p. 281, also J.L. Palache, *Semantic Notes on the Hebrew Lexicon* (trans. R.J. Werblowsky; Leiden: E.J. Brill, 1959), p. 45 (נבט).

85. Morag, '"ומתערה כאזרח רענן" (Psalms XXXVI, 35)'.

86. *HALOT*, pp. 881-82.

woman'.[87] According to *HALOT*, the phrase ערות הארץ, which appears in the Joseph Narrative (42.9, 12), is a metaphor for the bare and undefended places in the land. Joseph accuses his brothers of coming to see 'the nakedness of the land'—in other words, of spying, or exposing its secrets. There is a similar root in Akkadian, *ūru*, which means nakedness, or the feminine pudenda.[88]

2.3.4.4. עֵירֹם/עירם, עָרוֹם/ערם. According to the BDB, these nouns are derived from the root עור II, which is akin to the root ערה. According to *HALOT* it derives from ערה or ערם III.[89] The root ערה has been discussed above. The meaning of the adjective עירם is naked, completely naked. This lexeme is found in the story of the Garden of Eden at Gen. 2.25; 3.7, 10, 11. The form עָרוֹם/ערם occurs fifteen times in the Bible, and the form עירם/עֵרם occurs ten times: three in Genesis, one in Deuteronomy, and six in Ezekiel.

2.3.4.5. מחשׂף. This noun is derived from the root חשׂף, which means 'to strip, make bare'.[90] The dictionaries interpret מחשׂף as a peeling, stripping of the bark of the tree, when the wood is left bare.[91] This is a *hapax legomenon*, and appears only at Gen. 30.37.

2.3.4.6. חבא. This verb appears in Genesis once in the hithpael (3.8), and twice in the niphal (3.10; 31.27). It means 'to hide oneself' (niphal), 'to keep oneself hidden' (hithpael).[92] This idea of hiding is close to the notion of the abstract schema 'creation of conditions for not-seeing'; hence, it is included as a category in the SF.

2.3.4.7. כסה. The verb כסה is found seven times in Genesis, and its meaning is 'to cover'. Balentine treats it as part of a separate field, the field of Cover or Veil.[93] I, however, treat it as part of a sub-group of the SF, since covering is an act whereby a person covers something in order that it shall not be seen. It is connected with the SF since its semantic definition includes the abstract schema 'creation of conditions for not-seeing'.

The verb כסה appears twice in Genesis in the pual, at 7.19, 20. In these verses the context is the Flood, in the course of which the hills were *covered* with water. It also appears in the piel, at 9.23, where the sons of Noah *cover*

87. *HALOT*, p. 882.
88. *AHw*, p. 1435; *CAD*, U–W, p. 265.
89. BDB, p. 735; *HALOT*, p. 823.
90. BDB, p. 362.
91. BDB, p. 362; *HALOT*, p. 572.
92. *HALOT*, p. 284; BDB, p. 285.
93. Balentine, *The Hidden God*, p. 14.

their father's nakedness, which is almost revealed to their eyes, and at 38.15. In this latter context, the motif of covering is found when Tamar, Judah's daughter-in-law, *covers* her face. In the previous verse (38.14) the verb כסה appears in the qal, when Tamar is mentioned covering her face with a veil (ותכס בצעיף).[94] Tamar does this so that her father-in-law shall not recognize her. Another use of the piel is found at 37.26, when Judah, Joseph's brother says: 'What profit is it if we slay our brother and *conceal* (וכסינו) his blood?' The verb is found as a qal participle in Gen. 18.17, when God asks himself, 'Shall I *hide* (המכסה) from Abraham what I am about to do'. Here, God means to ask whether he is concealing information from Abraham. This concealment is not concrete, but rather abstract.

כסה is found once in Genesis in the hithpael, ותתכס, when Rebekah covers herself with a veil in order not to expose herself before Isaac, who is about to marry her (24.65).

2.3.4.8. כסות עינים. See the discussion of the phrase under the noun עין in §§2.3.2.1.1, 9.

2.3.4.9. מכסה. The root כסה also appears in the form of a noun, מכסה (cover, overlay), in Gen. 8.13. There we read that Noah took off the covering of the ark at the end of the Flood: that is to say, Noah revealed himself anew to the world. The cover is a means of creating conditions for not seeing. This lexeme appears again in the Bible only in connection with the tabernacle and the Temple, in Exodus 26; 35; 36; 39; 40 and Numbers 3; 4.

2.3.4.10. סתר. The verb סתר (to hide) is found in Genesis only twice, in the niphal. In both instances a person is described hiding from someone else. The meaning of hiding can be described as the creation of conditions by one party whereby the other party will not see him. This verb then contains the schema 'creation of conditions for not-seeing'; hence it is included in the SF. In the first context of its occurrence, Cain hides from God: 'from thy face I shall be hidden' (Gen. 4.14). This use of the verb סתר is of particular importance, since it expresses the concept of a man hiding from God, an act with theological implications.[95] The second occurrence of the verb סתר in Genesis is at 31.49, when Laban says to Jacob: 'when we are *absent* (נסתר) one from the other'.

94. Westermann corrects the form ותכס into the hithpael ותתכס, which is found in the Samaritan Pentateuch, probably assuming haplography in the Hebrew version (Westermann, *Genesis 37–50*, p. 48). This is also one of Skinner's suggestions (Skinner, *Genesis*, p. 453), in addition to another suggestion to read וַתִּכָּס, in the niphal.

95. Balentine's study (*The Hidden God*), which focuses on the syntagm הסתר פנים (hide the face) in situations in which God hides his face, discusses a situation opposite to many syntagms in the SF, in which God is revealed to the Fathers.

2.3.4.11. עלף.[96] Balentine treats this verb as one of those belonging to the Cover field.[97] According to BDB and *HALOT*,[98] it means 'to cover', and, in the hithpael, 'to wrap oneself up'. In this sense it is included in the schema 'creation of conditions for not-seeing'. The second meaning of the verb עלף, as in Modern Hebrew, is 'to become faint', and is also found in Rabbinical Hebrew, but it is not found in this sense in Genesis. The root עלף appears once in Gen. 38.14, describing Tamar's actions: 'She put off her widow's garments, and put on a veil, *wrapping herself up* (ותתעלף)'. Here the verb means to cover oneself up.

This verb appears outside of Genesis only once in the sense of covering oneself up in Song 5.14 (in the pual), and three more times in the sense of exhaustion leading to loss of consciousness: Isa. 51.20 (in the pual); Amos 8.13 (in the hithpael); Jon. 4.8 (in the hithpael).

2.3.4.12. צעיף. The article of clothing צעיף (veil), is also part of the SF since it is a means of creating conditions of not-seeing. In its occurrences in Genesis the veil is put on in order to hide the body, and prevent another party from seeing it. צעיף appears three times in the Bible, with the occurrences concentrated in two chapters of Genesis (Gen. 24.65; 38.14, 19). In Genesis 24 Rebekah covers herself with a veil in order to conceal herself from Isaac, and in Genesis 38 Tamar tries to hide her identity from Judah by covering herself with a veil.

2.3.5. *Lexemes Which Contain the Schema 'Objects Which Fulfil their Function by Being Seen'*

This category concerns a schema which contains objects intended to influence the consciousness of those who look at them, on condition that the text refers to this explicitly: in other words, the objects have influence as a result of being looked at. It could be said that in the syntactical neighbourhood of these objects there is a participant who is not explicitly mentioned, but is included in the semantic definition of these objects. Rubinstein calls this participant the 'hidden perceiver'.[99]

96. In certain contexts the verb עטף, which also occurs in Genesis, could be added. Sometimes עטף means 'to cover oneself', which is close to לבש (to dress). Thus, for instance, in Ps. 65.13: 'The meadows clothe themselves (לבשׁו) with flocks, the valleys deck themselves (יעטפו) with grain'. This verb is derived from the root עטף II (BDB, p. 742). But in Genesis the verb עטף is derived from the homonymous root עטף III (BDB, p. 742), which means 'be feeble, faint', or 'to be sickly' (*HALOT*, p. 814). Thus, the instances of the verb עטף in Genesis do not form part of the structure of the SF.

97. Balentine, *The Hidden God*, p. 14.

98. BDB, p. 763; *HALOT*, p. 836.

99. Rubinstein, 'The Hidden Perceiver', pp. 63-68.

2.3.5.1. אות. The Mark of Cain (אות) is mentioned in the story of Cain and Abel in Genesis 4. After Cain kills Abel, God punishes him by making him 'a fugitive and a wanderer on the earth' (4.12). Cain finds himself persecuted by people who want to take vengeance for Abel (4.14): 'from your *face I shall be hidden* (ומפניך אסתר); and I shall be a fugitive and a wanderer on the earth, and whoever *finds* (מצאי) me will slay me'.

God reduces the cruel punishment slightly and threatens to punish anybody who tries to avenge Abel. He puts a mark on Cain, so anybody who finds Cain will recognize some bodily mark with which God has marked him, and will refrain from killing him. This bodily sign is intended to influence the consciousness of whoever looks at him, and prevent him from injuring Cain. This is Rubinstein's 'hidden perceiver'.[100] Although the text does not explicitly say that somebody sees the mark, the terms concerning hiding and finding which appear in the vicinity emphasize the act of seeing connected with the mark. The implicit perceiver is the semantic element which does not appear explicitly in the clause, but is part of the semantic definition of the lexeme אות. Thus, when God puts the mark on Cain and somebody *finds* him we can assume that Cain's mark is visually perceived.

2.3.5.2. קֶשֶׁת. The Rainbow: A Sign of the Covenant. The rainbow in the clouds is described as a sign (אות) of the covenant between God and the living on earth, which God grants at the end of the story of the Flood, in Gen. 9.12. According to God's words the rainbow is there first of all for him to see, and as a result of this sight he will remember the covenant and will not cause another Flood (Gen. 9.14-16). Thus, the rainbow is an object designed to influence the consciousness of God, and, specifically, his memory. After the rainbow influences his consciousness; it influences his action, in that he does not bring about another Flood.[101] The rainbow may

100. Rubinstein, 'The Hidden Perceiver', pp. 63-68.

101. The majority of commentators understand the bow in the clouds to maintain military connotations, and thus to represent God's war bow. Rabbinic commentators such as the Ramban saw the rainbow as symbolizing a war bow turned upwards so that arrows would be shot away from the earth, rather than towards it. Marduk's bow took its place among the Gods after his defeat of Tiamat, and Gen. 9 has been taken to reflect this tradition (Skinner, *Genesis*, p. 173; *Enuma Elish*, VI.83-94 [Stephanie Dalley, *Myths from Mesopotamia: Creation, the Flood, Gilgamesh, and Others* (Oxford: Oxford University Press, 1989), p. 263]). Turner takes a different path and explains the rainbow as a sign that represents the firmament (רקיע), which according to Gen. 1 has been established to act as a barrier between the waters from above and the waters below. The firmament according to Ezek. 1.22-23, 26, 28 separates the creatures below from God's throne, and thus this may be understood to be the function of the bow (Laurence A. Turner, 'The Rainbow as the Sign of the Covenant in Genesis ix 11-13', *VT* 43 [1993], pp. 119-24).

also be considered as a constituent in the category of symbols, since it symbolizes the covenant between God and humanity.

2.3.5.3. מול. Circumcision: A Sign of the Covenant. The precept of circumcision is given at Gen. 17.11, where it is explicitly stated that it is a covenantal sign (אות ברית).[102] So, circumcision is an external bodily sign, whose purpose is to show that the man who bears it has entered into a covenant with God. Although the lexeme אות (sign) does not appear in Gen. 21.4 (the circumcision of Isaac), or in ch. 34 (circumcision of the men of Shechem), it is clear that, just as in ch. 17, circumcision is a bodily sign which fulfils its function when seen. Circumcision includes the abstract schema 'objects which fulfil their function by being seen'. Hence, we may say that it is connected to the SF. Circumcision may also be considered as a constituent in the next category, that of symbols in the SF, since it is an entity which represents another entity, that of the covenant between God and Israel.

2.3.5.4. פצלה. The definition of פצלה in Ben Yehuda's dictionary is 'an area in the wood from which the bark has been stripped and the white undercoat revealed'.[103] *HALOT*'s definition of פצלות is similar: 'stripped sections (of the sticks)'.[104] The noun פצלות appears once only in the Bible, in the plural, at Gen. 30.37. Here it refers to the stripped sticks Jacob puts in front of his flock, an action which is intended to increase the birth-rate within the enclosure.

2.4. *Symbols in the Sight Field*

When using the term 'Symbol', I refer to its very wide sense of one entity which stands for and represents another entity.[105] Circumcision and the rainbow, which are constituents in the former category, may also be considered as symbols, both representing covenants between God and Israel (circumcision), and God and humankind (the rainbow).

102. Wyatt refers to the apotropaic value of circumcision, and analyzes instances of circumcision in the Bible (Nick Wyatt, 'Circumcision and Circumstance: Male Genital Mutilation in Ancient Israel and Ugarit', *JSOT* 33 [2009], pp. 405-31 [426]).

103. Ben Yehuda, *A Complete Dictionary*, p. 5085 (my translation from the Hebrew).

104. *HALOT*, p. 954.

105. Ake Viberg, *Symbols of Law: A Contextual Analysis of Legal Symbolic Acts in the Old Testament* (Stockholm: Almqvist & Wiksell International, 1992), p. 3. Viberg also mentions Geertz, who defines the term 'symbol' as 'any physical, social, or cultural act or object that serves as the vehicle for a conception' (C. Geertz, *The Interpretation of Cultures* [New York: Basic Books, 1973], p. 208 n. 19).

2.4.1. נחש

The serpent (נחש) is connected with the SF both in the concrete sense of visual perception and in the sense of the more abstract cognitive perception. I shall begin by recalling the appearance of the serpent outside Genesis, in the story of the bronze serpent in Num. 21.4-9, since here there is a connection between visual perception and the serpent.[106] In this short story the Israelites complain to Moses that they do not have enough bread and water in the desert, and that they are being led to their death (Num. 21.5). God's reaction is to send fiery serpents, which bite the people, many of whom die (21.6). Moses prays to God, who tells him to make a serpent of bronze. In v. 9, the biblical story tells of Moses' actions: 'So Moses made a bronze serpent, and set it on a pole; and if a serpent bit any man, *he would look at the bronze serpent and live*' (Num. 21.9). The function of the object, the bronze serpent, is fulfilled when it is looked at.[107] According to this story, the snake may be linked to the SF through the schema 'things which fulfil their function by being looked at'. Joines finds the serpent in Genesis 3 connected to the notion of life and death through its denial of the validity of the divine warning that death will follow eating from the tree in the midst of the garden (לא־מות תמתון, Gen. 3.4). By this the serpent has set itself in direct opposition to God as an authority in the subject of life.[108]

In addition to the notion of life and death, the serpent mentioned in the story of the Garden of Eden is connected to the SF, from the aspect of cognitive perception. The serpent is mentioned for the first time in Gen. 3.1, where it is said to be עָרוּם (crafty, cunning). The serpent in Genesis is a clever and sophisticated being, who tempts the woman to take the fruit of the forbidden tree of knowledge. It is the cunning attributed to the serpent that constitutes its link to the SF. It may be recalled that the result of the temptation is that the *eyes* of Adam and Eve are *opened*, and they enter into their new way of life, in which they *know* that they are *naked* (Gen. 3.7).

Thus, the serpent is a variegated character who symbolizes cleverness and guile, as well as killing and healing, life and death, which are activated when it is looked at. I propose that it is because of this symbolic meaning of the

106. For a summary concerning the character of the snake-serpent in other cultures, such as India, Mesopotamia, Mari and Egypt, see Leslie S. Wilson, *The Serpent Symbol in the Ancient Near East* (Lanham, MD: University Press of America, 2001), pp. 11-18. See also H.J. Fabry, 'נחש', in *TDOT*, IX, pp. 356-69.

107. According to Joines the most prominent element in the tradition of Moses and the bronze serpent seems to be that of sympathetic magic, that is, the belief that the fate of an object or person can be governed by the manipulation of its exact image. By means of sympathetic magic an adversary could be controlled by manipulation of his exact image (Karen Randolph Joines, 'The Bronze Serpent in the Israelite Cult', *JBL* 87 [1968], pp. 245-56 [251]).

108. Karen Randolph Joines, 'The Serpent in Gen 3', *ZAW* 87 (1975), pp. 1-11.

serpent in the fields of Cognitive and Visual Perception that in 1 Samuel 11 Nahash the Ammonite threatens to hurt the organ of sight of the people of Jabesh Gilead. In this story the Ammonite king, whose name is 'Nahash', literally meaning 'serpent', suggests partly blinding the men of Jabesh Gilead by plucking out their right eye (1 Sam. 11.1-2). It appears that in this incident, too, there is a connection between the serpent and the SF.

2.4.2. עין

The lexeme עין, in the sense of 'a spring of water' forms part of the SF through polysemy.[109] The lexeme עין in BDB is divided into two separate entries, in which it is stated that the connection between עין I (the organ of sight) and עין II (spring) is dubious.[110] In other words, it is unclear whether there was a semantic shift of עין in the sense of the organ of sight, to the meaning of spring of water (or the other way around), or whether these are two different lexemes with different etymologies.

Stendebach suggests that עין as a source of water is a metaphorical development from עין, the organ of sight. He proposes that the usage of עין as the source of water is connected with the actual and mental image of the spring rising from the surface of the earth, which is similar to the eyes in the human face,[111] or rather that it is based on an image of the eyes of the subterranean monster.[112] I wish to take this idea forward and suggest that in certain contexts in Genesis עין (spring) symbolizes the presence of God.[113] This is the case in the stories of Hagar (Gen. 16; 21). The angel finds the lost Hagar 'by a spring of water in the wilderness, the spring on the way to Shur' (16.7). Then, in 21.19, God saves Hagar from death in the wilderness by opening her eyes to see a well of water. The water of course saves Hagar from dying of thirst, but Hagar needs her eyes to be opened in order to see them. I think there is more to this water, and it symbolizes God's presence.

Continuing the etymological character of the lexeme, Song 7.4 exemplifies the similarity between עין as a source of water and as a body organ:

109. Amos Frisch suggests that place-names such as העין (spring) and עין המים (spring of water) belong to the SF (Frisch, 'שמע and ראה as a Pair of *Leitwörter*').

110. BDB, pp. 744-45.

111. Stendebach refers here to A. Schwarzenbach, *Die geographische Terminologie im Hebräischen des Alten Testamentes* (Leiden: Brill, 1954), p. 55. See F.J. Stendebach, 'עין', in *TDOT*, XI, pp. 28-44.

112. T.J. Jones, *Quelle, Brunnen und Zisterne im Alten Testament* (Leipzig: E. Pfriffer, 1928), p. 2.

113. According to Zakovitch, God expresses punishment, rebuke, and compassion through water images (Yair Zakovitch, '"The voice of the LORD...upon many waters"—The God Who Leads his World and People in the Water' [Hebrew], in Yair Zakovitch and Avigdor Shinan [eds.], *"...Like Watercourses in the Negeb": Water in the Bible and Rabbinic Literature* [Jerusalem: The Presidential Residence, 1998], pp. 13-23).

'Your neck is like an ivory tower. Your eyes are pools in Heshbon.' In Akkadian, too, the lexeme *īnu*, which is derived from the same root, means both an organ of sight and a source of water.[114]

The word עין in the sense of a source of water occurs ten times in Genesis, at 16.7 (twice); 24.13, 16, 29, 30, 42, 43, 45; 49.22—that is, in three contexts only. I shall discuss the place-name עין משפט (Gen. 14.7) separately, in the section on place-names (§2.8.1.13).

2.4.3. מעין

The form מעין derives from the same root as the previous lexeme עין, in the sense of a spring of water, and according to the dictionaries has a similar meaning, though *HALOT* defines the term as 'place of origin, source, head-waters'. מעין is found twice in Genesis, only in the story of the Flood: Gen. 7.11; 8.2.

2.5. *Lexemes Which Participate Both in the Sight Field and in the Field of Cognitive Perception*

This category consists of lexemes whose semantic definitions include the act of sight but also include elements from the neighbouring field of Cognitive Perception. These lexemes, therefore, lie on the border between the two semantic fields.

2.5.1. בקש

The verb בקש often means 'to seek' or 'to find'. In BDB it is translated as 'seek to find', and in *HALOT*, 'to discover', 'to find', 'to search for'. In Prov. 2.4 there is parallelism which stresses the close meaning of בקש and חפש. בקש appears five times in Genesis: 31.39; 37.15, 16; 43.9, 30.

2.5.2. חפש

In the verb חפש there are semantic elements both of the SF and of the field of Cognitive Perception. The meaning of the verb is seeing with the intention of finding something, directed seeing. It is translated 'search out/for', 'examine'. In Akkadian the verb *še'ûm* means to look for, to seek,[115] and this verb is to be found in Hebrew in the form of the verb שעה, as has been pointed out above. Twenty-three instances of the verb חפש are found in the Bible, two of them in Genesis, at 31.35, where Laban seeks his idols in Rachel's tent, and at 44.12, where Joseph's house-steward looks for the missing cup in Joseph's brothers' belongings.

114. *CAD*, I–J, p. 153.
115. *AHw*, pp. 1222-24; *CAD*, Š/2, p. 359.

2.5.3. מצא

This verb is the antonym of חפש. It is found frequently as part of the expression מצא חן בעיני (to find favour in the eyes of). The overall meaning can be translated as 'find, reach'.

2.5.4. נכר

This lexeme contains both a semantic component of visual perception and of cognitive perception. But the comprehension may come about not only as a result of visual identification but as the result of auditory identification. Therefore, not all the occurrences of the root נכר are considered—only those which are connected with visual perception. The root נכר is found ten times in Genesis: 27.23; 31.32; 37.32, 33; 38.25, 26; 42.7 (twice), 8 (twice).

It may be pointed out that this root appears for the first time only in Genesis 27, which shows that it has a strong connection with the Jacob Narrative. Daube surmises that the occurrence of the verb הכיר (to recognize) in the Joseph Narrative in ch. 37, signifies actual legal recognition of the death of Joseph. In other words, Joseph's brothers brought legally valid proof of the fact that their brother was dead in order to clear themselves of the charge of murder. Bringing Joseph's blood-stained garment from the field constituted valid legal proof.[116] Daube says that when Jacob states at 37.33, 'And he recognized it, and said, "It is my son's robe"', the recognition is formal. The fact that later in this chapter he does not willingly send Benjamin with them shows that he is afraid that Benjamin will disappear, like Joseph.[117]

2.5.5. *Clothes and Other Supplementary Appurtenances which Serve to Identify their Owners*

Clothes and articles of attire may be connected to the SF. Matthews's remarks about the connection between clothes and sight are noteworthy:

> However, on the symbolic level, clothing always serves as *a means of visual communication*. The message conveyed may be artistic..., but very often it is also relevant to power relationships.[118]

Clothes and other articles of attire hide the different parts of the body. Palache writes about the connection between the concept of concealing and covering, which is expressed by the root בגד, and the CPF, from the aspect

116. D. Daube, *Studies in Biblical Law* (New York: KTAV; Cambridge: Cambridge University Press, 1969 [reprint of 1947]), pp. 3-10. Malul maintains that the verb הכיר in 2 Sam. 3.36 has a similar meaning (Malul, 'Law in the Narratives', pp. 23-36).

117. Daube, *Studies in Biblical Law*, pp. 8-9.

118. Matthews, 'The Anthropology of Clothing', pp. 25-26 (my emphasis).

of concealment of truth, lying, and so forth, which is expressed by exactly the same root.[119]

This, however, is not the only function of clothing. Sometimes it serves as protection against heat or cold, and sometimes as ornamentation. It can also be a means of identification of the wearer, or to signify his/her social status or authority. Included in the SF are only those articles of clothing which serve to identify the person who wears them, on condition that this is explicitly mentioned in the text.

Matthews maintains that clothing is a recurrent motif in the Joseph Narrative, which constitutes the connecting link between the secondary plots. According to him, Joseph's stay in the house of Potiphar, and his imprisonment (Gen. 39.1–41.23), are linked by the motif of clothing to the main plot line, having to do with Joseph and his brothers. The motif of clothing emphasizes the central theme of the Joseph Narrative: his elevation to the status of favourite son, and, after his fall, his further elevation to the status of the king's deputy, through which he saves his family. The changes of clothing accompany the turning-points in Joseph's changing status. At the beginning of the story his father gives him the long-sleeved garment (37.3).[120] Later, his brothers take it from him (37.23). As the plot evolves, Pharaoh dresses him in 'garments of fine linen' (41.42), and at the end of the narrative Joseph gives his brothers 'festal garments' (45.22).[121]

In the culture of the Middle East the giving of clothing is a symbolic act; in Mari it was customary to send garments as a royal gift. Emissaries, ambassadors and military leaders often receive a gift of clothing as a symbol of esteem.[122] In connection with the importance of clothing Matthews cites Gen. 3.21, where God sews a leather garment for Adam and Eve.[123]

2.5.5.1. בגד. The lexeme בגד (garment, covering) is found in the story of Joseph and Potiphar's wife at Gen. 39.11, 12, 15, 16, 18. In this story clothing is used by Potiphar's wife as evidence that Joseph tried to rape her. This object is connected with the SF, since it serves to identify a particular person, and it is meant to be seen and identified as the 'sinner's' garment. In other words, in this instance it is the function of the object in the text, which is decisive in relation to the question of whether it belongs to the SF. On the

119. Palache, *Semantic Notes on the Hebrew Lexicon*, p. 10.

120. Matthews ('The Anthropology of Clothing', pp. 25-36 [30]) cites 2 Sam. 13.18, where it is said that כתנת פסים was worn by the king's virgin daughters. Matthews supports the proposal that it was probably a long-sleeved coat.

121. Matthews, 'The Anthropology of Clothing', pp. 28-29.

122. J. Schneider and A.B. Weiner (eds.), *Cloth and Human Experience* (Washington, DC: Smithsonian Institution Press, 1989), p. 2.

123. Matthews, 'The Anthropology of Clothing', p. 30.

other hand, Tamar's 'garments of her widowhood' mentioned in Gen. 38.14, 19 do not belong to the SF, since they are not objects whose specific function is to identify Tamar; rather, they indicate her social status as a widow.

2.5.5.2. כתנת פסים. Joseph's long-sleeved garment, mentioned several times in Genesis 37 (vv. 3, 23, 32), is connected to the SF since, in addition to the function of all articles of clothing—to cover the body—it serves as an identifying sign of Joseph. The garment is mentioned in collocation with the verb להכיר (to recognize). In 37.32 the blood-stained garment is brought to Jacob in order that he may recognize it as Joseph's. Thus, the garment is part of the SF, since it is not only an article of clothing but an object which Jacob must identify and recognize. Recognition and identification are mental processes which are often connected to the SF, since they often involve seeing the object.

2.5.5.3. חותם, פתילים, מטה, שני. The seal (חותם), cord (פתיל), staff (מטה), and the thread of scarlet (חוט] שני]) in the story of Judah and Tamar serve as identifying items of their owners. But, they are not included in the category of articles of clothing, since they do not constitute the meanings 'concealing, covering'. The seal, cords and staff are objects that belonged to Judah, and which he had to recognize, that is, to look at them and realize that they were his (38.25-26). Such objects mark their owners, and are, therefore, included in the SF.

The scarlet thread (שני) which the midwife ties to the hand of the child emerging first in the birth of the twins (38.28) is connected with the SF, because it functions as a sign of recognition of the child, just as did Judah's seal, cords and staff. When Zerah emerges second, after Perez, he is identified as the child with the scarlet thread on his hand (38.30). On the one hand, the schema 'objects which fulfil their function by being seen' (§2.3.5) is part of the semantic definition of these identifying objects. And, once again, the hidden perceiver is a participant in the semantic definitions.[124] On the other hand, these objects influence the cognition of the observer in that they indicate the identity of their owners. As soon the objects discussed in this paragraph are looked at, it is immediately understood to whom they belong, and their basic function is to bear evidence to their owner's identity.

2.5.5.4. *Articles of Clothing Which Are Not Included in the Sight Field.* Not all instances of articles of clothing in the Joseph Narrative are explicitly connected with the SF, and they will not always be included in it. For example, Joseph's long-sleeved garment (כתנת פסים) stands in contrast to

124. Rubinstein, 'The Hidden Perceiver'.

the שׂמלה (garment, clothing) which Jacob tears when he discovers that the-blood stained garment belongs to his son (37.34). It also stands in contrast to the clothes Reuben tears when he returns to the pit and does not see Joseph in it (ויקרע את־בגדיו, 37.29). Although the garment (בגד, שׂמלה) is an article of clothing, it is not connected with the SF, since it serves no function of seeing or identifying. The function of the clothes in these instances is to indicate mourning, not sight.

Another instance of 'garments' which are not included in the SF is when Joseph comes out of the pit and changes his garments (41.14). These garments are not included in the SF since they are not accompanied by verbs denoting sight, concealment, covering, or identification, which could have connected them with the field. In other words, they do not fulfil any explicit function in the SF.

Moreover, the 'garments of linen' with which Pharaoh clothes Joseph, and the special jewels he is given, are not included in the SF in this study, since their function is not to identify Joseph specifically, but to represent authority. The dressing of Joseph in these clothes, giving him the ring, and the gold chain put on his neck do not mean that these objects should be included in the SF; this is because there is no explicit mention of sight. In other words, although articles of clothing, or a jewel which is meant to be looked at, are mentioned, the aspect that is emphasized is the transfer of sovereign power to Joseph. The clothes and jewels here represent authority, and not the identity of the person who wears them.

2.6. *Lexemes from Nearby Fields*

2.6.1. *Lexemes from the Field of Cognitive Perception Alone*

As was said in the introduction, Sovran maintains that in addition to the natural aspect of the structure of the semantic field, there is a considerable degree of arbitrariness in defining its borders.[125] This also applies to the SF. The semantic field closest to the SF is the CPF, and sometimes the verb ראה (see) itself refers to thinking and understanding rather than perceiving visually, and it could be replaced by lexemes from the CPF.[126] I shall now enumerate lexemes from the CPF which are connected with the SF.

2.6.1.1. **אמן**. According to Ben Yehuda, the meaning of the verb האמין, in the hiphil (found in this conjugation at Gen. 15.6; 45.26) is 'to think that in one's opinion it is so'.[127] He says that the niphal form (42.20) means 'is

125. Sovran, *Semantic Fields*, p. 24.
126. On the proximity of the SF and the CPF, see §1.1.2.
127. Ben Yehuda, *A Complete Dictionary*, p. 283.

found and revealed to be true, its existence is confirmed'. *HALOT* translates the verb as 'to prove to be firm, reliable, faithful'.[128] The instance found in 15.6 is translated there as 'to have trust in, to believe in God'.

2.6.1.2. בין. Generally speaking, the meaning of the verbal form בין is 'understanding'. In certain contexts it has the sense of understanding by means of the eyes—that is to say, seeing. In such instances it is hard to say which is referred to—cognitive or visual perception. Thus, for instance, in Prov. 7.7: 'And I have *seen* (ואראה) among the simple, I have *perceived* (אבינה) among the youths'. Sometimes the meaning is perceiving by means of the ears—hearing (Prov. 29.10). It sometimes refers to perceiving by touch (Ps. 58.10), and perceiving as a result of tasting (Job 6.30).[129] The root, בין has been suggested to be etymologically connected with the Akkadian verb *barû*, meaning 'to see', on the supposition of the interchanging between the consonants *resh* and *nun*.[130]

In Genesis the root בין is found as a participle in the niphal, in the form נבון, only twice, each time describing a characteristic of Joseph. At 40.33 Joseph is described as נבון (discerning) and חכם (wise). This description is repeated in 40.38. Joseph is perceived as a wise man who has unusual powers of comprehension; according to the story, this is connected with his power to interpret dreams. This characteristic, Joseph's wisdom, is linked to the spirit of God within him, and it is this that gives him the ability to interpret dreams.

2.6.1.3. זכר. This verb appears ten times in Genesis, at 8.1; 9.15, 16; 19.29; 30.22; 40.14 (twice), 23; 41.9; 42.9. In most cases it is found in the qal, but appears twice in the hiphil (40.14; 41.9), where the meaning is 'to mention', to notify verbally another person. Elsewhere in Genesis and other places it means 'to remember, to call to mind'.[131]

128. *HALOT*, p. 63.

129. BDB, p. 106.

130. This has been suggested in *HALOT*, p. 122. For the meanings of *barû*, see *CAD*, B, p. 115.

131. On remembering and memory in the Bible, see Athalya Brenner and Frank Polak (eds.), *Performing Memory in Biblical Narrative and Beyond* (The Bible in the Modern World, 25; Sheffield: Sheffield Phoenix Press, 2009). When analyzing narratives of the daughters in Judges, Bal suggests a connection between the noun זכר (male) and the verb זכר (remember) in the qal (perfect, third person, singular, masculine), saying that to remember is a male prerogative, denied to women (Mieke Bal, 'Dealing/With/ Women: Daughters in the Book of Judges', in Regina M. Schwartz [ed.], *The Book and the Text: The Bible and Literary Theory* [Oxford: Basil Blackwell, 1990], pp. 16-39 [25]).

2.6.1.4. חשב. This verb has many meanings, and it is found in Genesis at 15.6; 31.15 (twice); 38.15; 50.20 (twice). According to *HALOT* (p. 360), at 38.15 it means 'to assume', whereas at 15.6 and 50.20 it is translated 'to impute, to reckon'. There is an interesting link between the roots ידע and חשב at, for instance, Ps. 144.3: 'O LORD, what is man that you do regard him (ותדעהו), or the son of man that you do think of him (ותחשבהו)?' The verb ראה is also found nearby the verb חשב in Gen. 38.15: 'When Judah saw her (ויראה), he thought her (ויחשבה) to be a harlot'.

2.6.1.5. ידע. According to *HALOT*, the main meanings of ידע are 'to notice, hear of, learn, know (also sexually), take care of someone'. Since the CPF is close to the SF, and ראה often has the meaning of ידע, in the sense of learning, knowing, I include this verb as part of the SF.

The verb ידע at Gen. 18.19 has a unique meaning. Westermann claims that this is the only place in the patriarchal narratives that the verb ידע means 'to choose': God chooses Abraham.[132] Talmon points out that sometimes the verbs ידע and ראה serve to represent a single complex concept, one which indicates visual perception followed by psychological processes of cognitive perception and thought. He illustrates this by the passages such as Deut. 11.2: 'your children who have not *known* or *seen* it'; 1 Sam. 23.22: '*know* and *see* the place where his haunt is' (cf. 24.12; 25.17). Sometimes the components of the complex concept are divided between two parallel parts of the verse (Exod. 2.25; Jer. 2.23).[133]

Talmon says that the syntactic linkage and semantic propinquity between these two verbs may lead to interchange between them: Josh. 24.31, in comparison with Judg. 2.7. A similar phenomenon may be found in the differences between the Masoretic text and parallel versions and translations. In Isa. 47.8 the Masoretic text reads: 'know (אדע) the loss', whereas the Isaiah scroll from Qumran reads: 'see (אראה) the loss'.[134] In Josh. 24.31 the Masoretic reading is ידעו (had known), while the Septuagint reads εἴδοσαν (saw). Similarly, the Masoretic text reads ראו in Judg. 2.7 (had seen), while the Septuagint has ἔγνωσαν (knew).

2.6.1.6. דעת. The noun דעת (knowledge) is derived from the root ידע. This lexeme occurs in the Garden of Eden narrative, in the syntagm עץ הדעת (the tree of knowledge), found at Gen. 2.9 and 17.

132. Westermann, *Genesis 12–36*, p. 288.

133. Talmon, 'Synonymous Readings', pp. 340-42.

134. See the Isaiah scroll from Qumran in M. Burrows (ed.), *The Dead Sea Scrolls of St. Mark's Monastery*. I. *The Isaiah Manuscript and the Habakkuk Commentary* (New Haven: The American Schools of Oriental Research, 1950).

2.6.1.7. עָרוּם. The adjective עָרוּם (crafty, shrewd) is found in Genesis once, at 3.1. This lexeme is also found twice in Job, and eight times in Proverbs; it is, therefore characteristic of the wisdom literature. In Proverbs this adjective does not have the negative connotation which it has in Genesis and Job. In Proverbs the עָרוּם is contrasted with the foolish (אויל), the stupid (כסיל) and the naive (פתי), and refers to a wise person.[135]

2.6.1.8. פקד. The verb פקד is found in Genesis nine times, at 21.1; 39.4, 5; 40.4; 41.34; 50.24 (twice), 25 (twice). This verb has a variety of meanings in the Bible, including Genesis: 'attend to, visit, muster, appoint, pay attention to, observe'. According to *HALOT*, in Gen. 21.1 and in Genesis 50 it means 'to look at', or 'to see to something'. In 39.4, 5 and in 41.34 it means to appoint, install as superior.

2.6.1.9. שׁכח. This verb appears three times in Genesis, at 27.45; 40.23; 41.30. In Biblical Hebrew dictionaries this verb is translated 'to forget'. In Gen. 40.23 it sums up the preceding clause, in which the verb לא־זכר (did not remember) appears.

2.6.2. *Lexemes from the Field of Emotion*

2.6.2.1. ירא. ירא (to fear) is linked to the SF because it belongs to the field of Emotion, which is close to visual perception. A further reason for including this lexeme in the SF is its auditory similarity to the root ראה/י.[136] De Saussure, who discusses the semantic field of Teaching, also speaks of words connected to the field by sound similarities.[137] The sound similarity between ירא and ראה is particularly striking in the places where the two roots are found close to each other, for instance in Gen. 26.24: וירא (appeared), תירא (fear); Gen. 42.35: ויראו (they saw), וייראו (they feared). Apart from Genesis, there are further examples of the use of sound plays in the verbs ירא and ראה by narrators and poets: Exod. 14.31; Deut. 28.10; 1 Sam. 28.5; Isa. 41.5; Zech. 9.5; Ps. 40.4; Job 6.21. In addition, Frisch adduces the example of 1 Sam. 28.13.

2.6.3. *A Lexeme from the Field of Education*

Since learning and teaching are activities which strongly involve cognitive perception, I consider them close to visual perception, hence, to the SF.

135. BDB, p. 791.

136. Frisch, 'שׁמע and ראה as a Pair of *Leitwörter*', p. 91.

137. Ferdinand de Saussure, *Course in General Linguistics* (ed. Charles Bally and Albert Sechehaye with the collaboration of Albert Reidlinger; trans. Wade Baskin; New York: Philosophical Library, 1959 [based on de Sussure's lectures given between 1906 and 1911, first published 1916]), pp. 125-27.

2.6.3.1. ירה. The root ירה is found in the noun תורתי (my instructions) at Gen. 26.5, and in the verb להורת (to instruct, 46.28).[138] The meaning of the root is 'to instruct, teach'; thus it belongs to the field of Education, which is a branch of the CPF. The root appears in the place names מוריה (Gen. 22.2) and אלון מורה (12.6), which I shall discuss separately in §2.8. The root appears in Genesis five times: twice in place names, once in a noun and twice in verbs. In 12.6 and 22.2 it appears close to ראה, which emphasizes the sound similarity between them. In 40.28 the situation is rather similar, but the verb ראה (48.29) stands somewhat further from ירה (48.28). It is only in the case of the noun תורתי (my laws or instructions) at 26.5 that the verb ראה does not stand close by to stress sound play. Still, I include תורתי in the SF due to its close semantic relations.

2.7. *Peripheral Lexemes*

On the periphery of the SF there are a number of lexemes indirectly linked to the centre, through the mediation of lexemes belonging to the first circle of the field. Peripheral lexemes can also be those which their semantic definition includes a component from the SF. The question of whether any peripheral lexeme is connected to the field or remains outside it is frequently determined by the context.

2.7.1. פנים

The lexeme פנים (face, front, surface) is connected to the lexeme עין (eye), from the SF, by meronymy, that is, part–whole semantic relations. The eye is part of the face, and can sometimes represent it (Isa. 5.21). Here, too, as in the case of ראשׁ (head, see later on), the connection is secondary and indirect, since it is made through the lexeme עין. The word פנים is found frequently in Genesis, and will be discussed in the framework of the phrase ראה פנים (see the face), which appears from Gen. 31.2 onwards, as well as in particular contexts where it is found in collocation with a verb of sight.

2.7.2. פני

The word פני is not included in the SF, since it is emptied of the concrete meaning of פנים (face—see above) and functions as a preposition. There are, however, particular contexts in which the concrete sense of the lexeme is echoed—contexts in which it is understood to mean 'face, front' or 'surface'. This word is mentioned in the literary analysis in relation to the particular contexts, where it appears in collocation with other lexemes of sight.

138. There is also ירית׳ in 31.51, but this verbs stems from the polysemic verb ירה, which also means 'to shoot, set up' (*HALOT*).

2.7.3. ראש

The lexeme ראש (head) is metonymously connected with עין (eye), since the eye is situated in the head, and they are physically close to each other. Thus, ראש joins the SF through the intermediary lexeme עין. At various places in the Bible this connection between the eyes and the head is recalled, and parallelisms even show that ראש can serve as an exact substitute for עין: Isa. 29.10, Jer. 8.23 (RSV 9.1).

Thus, as a result of these connections this lexeme is linked to the SF, but only secondarily, since it is not connected directly with the centre of the field. This lexeme appears 21 times in Genesis, twice in the form מראשתיו (28.11, 18), which means 'place at the head, head-place' (BDB, p. 912).

In Gen. 2.10, it is said that the river goes out of Eden in 'four units' (ראשים). Although the meaning of ראש here is not exactly 'head', the general context which includes a great concentration of words from the SF, may echo the meaning 'head', and thus the lexeme may be considered as belonging to the SF.

2.7.4. *Lexemes Which Include the Semantic Component 'Light'*

2.7.4.1. אש. The noun אש (fire) appears in Gen. 15.17 (a flaming torch); 19.24; 22.6, 7. According to Ben Yehuda (p. 405), אש is the natural activity which gives off both heat and light. Since its semantic definition includes the component 'light', this lexeme belongs to the periphery of the SF.

2.7.4.2. לפיד. The noun לפיד (torch) appears in Genesis only in the story of the 'covenant between the divided parts' in 15.17, as part of the phrase לפיד אש (a flaming torch). לפיד is wood or some other substance dipped in inflammable material, which burns in order to give light.[139] Since its semantic definition includes the component 'light', לפיד belongs to the periphery of the SF.

2.7.4.3. תנור. The noun תנור (oven) is an appliance in which a fire is lit for warmth, baking bread, or smelting metals.[140] In Genesis it is found only as part of the phrase תנור עשן (15.17), in the sense of 'fiery brazier'. According to *HALOT* this is an Akkadian loanword *tinūru(m)*, meaning an appliance for making fire.[141] Further, the root נור, which means 'to dawn, to shine, illuminate', occurs in Akkadian *(nawāru/namāru)*.[142] In Aramaic and Hebrew it means 'light' and 'to illuminate', and in Rabbinical Hebrew נור means 'fire'. תנור is part of the SF, since its semantic definition contains the components of 'fire' and 'light'.

139. Ben Yehuda, *A Complete Dictionary*, p. 2717.
140. Ben Yehuda, *A Complete Dictionary*, pp. 7822-23.
141. *AHw*, p. 1360; *CAD*, T, p. 420.
142. *CAD*, N/1, p. 209.

2.7.5. *Lexemes Which Include the Schema: 'States of Consciousness Which Can Be Determined Mainly by the Closing or Opening of the Eyes of their Experiencer'*

2.7.5.1. יקץ. *HALOT* translates the verb יקץ as 'to awake'. It appears in Gen. 9.24; 28.16; 41.4, 7, 21. In 28.16 Jacob wakes from his sleep, and in ch. 41 Pharaoh wakes and dreams intermittently. Hence we learn that waking involves opening the eyes, when it follows a state of sleep. On the other hand, in 9.24 Noah awakens from his wine. After his awakening he understands what his youngest son has done to him. It seems that this word refers here to a state of drunkenness likened to a state of sleep, in which the sleeper is not wholly aware of his deeds (see §4.4). In most of the references in the Bible (eleven in all) it is sleepers who awaken. In Ps. 78.65 he who awakes from his sleep is likened to him who wakes from wine: 'Then Yhwh awoke as from sleep, like a strong man shouting because of wine'.

2.7.5.2. ישן. *HALOT*'s translation (p. 447) is 'to fall asleep'. This verb appears in Genesis twice, 2.21; 41.5.

2.7.5.3. שנה. This noun means 'sleep', and occurs in Genesis twice at 28.16; 31.40.

2.7.5.4. לין. This verb appears nine times in Genesis: 19.2 (twice); 24.23, 25, 54; 28.11; 31.54; 32.14, 22. Its meaning in Genesis is 'to spend the night, stay overnight' (*HALOT*). However, the context indicates that the semantic definition of the verb includes a presupposition of sleeping in the place indicated. This is pronounced in an instance such as Gen. 24.54: 'and they spent the night there (וילינו). When they arose in the morning.' Hence, the men get up in the morning after they sleep (וילינו) in the night. In Gen. 28.11 it is said of Jacob: 'and stayed there (וילן) that night, because the sun had set'; after this, he dreams. Thus, sojourning (לין) involves sleeping in the place indicated. And, again, immediately after 'and tarried all night on the mountain' (וילינו בהר, 31.54), come the words: 'early in the morning Laban arose' (32.1).

2.7.5.5. מלון. This noun is found twice in Genesis, at 42.27 and 43.21. It means 'lodging-place, inn, khan' (BDB).

2.7.5.6. שכר. The verb שכר (to be, become drunk) is a special lexeme which does not accord exactly with the above schema; but here, too, there is a state of consciousness which is expressed in the behaviour of the person who is under the influence of wine, and also in the look in his/her eyes (a confused or opaque look). On the look, see Gen. 49.12: 'His eyes shall be red with wine, and his teeth white with milk'. Here again, a connection between cognitive perception (the state of drunkenness) and the eyes can be seen. Genesis 9.24 says of Noah: 'When Noah awoke from his wine and knew what his youngest son had done to him'. Hence, intoxication is considered to be a state of consciousness, like sleep, during which the eyes are closed. It could also be that the state of drunkenness leads to sleep, but in this case also, there is a connection between the cognitive state and the opening of the eyes later on.

2.7.5.7. תרדמה. This noun means 'deep sleep', and it is found at Gen. 2.21, 15.12.

2.7.6. *Colour Terms*
Since the phenomenon of colour involves the eyes of an observer, I linked it to the SF (see §1.2.7). Yet, as stated in §1.2.7, I shall not elaborate on the Colour field since this has already been done by Brenner,[143] and because of its indirect connection to the SF.

2.7.7. הנה
Loewenstamm and Blau define הנה (*hinneh*) as a deictic or emphasizing term. It may appear before a single-membered clauses, such as exclamations: הנה אשתך ('here is your wife', Gen. 12.19), or in indicative clauses, such as Gen. 16.14: '...it lies between (הנה בין) Kadesh and Bered'. It frequently appears after verbs of sight to indicate surprise, as for instance in 1 Kgs 19.6, or to indicate simple declaratives, such as Gen. 1.31; 37.7.[144]

Waltke and O'Connor point out that the word הנה functions as a 'presentative particle' in presentative clauses which express a variety of meanings: urgency, perception, causation, and so on.[145] Since הנה does not only serve to present clauses of content, that is, the sight which the character sees in the case of verbs of visual perception, it is not included independently in the SF. Nonetheless, in certain contexts it may strengthen the idea of sight, which is expressed independently in the clause, when it appears alongside other lexemes of Sight; for instance: 'I lifted up my eyes, and *saw* in a dream that (והנה) the he-goats...' (Gen. 31.10).

143. Brenner, *Colour Terms in the Old Testament.*

144. Loewenstamm and Blau, *Otzar Leshon haMikra*, p. 412.

145. B.K. Waltke and M. O'Connor, *An Introduction to Biblical Hebrew Syntax* (Winona Lake, IN: Eisenbrauns, 1990), §40.2.1. On the uses of the word *hinneh*, see Adele Berlin, *Poetics and Interpretation of Biblical Narrative* (Sheffield: Almond Press, 1983), pp. 91-95, and C.H.J. van der Merwe, 'A Cognitive Linguistic Perspective on הִנֵּה in the Pentateuch, Joshua, Judges, and Ruth', *Hebrew Studies* 48 (2007), pp. 101-40.

2.8. *Place Names, Personal Names, Words Denoting Time and the Heavenly Bodies*

One of the most important characteristics of a dominant semantic field in a text is the existence of personal names, place names or indications of time containing roots of lexemes from the field. In effect, this is a typical category of the dominant semantic fields in a text. Personal names, place names and indications of time belong to the background details of the plot, and are the kingpins of the biblical narrative; hence their importance when they consist of lexemes from a certain semantic field. When the semantic discussion is not purely linguistic and involves a specific text and plot, then the category of names and time references are central rather than peripheral; they are of great importance for the delineation of the field.

A lexeme belonging to the field may serve as one of the components of a name consisting of a number of components; for example, ראובן (Reuben, ראה + בן). There are also instances in which the whole of the name consists of a single lexeme belonging to the field: for instance, the place name עינים (Enaim, also understood literally as 'eyes' or 'springs'). I shall enumerate personal names and place names in Hebrew alphabetical order, and discuss indications of time after them.

2.8.1. *Personal Names and Place Names*

2.8.1.1. אוּר כשׂדים. The place name אוּר (Ur) is etymologically connected with the Sumerian URU, meaning 'city',[146] but it is included in the SF because of the sound resemblance between אוּר and אוֹר, and because in the Mishnah אוּר means 'fire'. Accordingly, in the semantic definition of the word there is an echo of the component אוֹר (light). In Genesis this place name is found at 11.28, 31; 15.7.

2.8.1.2. אל ראי *(God of seeing).* Genesis 16 tells of Hagar's flight to the desert because of Sarah's abuse. The angel finds her by a spring of water, tells her to return to her mistress, and promises her a son and many descendants. She points out the special event to which she was witness by naming the God who spoke to her; she calls him אֵל רֳאִי (God of seeing): 'So she called the name of Yhwh who spoke to her, "You are a God of seeing" (אֵל רֳאִי); for she said, "Have I really (הגם הלם) seen (ראיתי) God and remained alive after seeing him (רֹאִי)?"' (Gen. 16.13). In the Septuagint and

146. Karl Oberhuber, *Innsbrucker sumerisches Lexicon* (Innsbruck: Institut für Sprachwissenschaft der Universität Innsbruck, 1990), p. 516. See also Th.J.H. Krispijn, 'The Sumerian Lexeme URUM, a Lexico-Etymological Approach', in W.H. van Soldt *et al.* (eds.), *Veenhof Anniversary Volume: Studies Presented to Klaas R. Veenhof on the Occasion of his Sixty-fifth Birthd*ay (Leiden: Nederlands Instituut voor het Nabije Oosten, 2001), pp. 251-61.

the Vulgate the verbal form רֹאִי is reflected in the name אל ראי. Thus, according to these translations, the preferred form is the participle (רֹאִי), meaning 'the God who sees me', rather than an infinitive form (רֳאִי) meaning 'God of sight'.[147] Westermann and Skinner, following Wellhausen, prefer to read אלהים, instead of הלם. In that case, the meaning is that Hagar gives thanks for having seen God after he had seen her.[148] This means that the angel, who represents God, saw Hagar and protected her, and she thanks him for this. This divine name belongs to the SF, because it contains the verb ראה (see). Garsiel emphasizes the broader context of this chapter, in which matters connected with sight are repeatedly mentioned.[149]

2.8.1.3. אלון מרה *('the oak of Moreh' or 'Elon Moreh')*. The place name Elon Moreh is found at 12.6.[150] The root of the name מרה is ירה, meaning 'to instruct, teach' belongs to the field of Education, which is close to the SF (§2.6.3); it is also connected to the SF by sound similarity to the roots ירא (fear) and ראה (see).[151] Moreover, the context emphasizes the sound resemblance between the roots. The name of the place is mentioned in 12.6, and immediately afterwards, in 12.7, the verb ראה occurs twice: 'Then Yhwh *appeared* to Abram (וירא), and said, …So he built there an altar to Yhwh, *who had appeared* (הנראה) to him. It is in that place that God was revealed to Abraham. The name אלוני מורה appears once more, but not in Genesis, rather in Deut. 11.30. According to this reference, Elon Moreh was in the Arabah region, opposite Gilgal.

2.8.1.4. אלני ממרא *(Elonei Mamre)*. This place is mentioned three times in Genesis, at 13.18; 14.13; 18.1. The place name is connected to the SF, first of all since it derives from the root ירא (fear), which belongs to the field of

147. Westermann, *Genesis 12–36*, pp. 234, 246-49.

148. J. Wellhausen, *Prolegomena zur Geschichte Israels* (Berlin: G. Reimer, 1905), pp. 323-24. Westermann discusses the suggestion, reading הגם אלהים ראיתי ואחי אחרי ראי, in which case the verse matches the description of the name of the well in v. 14: באר לחי ראי (Beer Lahai Roi). That is to say, the verse aims to explain that Hagar saw God and stayed alive (Westermann, *Genesis 12–36*, p. 248). See Skinner, *Genesis*, p. 289.

149. Garsiel, *Biblical Names*, p. 183.

150. There are variant readings of this place name; the Septuagint has τὴν δρῦν τὴν ὑψηλήν, which may be a derivation from מרום (Skinner, *Genesis*, p. 245). Onkelos translates מישרי מורה (the plains of Moreh) instead of אלון מורה. Skinner suggests that this change in Onkelos was probably intended to eliminate any connections between Abraham and idolatrous associations with a sacred tree. Both Symmachus and the Peshitta read אלון ממרא (Elon Mamre, as in Gen. 13.18; 14.13; 18.1). On the tradition relating to the 'tree of Abraham', see Roland de Vaux, *Ancient Israel* (trans. John McHugh; London: Darton, Longman & Todd, 1961), II, pp. 278-79, 292-93.

151. Garsiel, *Biblical Names*, pp. 193-94.

Emotion, close to the SF, and also because of sound resemblance between the roots ראה (see) and ירא (fear). After parting from Lot, Abraham settled in Elonei Mamre, which, according to the context in Gen. 13.18, was in the vicinity of Hebron.[152]

2.8.1.5. ארץ המֹּריה *(the land of Moriah)*. This place name, the site of the sacrifice of Isaac, is found in Gen. 22.2. God tells Abraham to take his only son, Isaac, to the land of Moriah, and to sacrifice him there on one of the mountains. Frisch claims that the leading word in this episode is ראה (see). He also connects it with the root ירא (fear), which has a similar sound, and to the place where the episode takes place—the land of Moriah. The root ירה, which constructs the name מוריה, resembles in its sounds to that of ראה and ירא, but it is also a constituent in the nearby semantic field of Education (§2.6.3). After the appearance of the angel, the place is linked to the act of seeing which takes place there by a Midrash on its name: 'So Abraham called the name of that place *Yhwh* will provide (יִרְאֶה); as it is said to this day, "On the mount of Yhwh it shall be provided (יֵרָאֶה)' (Gen. 22.14).[153] In 2 Chron. 3.1 the place name הר מוריה (Mount Moriah) is mentioned. This verse links the place with the act of sight: 'Then Solomon began to build the house of Yhwh in Jerusalem on Mount Moriah, where Yhwh had *appeared* to David'.[154]

152. With regard to the component 'Elon' (אלון) in the place names Elon Moreh and Elonei Mamre, some scholars maintain that the אלון and the אלה were holy trees, and that there were such trees in the vicinity of Shechem. אלון is apparently a synonym of אלה, and various biblical references indicate that the אלה was connected with various types of cult. See, e.g., Isa. 57.5 (U. Cassuto *et al.*, 'אלון, אלה' [Hebrew], *Encyclopedia Biblica*, I, cols. 294-95). Abraham also built altars in Elonei Mamre and Elon Moreh (Gen. 12.6; 13.18).

153. Frisch, 'The Conveyance of the *Leitwort* in English Translations', p. 247. Polak also discusses the word play between the name Moriah and the verb ראה (Polak, *Biblical Narrative*, p. 231). According to Amit, there is sound resemblance between מורא (fear), which derives from the root ירא and the name Moriah (Amit, 'The Multi-purpose "Leading Word"', p. 108). In other words, the connection of Moriah to the SF runs through מורא.

154. Amit points out that 2 Chron. 3.1 connects the land of Moriah and the place named ה' יראה ('The Lord will provide') mentioned in the Akedah with Mount Moriah, which is an alternative name for Jerusalem. She adds that this interpretation of the place of the sacrifice is found in Josephus, *Ant.* 1.224 and *Jub.* 18.14, as well as in the rabbinical literature. In the *Midrash Tehillim* 76 the commentator links Gen. 14 to Gen. 22; this is also found in *Sifre* (Midrash on Deuteronomy) 352, and in the *Tosefta*, *Berakot* 81 (Yairah Amit, 'The Function of Topographical Indications in the Biblical Story' (Hebrew), *Shnaton: An Annual for Biblical and Ancient Near Eastern Studies* 9 (1985), pp. 15-30 (22).

2.8.1.6. באר לחי ראי *(Beer Lahai Roi)*. This place name appears only in Genesis, at 16.14; 24.62; 25.11. In the story of Hagar's flight she calls the place where the angel appeared to her by this name (16.14). The name is included in the SF because it consists of the root ראה (see). According to Westermann, by giving this name Hagar meant to acknowledge the well of the living being (God or his angel) who saw her, or, alternatively, the well of the person who saw him (God) and remained alive.[155]

If we consider the context, this name appears on a wider background of sight terms (see the discussion in §3.2.4). In the previous verse, Hagar calls the god who speaks to her 'God who sees' (16.13). Garsiel connects this name with other contexts of sight in vv. 6 and 7 of this chapter.[156] It seems probable, therefore, that the name Beer Lahai Roi itself is connected with seeing, as Westermann says.

Moreover, as has been said, the place name Beer Lahai Roi is also found at 24.62, at a place where there is a large accumulation of SF terms. After Abraham's slave has taken Rebekah with him to Canaan, she meets Isaac for the first time as he journeys from the vicinity of Beer Lahai Roi and settles in the region of the Negev. Their meeting is described thus: 'And Isaac went out to meditate in the field in the *evening*; and *he lifted up his eyes* and *looked*, and *behold*, there were camels coming. And Rebekah *lifted up her eyes*, and when *she saw* Isaac, she alighted from the camel' (24.63-64). Seeing is emphasized by means of the long formulae of sight, that is, the lifting of the eyes followed by the verb of sight, as well as the mention of the time of day (it was evening, when conditions of sight are poor). The next verse tells of Rebekah covering herself with a veil (צעיף) as a response to the realization that the man she sees is Isaac (24.65). The veil is a lexeme which belongs to the SF, since it is a means of concealment; and the verb ותתכס (covered herself) also belongs to this field. The mention of the place name Beer Lahai Roi strengthens the impression that the author is making intentional use of this name, one of whose components is the verb ראה (see), which is at the nucleus of the SF.

2.8.1.7. שׁור *(Shur)*. This place is mentioned for the first time in Genesis in the story of Hagar's flight, 16.7: 'The angel of Yhwh *found* her by a *spring* (עין) of water in the wilderness, the *spring* on the way to *Shur*'. It is also mentioned at 20.1; 25.18; 49.22. On its appearance at 16.7, Garsiel comments that שׁור may be interpreted as a term of sight: the word עין occurs twice in this verse, and its sense as the organ of sight is echoed. שׁור can be interpreted as an act of seeing or looking. In this connection, Garsiel quotes

155. Westermann, *Genesis 12–36*, p. 248.
156. Garsiel, *Biblical Names*, p. 183.

Job 7.8, in which שׁור has the meaning of 'to look at': 'The eye of him who sees me will behold me (תשׁורני) no more; while your eyes are upon me, I shall be gone'.[157]

2.8.1.8. ה' יראה *(Yhwh sees)*.[158] This place name is found at Gen. 22.14. It is the name of the place where the sacrifice of Isaac almost takes place. Wenham considers that there is sound resemblance between the name ה' יֵרָאֶה and Moriah, which is mentioned in 22.2.[159]

2.8.1.9. זרח *(Zerah)*. This appears as a personal name in an Edomite dynasty at Gen. 36.13, 17, 33. In Gen. 38.30 and 46.12 it refers to the son of Judah and Tamar. The name is derived from the root זרח, which means both 'to shine' and 'to come out, to appear'.[160]

2.8.1.10. לוט *(Lot)*. Lot is found as a personal name at Gen. 11.27, 31; 12. 4, 5; 13.1-14; 14.12, 16; 19.1, 2, 5, 6, 9, 10, 12, 14, 15, 18, 23, 29 (twice), 30, 36. Outside Genesis the sons of Lot (בני לוט) are mentioned, referring to the Moabites in Deut. 2.9, the Ammonites in Deut. 2.19, and both of these in Ps. 83.9.

The root לוט appears as a verb in 1 Sam. 21.10, 2 Sam. 19.5 and possibly in Isa. 25.7. According to *HALOT*, it means 'to wrap, wrap up'. In Isa. 25.7 there may be a metaphorical sense of 'covering'. Because of this sense—covering, hiding from the eyes—this name is included in the SF.

2.8.1.11. ממרא *(Mamre)*. In addition to the name אלוני ממרא, the place name ממרא appears by itself six times in Genesis, at 23.17, 19; 25.9; 35.27; 49.30; 50.13. It is found once as a personal name, at 14.24. From these references it appears that Mamre is Hebron (Kiriath-arba). The name is connected to the SF because of sound resemblance to the roots ראה (see) and ירא (fear).

157. Gersiel, *Biblical Names*, p. 183; see also BDB, p. 1003. According to *HALOT*, שׁור means 'to look at from a bent position'; but it may be that, under the influence of Akkadian, it bears the nuance of 'to look from a leaning position' (*HALOT*, pp. 1449-50). In Akkadian, *šurru(m)* in the D conjugation means 'to go down, descend', 'to lean down over a wall into a window, to lean' (*CAD*, Š/3, p. 356).

158. Speiser, *Genesis*, p. 162.

159. On the form יֵרָאֶה (also in 22.14), which is derived from the root ראה in the niphal, Wenham says that this is the characteristic inflection of descriptions of divine appearance (see Gen. 12.7; 17.1; 18.1). In this way links are created to Abraham's past experiences and to the future experiences of Israel, when God is revealed on Horeb, the mountain of God (for instance, Exod. 3.1-2). See G.J. Wenham, *Genesis 16–50* (WBC, 2; Dallas, TX: Word Books, 1995). pp. 110-11.

160. *HALOT*, p. 281.

At Gen. 14.24, Mamre is mentioned as one of the men who accompanied Abraham when he freed Lot from his captors, Chedorlaomer, king of Elam, and the three kings who accompanied him.

2.8.1.12. מצפה *(Mizpah)*. The place name מצפה is found only in Gen. 31.49: 'And the pillar Mizpah, for he said (והמצפה אשר אמר), "*Yhwh* watch (יצף) between you and me, when we are absent one from the other"'. The first three words of the verse do not appear in the Vulgate. The Samaritan Pentateuch has מצבה instead of מצפה. In any case, the name which appears in the Masoretic text is derived from the verb of sight צפה (to look, spy, examine), and is, therefore, included in the SF.

2.8.1.13. עין משפט *(En-mishpat)*. This place is mentioned in the episode of the war of the four kings against the five kings at Gen. 14.7. After Chedorlaomer and the kings who accompanied him have smitten the Rephaim, the Zuzim, the Emim and the Horites, they return to En-mishpat, which is Kadesh (Gen. 14.7). This place name belongs to the SF, since the lexeme עין (spring/eye) is one of its components.

2.8.1.14. עינים *(Enaim)*. This place name is mentioned in the story of Judah and Tamar, at Gen. 38.14, 21. It is connected to the SF because the lexeme עין (spring/eye) is one of its components.

2.8.1.15. ער *(Er)*. Er, Judah's eldest son, is mentioned at Gen. 38.3, 6, 7, 46.12 (twice). This name is at the periphery of the SF, since it belongs primarily to the CPF. The name denotes a cognitive state of wakefulness and sobriety, as against a cognitive state of confusion, sleep or fainting. In a state of wakefulness one can see accurately. A state of lack of consciousness is opposite to this, and is described, for instance, in the story of Lot's daughters lying with him (Gen. 19.30-38). This occurs when Lot was under the influence of wine and *did not know* that his daughters lay with him (19.33-36).

This meaning of the name of Judah's eldest son ער (wakefulness) is particularly significant in light of the fact that in the course of the narrative Judah himself was not conscious of the wrong he had done to his daughter-in-law, Tamar. At the climax of the story, Tamar asks to show him his signet, the cord and the staff, hoping that he will *recognize* (הכר־נא) them (38.25). It is said of Judah that he had indeed recognized (ויכר) them as his. The occurrences of the verb הכיר (recognized) and ידע (know, though here in the sense of sexual intercourse) emphasize that the personal name Er belongs to the CPF, which is close to the SF.

2.8.1.16. ערי *(Eri)*. This personal name is one of the names of those who went down to Egypt, the son of Gad (Gen. 46.16). It may be that the name echoes the meaning of the lexeme ער (Er), the cognitive state of wakefulness, as was said of the personal name Er in the above paragraph (§2.8.1.15). Eri also occurs in Num. 26.16.

2.8.1.17. פניאל/פנואל *(Penuel/Peniel)*. This name is mentioned at Gen. 32.31, 32. One of its constituents is the peripheral lexeme פני (face—§§2.7.1–2). The name is explicitly connected with the act of seeing: 'So Jacob called the name of the place Peniel, saying, "For I have *seen* God *face to face*, and yet my life is preserved" (Gen. 32.31).

2.8.1.18. ראובן *(Reuben)*. Reuben is the name of Jacob's eldest son, by Leah. Leah herself is described as 'soft-eyed', a description which links her to the SF.[161] The name ראובן is linked explicitly to the verb ראה by a word-play appearing in the explanation of his name: 'and she called his name Reuben; for she said, "Because Yhwh has *looked* upon my affliction; surely now my husband will love me"' (Gen. 29.32). The name Reuben is found frequently in Genesis—thirteen times in all, at 29.32; 30.14; 35.22, 23; 37.21, 22, 29; 42.22, 37; 46.8, 9; 48.5; 49.3.

2.8.2. *Lexemes Denoting Time*

Lexemes denoting time may also be connected to a semantic field. Some lexemes denote the time of day as a function of the amount of light to be seen: for instance, לילה (night), ערב (evening), בקר (morning), or through the mention of the luminaries—for instance: 'As the *sun* was going down' (Gen. 15.12). These words of time are linked to the SF because they contain observations connected with the amount of light to be seen, and this has implications for the way in which the characters see.

Thus, for example, in the story of Laban's deception of Jacob in Genesis 29, when Laban gives Leah to Jacob instead of Rachel, it is said that Laban takes Leah *in the evening*, and gives her to Jacob (29.23). Only *in the morning* Jacob realizes that it is Leah by his side (29.25). Thus, in this situation morning and evening are important from the point of view of their implications for the conditions of sight and the cognitive state of alertness of the characters. Lot's daughters, too, lie with him *at night* (19.33, 35). Sometimes when it is explicitly stated that a particular act takes place in the morning, this indicates that the character performs its action in a state of the greatest possible awareness.

161. Leah's soft eyes (or weak eyes) are connected to a more general motif, the beauty of the matriarchs, which is also connected to the SF (see discussions in Chapter 5, and §2.3.2.1).

Polak claims that remarks about the time of day may be significant to the understanding of the plot. Instances are: 'in the heat of the *day*' (Gen. 18.1), 'And Isaac went out to meditate in the field *in the evening*' (24.63), 'in the cool of the *day*' (3.8). Polak explains that the night is the appropriate time for the appearance of God (15.1-5; 28.11-12; 1 Sam. 5.2-15). Only after sunset was Abraham permitted to see the smoking fire pot and a flaming torch that passed between the divided pieces (Gen. 15.17). Abraham sees the fire and the smoke against the background of the darkness of night, which increases the awe caused by the sight.[162]

2.8.2.1. בקר *(morning)*. The morning constitutes the earliest hours of the day, when the sun shines. Sunlight is taken as a constituent in the semantic definition of the lexeme 'morning'. Palache remarks that the basic meaning of the word is 'rising, appearing' of light—that is to say, first light.[163] The lexeme בֹּקֶר also acquires the meaning of the first of the two parts of the day: morning and evening (Gen. 1.5, 8, 13 etc.). The fact that there is light in the morning becomes a presupposition, whenever the lexeme בקר appears in the text, but I preferred to set a limit here, considering only those cases in which 'light' is explicitly mentioned.[164] Hence, the phrase בֹּקֶר אוֹר (the morning lit up) in Gen. 44.3 is the only case in which it may be said that the lexeme בֹּקֶר belongs to the SF. In this case the element of light appears in the context, and is not only a presupposition.

2.8.2.2. יום *(day, daylight)*. The semantic definition of the lexeme יום (day) consists of the presupposition of sunlight.[165] In other words, the basic meaning of יום is that part of the day in which there is light.[166] This presupposition is formulated as new information in Gen. 1.5: 'God called the *light Day*, and the *darkness* he called *Night*'. In most cases, however, this lexeme is found in its calendric meaning,[167] and its meaning as the light part of the day is no more than a presupposition, such as in: 'And there was *evening* and there was *morning*, one *day*' (1.5). For this reason, in most cases the lexeme יום is not included in the SF. In certain textual environments, however, the matter of sight is particularly prominent in itself, and then the link of this lexeme to the SF stands out. This is the case, for instance, in the story of the sacrifice

162. Polak, *Biblical Narrative*, pp. 232-43.

163. Palache, *Semantic Notes*, p. 16. Also *HALOT*, p. 151.

164. On presuppositions, see Knud Lambrecht, *Information Structure and Sentence Form: Topic, Focus and the Mental Representations of Discourse Referents* (Cambridge: Cambridge University Press, 1994), pp. 52-65.

165. On presuppositions see the preceding note.

166. *HALOT*, p. 399, יום I, 1.

167. *HALOT*, p. 399, יום I, 2.

of Isaac, in which matters of time and place are repeated alongside lexemes of sight. In 22.4 we find: 'On the third day Abraham *lifted up his eyes* and *saw* the place afar off'. Here, the use of the long formula of seeing 'and he lifted up his eyes and saw', in addition to the repetition of lexemes of time, brings the presupposition of light in the lexeme יום to the surface. Even so, the lexeme יום is not included in the general list of the words of the SF, apart from its appearance in the creation account in Genesis 1. This lexeme is found outside Genesis in contexts emphasizing the element of light in it. Thus, in Amos 5.18: 'Woe to you who desire the day of Yhwh! Why would you have the day of Yhwh? It is darkness, and not light.' Proverbs 4.18: 'But the path of the righteous is like the light of dawn, which shines brighter and brighter until full day'. Nehemiah 8.3: 'And he read from it facing the square before the Water Gate from early morning (מן־האור) until midday (עד־מחצית היום)'.

2.8.2.3. לילה *(night)*. Unlike the lexeme יום (day), the lexeme לילה has no calendric significance. It refers to that part of the day in which there is no light—'night'.[168] Therefore, wherever it appears this lexeme belongs to the SF. It is found 25 times in Genesis. Night and evening are characterized by darkness, and always imply poor conditions of visibility.

2.8.2.4. שׁחר *(dawn)*. The lexeme שׁחר belongs to the SF because it means 'the rise of morning light',[169] or dawn. In Genesis the lexeme appears three times: 19.15; 32.25, 27. When this lexeme appears in the text it is assumed that this is the part of the day in which the sun begins to shine, and the light begins to appear. Thus, a necessary condition for visual perception is fulfilled.

2.8.3. *The Heavenly Luminaries*

2.8.3.1. מאור *(luminary)*. The luminaries provide light, which is a necessary condition for visual perception: 'and let them be lights in the firmament of the heavens to give light upon the earth' (Gen. 1.15). The lexeme מאור is found in Gen. 1.14, 15, 16 (3 times). In v. 16 the two great luminaries are mentioned—the greater light and the lesser light. See the discussion below.

168. Nevertheless, Galinier *et al.* suggest that night has a lot more to it, and should be investigated as an anthropological object. They discuss different notions connected with the night, such as sleeping, dreaming, and myths about the creation of the night (Jacques Galinier *et al.*, 'Anthropology of the Night: Cross-Disciplinary Investigations', *Current Anthropology* 51 [2010], pp. 819-47).

169. Ben Yehudah, *A Complete Dictionary*, p. 7038.

2.8.3.2. המאור הגדל *(the greater light)*. The sun is called 'the greater light' once in Gen. 1.16. The expression 'the two great lights' in this verse includes both the sun and the moon. 'The greater light' refers to the greater light in comparison with the smaller light, mentioned below.

2.8.3.3. שמש *(sun)*. The sun is the 'greater light' which gives light in the heavens. It is mentioned in Genesis six times: 15.12, 17; 19.23; 28.11; 32.32; 37.9. When the sun is mentioned in the text there is a presupposition that the sun gives out light; hence the link to the SF. When the sun is present, a necessary condition for visual perception—the presence of light—is fulfilled.

2.8.3.4. ירח *(moon)*. The lexeme ירח (moon) is mentioned once in Genesis, at 37.9. It belongs to the SF because of the presupposition that it emanates light at night, and when it is present, as in the case of the sun, a necessary condition for visual perception is fulfilled. This presupposition is expressed explicitly, for instance, in Isa. 13.10: 'For the stars of the heavens and their constellations will not give their light; the sun will be dark at its rising and the *moon* will not shed its light'.

2.8.3.5. המאור הקטן *(the smaller light)*. This term is found at Gen. 1.16, and is a term referring to the moon (see §2.8.3.4).

2.8.3.6. כוכב *(star)*. The lexeme כוכב is found five times in Genesis, at 1.16; 15.5; 22.17; 26.4; 37.9. The stars, too, emanate light, and hence their connection with the SF. Outside Genesis there are explicit references to the stars as givers of light at, for instance, Joel 2.10: 'the sun and the moon are darkened, and the stars withdraw their shining'; Job 3.9: 'Let the stars of its dawn be dark; let it hope for light, but have none, nor see the eyelids of the morning'. Also, Ps. 148.3 mentions the phrase כוכבי אור ('shining stars', or 'stars of light'), which explicitly expresses this idea that the stars emanate light.

2.9. *Conclusion*

Up to this point I have described the structure of the SF, which is composed of a wide variety of lexemes from Genesis, as they are cognitively connected by semantic relations. I shall now continue to the next level of my discussion, the deployment of these terms of Sight in some individual plots of Genesis.

Chapter 3

The Deployment of the Sight Field in the Individual Narratives

3.1. *The Primeval History*

The stories analyzed in this chapter are the first story of creation and the story of the Garden of Eden. These narratives serve as the introduction to both the unit of Genesis 1–11 and to Genesis as a whole. Hence, they are strategic points for the unit and for the book. I shall also examine the story which closes this unit, the story of the Tower of Babel in Genesis 11, from the standpoint of the deployment of SF lexemes. The Flood narrative will be discussed in §4.4.

It should also be noted that the following discussion follows the deployment of SF lexemes in some individual narratives, whereas a detailed discussion concerning each lexeme is given in Chapter 2. Lastly, we have to bear in mind that a lot has been said and written about each of the individual narratives of Genesis, and the sections of the book as well. Nevertheless, since the present discussion is focused on the deployment of the SF in the narratives and its impact on their understanding, I will not be able to refer to many of the works that have been written regarding them.

3.1.1. *Sight in the First Story of Creation: Genesis 1.1–2.3*

In the first story of creation (Gen. 1.1–2.3), we find, at the end of almost every creation process, a distinctive rhetorical pattern, formed around the central lexeme of Sight: 'And God saw that X was good' (Gen. 1.4, 10, 12, 18, 21, 25, 31a). Furthermore, the first creation is the light, while prior to that, there had been only darkness in the world: 'And God *saw* that the *light* was good, and God separated the *light* from the *darkness*' (Gen. 1.4). As shown previously, the 'light' and the 'darkness' are lexemes belonging to the SF. The significance of this is that already at the outset of Genesis both aspects of the SF are presented, positive and negative. Additional lexemes from the SF continue to occur at key points in this creation account. The evening (ערב) and the morning (בקר) mentioned at the end of each day of creation also belong to the SF. So too do the day (יום) and the night (לילה) named by God in v. 5.

Many lexemes from the SF are concentrated in the account of the fourth day of creation; in this day the *luminaries* were created, whereby according to v. 14 they were intended to separate the *day* from the *night*, but also 'to give light' (להאיר) upon the land (vv. 15, 17). Hence, this passage in particular is dominated by Sight-related terms, because of the mention of the luminaries themselves, the lexemes 'day', 'night' and the verb 'to give light'.

Other lexemes of Sight, apart from those occurring in the concluding pattern in each day of creation, are mentioned in relation to the creation of humankind on the sixth day: 'So God created humankind in his own image (בצלמו), in the image (בצלם) of God he created him...' (v. 27). The first half of v. 27 consists of two clauses containing similar content. The first reads: 'So God created humankind in his image'; and the second: 'in the image of God he created it'. The first ends with 'in his own image' (בצלמו) and the second opens with 'in the image' (בצלם). This reversal emphasizes the lexeme in question. In this same day, in v. 26, the divine plan is mentioned: 'Then God said, "Let us make humankind in our image (בצלמנו), after our likeness (כדמותנו)"'. The lexemes 'in our image' and 'after our likeness' belong to the SF, and both have the masculine plural suffix. Polak calls attention to the rhetorical phenomenon of homoioteleuton or similar sound endings here, also noting the delicate play on repeating the Hebrew consonants ד, מ, and נ in this clause.[1] It may be observed that this is one of the few instances in the Bible in which God is referred to in the plural, thereby putting additional emphasis on the idea expressed by the Sight terms 'image' and 'likeness'.[2]

After the six days of creation, there is a concluding statement that also employs the formula of Sight: 'And God *saw* (וירא) everything that he had made, and behold, it was very good. And there was *evening* (ערב) and there was *morning* (בקר), a sixth day' (Gen. 1.31).

At the end of the description of God's rest on the seventh day, nothing at all is said of what God saw. The absence of the Sight formula is entirely in keeping with Longacre's theory of peaking, since according to him linguistic

1. Polak, *Biblical Narrative*, pp. 98-99.

2. Skinner notes that the most accepted explanation for referring to God here in the plural is that he is presented as one consulting with his entourage (Skinner, *Genesis*, pp 30-32). Speiser (*Genesis*, p. 7), on the other hand, says that the point at issue is one of grammar alone, without a direct bearing on the meaning. He explains that Elohim, the Hebrew term for 'God', is plural in form and is so construed at times (e.g. 20.13; 35.7). Hamilton is prone to accept the notion of 'plurality within unity' expressed by the use of plural in relation with God. He agrees with Hasel's idea of 'plural of wholeness', as well as Clines's 'duality within the Godhead' (G. Hasel, 'The Meaning of "Let Us" in Gn 1:26', *AUSS* 13 [1975], pp. 58-66 [75]; D.J.A. Clines, 'The Image of God in Man', *TynBul* 19 [1968], pp. 62-69 [68]; Victor P. Hamilton, *The Book of Genesis: Chapters 1–17* [Grand Rapids: Eerdmans, 1990], p. 134).

characteristics that appear throughout the story sometimes fade away at the peak itself, or near it (§1.4). Thus, it would seem that the narrative intends to emphasize that the seventh day is different, that is to say, by the absence of the repeated Sight formula for the Sabbath day. In any case, the Sight formula under discussion is significant in the first story of creation since it is repeated in the six days of creation, but also because of its absence in the seventh day.

3.1.2. *The Story of the Garden of Eden: Genesis 2.4–3.24*

The story of the Garden of Eden has a special status as far as the SF is concerned. Its climax entails the mental awakening of the main characters, stated in lexemes from the SF. Adam and Eve become fully aware after eating from the forbidden fruit: 'Then the *eyes* of both *were opened* (ותפקחנה עיני שניהם), and they *knew* (וידעו) that they were *naked* (עירמם)' (Gen. 3.7). The 'eyes' here are connected to the SF since they are the means of seeing; the nakedness belongs to the category of lexemes which contain the schema 'creation of conditions for seeing'; and their knowing and understanding relates to the SF, since they belong to the nearby CPF. After eating from the fruit of the tree of knowledge, they know something they did not know before. This knowledge changes the face of humanity from that moment forward. Now, to analyze the narrative in terms of the general deployment of Sight lexemes, we need to know where it begins. Scholars disagree as to the exact opening verse of the story of the Garden of Eden. The answer to this depends on the question of where exactly the first story of creation of ch. 1 ends. According to scholars such as Wenham and Cassuto,[3] the first account of creation ends at 2.3, while others maintain that it ends at 2.4a.[4] It could be that this blurring of the borders is not accidental, as it is meant to stress the direct connection between the two descriptions of creation, and that ch. 2, as some medieval exegetes see it, is a more detailed account of ch. 1.[5]

3. G.J. Wenham, *Genesis 1–15* (WBC, 1; Waco, TX: Word Books, 1987), p. 49. According to Wenham, the clause 'These are the generations of X' everywhere else in Genesis constitutes a heading to a cycle of narratives (e.g. 6.9; 11.27; 37.2) or to a genealogy (e.g. 5.1; 25.12). It seems preferable, he says, to regard 2.4 as fulfilling its usual function. According to Wenham, the same thing happens here; this formula is meant to function as the heading of a new section, the section comprised of chs. 2–4. Also see U. Cassuto, *A Commentary on the Book of Genesis* (trans. Israel Abrahams; Jerusalem: Magnes Press, 1965), p. 97

4. For example: Skinner, *Genesis*, p. 54; Speiser, *Genesis*, pp. 8, 12-13, 15; Amit, *Reading Biblical Stories*, p. 51.

5. This is the view of traditional commentators, such as Rashi and Rashbam, seen, for instance, in their commentary on Gen. 1.27. Van Wolde holds that the second story opens

Chapter 2 tells about background events for the Garden of Eden story. It focuses on the structure of the garden and on the creation of man, animals, and woman.[6] In ch. 2 there is also the prohibition against eating from the fruit of the tree of knowledge (2.17).

Within this chain of background events describing the idyllic life man lived in the Garden of Eden, as opposed to or as criticism of life on earth,[7] we find important connections to the SF. The first occurs only in 2.9 in a description of planting of trees by God. This verse describes God making every tree that is *pleasant to the sight* (נחמד למראה) and good for food grow out from the ground. While doing so, he makes the tree of life grow in the midst of the garden and also the *tree of the knowledge of good and evil.* Actually, it is the tree of knowledge that stands at the centre of the story, whereas the tree of life is peripheral and is recalled again only in the conclusion, in 3.22, 24. The appearance of the tree of life only in 2.9 and in the closing paragraph of ch. 3 led various scholars to conclude that, originally, the story was only about one tree, the tree that would give those who ate of its fruit the ability to distinguish between good and evil, while the second tree, the tree of life, was only a secondary motif.[8] As for the SF, the fact that the tree of knowledge and its fruit appear in the exposition, in the conclusion and in the climax, has special importance, since this supports the proposition that lexemes from the SF appear at key points in the narrative.

in 2.4b, and notes the syntactical parallel between the beginning of the story in ch. 1, 'In the beginning God created the heavens and the earth', and the beginning of the second narrative, 'In the day that Yhwh God made the earth and the heavens' (2.4b). In both cases the half-verse begins by noting the time factor, 'In the beginning', in the first case, 'In the day', in the second. This is followed by a verb of creation, 'created' (ברא), compared with 'made' (עשׂות), and finally, the object is noted, 'the heavens and the earth', compared with the transposition 'the earth and the heavens' (E.J. van Wolde, *Words Become Worlds: Semantic Studies of Genesis 1–11* [Leiden: E.J. Brill, 1994], p. 28). In her view, this parallel adds weight to the assumption that ch. 2 focuses on one point in time or on one day from the process of creation. Rabbi Yosef Bechor Shor had this to say regarding the words 'These are the generations of heavens' in his commentary on Gen. 2.4: 'Just as at the beginning, the description was concise, now the text returns and explains how things were carried out'. See also Tryggve N.D. Mettinger, *The Eden Narrative: A Literary and Religio-Historical Study of Genesis 2–3* (Winona Lake, IN: Eisenbrauns, 2007).

6. Amit assigns to ch. 2 the status of exposition of the story of the Garden of Eden. She refers to it as an exposition, consisting of 20 verses, of a narrative consisting of 24 verses (Amit, *Reading Biblical Stories*, p. 51). On the other hand, van Wolde thinks the story begins with the creation of man in Gen. 2.7 (van Wolde, *Words Become Worlds*, p. 29).

7. Amit, *Reading Biblical Stories*, pp. 52-53.

8. Westermann, *Genesis 1–11*, pp. 211-13.

The exposition contains an important background detail, connected to the SF, and that is the prohibition against eating *from the tree of knowledge* of good and evil (2.17). It is important to note that God only forbids eating from the tree of knowledge, whereas the tree of life is not even mentioned at this point.

At the next stage in the course of the exposition, we encounter a number of words related to the SF in different ways. God creates the beasts of the field and the birds of the air, and brings them to Adam *to see* (לראות) what he would call them (2.19). Still, even though animals now exist, God has *not found* (לא־מצא) a helper as yet for Adam (2.20). That being the case, God had put Adam to a *deep sleep* (תרדמה). Adam *slept* (ויישן, 2.21), and while he did, God took one of his ribs,[9] and from it made a woman (2.21-22). And indeed the lexemes 'deep sleep' and 'slept' connect to the SF in the broad sense, alluding also to the aspect of the cognitive perception of Adam. The verbs indicate that Adam, at that stage, was unaware of what was happening around him.

The end of the exposition brings us nearer to the narrative about Adam and Eve. At its end we learn that Adam and his wife were *naked* (עֲרוּמִּים, 2.25). The new story opens with a description of a new figure and a trait that characterizes it: 'Now the *serpent* (והנחש) was more *subtle* (עָרוּם) than any other wild creature that Yhwh God had made' (3.1a). Although the Hebrew root ערם is used for nakedness at one occurrence and the cunning of the reptile in the other, the two words are linked to the SF; the word עֲרוּמִּים (naked) is connected to the field because it expresses the idea of being in a state of physical exposure, revealed to the eye. The form עָרוּם (cunning, crafty) is linked to the field because it belongs to the category of lexemes from nearby fields—in this case, the CPF. In addition, the lexeme נחש (serpent) is a symbol in the SF (§2.4.1). In the present context, the lexemes עֲרוּמִּים and עָרוּם stand out because they are positioned near each other, and bear sound resemblance.[10] Wenham adds that Adam and Eve ate from the tree of knowledge seeking to be shrewd (cf. 3.6), but discovered instead that they are nude (3.7, 10).[11]

9. צלע in usually translated as 'rib', though medieval commentators such as Rashi and Ibn Ezra interpret it as 'side' based on Exod. 26.20 and others (Nahum Sarna, *The JPS Torah Commentary: Genesis* [Philadelphia: Jewish Publication Society, 1989], p. 22; R. Alter, *Genesis: Translation and Commentary* [New York: W.W. Norton, 1996], p. 9).

10. Wenham admits that the choice of the term עָרוּם, 'shrewd', here is one of the more obvious plays on words in the text, for the man and his wife have just been described as עֲרוּמִּים, 'nude' (Wenham, *Genesis 1–15*, p. 72).

11. Wenham, *Genesis 1–15*, p. 72.

These words from the exposition are background details on which the main events of the plot are based. Adam and Eve walking around without raiment, and not being ashamed on that account, is in absolute contradiction to the ramifications of eating from the forbidden fruit which were their awareness of being naked and their sewing fig leaves for themselves (3.7). It would seem that Rashi (on 3.1) grasped the importance of the comment about the nakedness of Adam and Eve for the events to come when he said that because the snake saw them naked, he sought to bring them to commit a sin. That is, according to Rashi, the nakedness of the human beings constituted a motive for the snake's deed, and thus, a word from the semantic field drives the plot forward.

The narrative about eating from the forbidden fruit opens with a transition to direct speech, within a dialogue between the snake and the woman. The snake turns to the woman and says something that has been interpreted as a question, or otherwise seems incomplete: 'Did God say, "You shall not eat of any tree of the garden?"' (3.1). The woman answers saying: 'We may eat of the fruit of the trees of the garden; but God said, "You shall not eat of the fruit of the tree which is in the midst of the garden, neither shall you touch it, lest you die"' (3.2-3). And the snake replied: 'You will not die. For God *knows* (ידע) that when you eat of it *your eyes will be opened* (ונפקחו עיניכם), and you will be like God, *knowing good and evil* (ידעי טוב ורע)' (3.4-5). The root ידע, belonging to the CPF and having a special affinity with the SF, appears in the text five times (2.9; 3.5, 5, 7, 22).[12]

In response, the woman *saw* that because the tree was good for eating, and that it was a *delight to the eyes* (תאוה־הוא לעינים), and that the tree was *to be desired to make one wise* (ונחמד העץ להשכיל), she took of its fruit and ate; and she also gave some to Adam, and he ate (3.6). Until this point in the complication, there is a large concentration of words from the SF, and now comes v. 7, mentioned above, which brings with it the turning-point, in which *the eyes of both were opened* and they *knew* that they were *naked*. The beginning of the resolution follows immediately in the same verse. The man and his wife sewed fig leaves together and made themselves aprons. In other words, the turning-point tells of a new cognitive situation into which the man and his wife have entered upon eating the forbidden fruit. But the story does not end here. Now they must account for their deeds, and it is time to relate to the matter of the violation of the divine taboo. The man and his wife heard the sound of Yhwh walking in the garden in the cool of the

12. Polak finds the CPF significant in the account of the Garden of Eden, and realizes the semantic connections between visual perception and cognitive perception. In his analysis he considers other terms of CPF, such as 'ashamed' (יתבששו, 2.25) and 'pain' (עצבון, 3.16) (Polak, *Biblical Narrative*, p. 97).

day, and they *hid themselves* (ויתחבא) from his presence among the trees of the garden (3.8). The act of hiding belongs to the SF since it includes the schema 'creation of conditions for not-seeing' (§2.3.4.6). But God called to the man, and said to him, 'Where are you?' (3.9). And Adam answers him: 'I heard the sound of you in the garden, and *I was afraid* (ואירא), because I was *naked* (עירם); and *I hid* (ואחבא) myself' (3.10). God asks the man who told him that he was *naked*, and if he has violated God's prohibition (3.11). The man blames the woman for giving the forbidden fruit (3.12), and when God turns to her, she transfers the blame to the serpent who enticed her to eat from it (3.13). Now, at the stage of resolution, the three receive punishments,[13] one after the other, punishments that are usually not connected with Sight.[14]

In any case, the punishments are over by v. 20, in which there is a conclusion in the form of a name aetiology. Adam calls his wife's name 'Eve' because she was the mother of all living things (3.20). Also God made for Adam and for his wife garments of skins, and clothed them (3.21). The phrase 'garments of skins' (כתנות עור) fits into the SF because the clothing is meant to hide the bodies of those who had in the past been naked and had not been aware of it. This is a kind of closure for the events that had been opened in 2.25 with the mention of the man and his wife's nakedness and the absence of shame accompanying that nakedness.

Verses 3.22-24 tell about the banishment of man from the Garden of Eden, and form another conclusion for the story, which some commentators would refer to as secondary.[15] Here the words from the SF are 'knowing (לדעת) good and evil' (3.22), and perhaps the lexeme 'flaming' (להט, 3.24), which hints of a connection to fire or to light—SF lexemes.

In sum, lexemes from the SF are scattered throughout every stage of the account, contributing to the understanding of its main theme. Adam and Eve turn into human beings able to see. Referring to the scale of Sight levels

13. Longacre calls the scene of hiding that comes after the first climax, a scene in which the punishments are meted out, a 'didactic peak' (Longacre, *The Grammar of Discourse*, p. 37; see §1.4).

14. Except, perhaps, for the punishment meted out to the snake. This punishment includes two appearances of the verb שוף: 'it will שוף your head and you will שוף its heel' (Hamilton, *The Book of Genesis*, p. 197). The first occurrence of this verb is often translated 'crush', while the second as 'strike at'. This verb occurs two more times in the Hebrew Bible: Job 9.17 and Ps. 139.11. Dahood appeals to the Arabic verb *šāfa*, 'he watches, looks', and translates both passages with 'observe' (Mitchell Dahood, *Psalms: Introduction, Translation, and Notes*, III [AB, 17; Garden City, NY: Doubleday, 1970], p. 291). The last meaning might be appropriate here too: 'He shall look for your head, and you shall look for his heel' (but also see Hamilton's suggestion 'lie in wait'; Hamilton, *The Book of Genesis*, p. 198).

15. Westermann, *Genesis 1–11*, pp. 212-13.

explained in the Introduction (also at §4.3), we may say that Adam and Eve undergo the experience of low-level sight, and an intermediate-level of sight, which includes not only concrete vision but also abstract seeing, that is, understanding and becoming aware. They see and understand, but the only knowledge they obtain relates to their nudity. Both humans at this point do not achieve sight of a high level.

3.1.3. *The Story of the City and Tower of Babel: Genesis 11.1-9—Humans Speak and God Intervenes by Sight*

In contrast to the stories analyzed above, the story of the City and Tower of Babel is an example of a narrative in Genesis in which SF lexemes do not contribute to the coherence of the unit. In this story, actually, another field is predominant—the field of Oral Communication. Many of the lexemes from this field appear in almost all its verses, with sound-plays to emphasize their presence. The words from the field of Oral Communication are: 'language' (שׂפה), 'words' (דברים, 11.1), 'and they said' (ויאמרו, 11.3), 'name' (שׁם, 11.4), 'and Yhwh said' (ויאמר, 11.6), 'language' (שׂפה, 11.6), 'their language' (שׂפתם, 11.7), 'understand' (literally: 'hear', ישׁמעו, 11.7), 'speech' (שׂפת, 11.7). The explanation for the name Babel at the end of the narrative is also connected with the field of Oral Communication, because there, 'God confused the language of all the earth' (בלל ה' את שׂפת כל־הארץ, 11.9).

It is important to note that the central verb of the SF, the verb ראה (see), has a single occurrence in this story, right at its middle: 'And Yhwh came down *to see* the city and the tower, which the sons of men had built' (11.5). The special construction of this story, from the point of view of the semantic fields working in it, emphasizes the contrast between God and humans: humans are engaged in speaking, whereas God sees them, in the sense of checking on their deeds. Hence, this contrast between humans and God is enhanced in this narrative by the unique deployment of the semantic fields of Sight and Oral Communication. The contrast between humans and the divine develops further on in Genesis, and will be dealt with in the coming sections.

Thus far we have seen that in selected narratives in the first section of Genesis[16] God is occupied with observing human beings, while they, for their part, do not see him, and sometimes even hide from him. The seeing of human beings is usually that of the physical sense, although it may sometimes include cognitive perception, but this is not an indication of Sight of the highest level which, as I have proposed, includes the awe of God and faith in him.

16. Since space and time are limited I am forced to choose some of the central episodes of Genesis, and analyze the deployment of the SF in them. The rest of the narratives of Genesis are briefly treated in Chapter 4.

3.2. *The Abraham Narrative*

I follow Buber in choosing to deal with Genesis 12, the opening to the Abraham section; Genesis 15, God's covenant with Abraham; and Genesis 22, the Sacrifice of Isaac, which serves as the climax of this section.[17] Then I shall discuss several additional narratives in which the SF is especially prominent: the stories about Hagar (Gen. 16; 21), the Sodom and Gomorrah narrative (Gen. 19), and the story of Abraham and Sarah in Egypt (Gen. 12.10-20). Other narratives in this section are discussed in Chapter 4 in connection with the coherence of Genesis as a whole.

3.2.1. *'Go from your country and your kindred': Genesis 12.1-9*

The final verses of Genesis 11, starting from v. 27, are usually seen as an introduction to the section of the Abraham stories that begin with God's command to 'go from your country' (12.1). In this introduction the name of the place Ur of the Chaldeans (אור כשדים) is mentioned (11.28, 31). This name has an indirect connection to the SF. The etymology of 'Ur' connects it with the Sumerian Urim (meaning 'city'), but the sound of the word also links it to the Hebrew lexeme אור ('light'), thus providing a connection to the SF. In addition, אור in Hebrew means 'firelight', which can form a semantic link to the field. Another name mentioned here that is connected with the SF is the name of Abraham's brother's son *Lot* (11.27, 31).

Genesis 12.1-9 tells of a number of short journeys. The first unit is constructed in the form of a command (12.1-3) and its implementation (12.4-5). The divine command requires that Abraham leave the place where he lives and move to another country 'to the land that I will *show* (אראך) you' (12.1).[18] Then God blesses Abraham (vv. 2-3). In describing the execution of the command, *Lot* is mentioned as accompanying Abraham (vv. 4-5). The clause 'when they had come to the land of Canaan' ends the account of the first journey.

In 12.6 Abraham is active again, renewed activity being a sign for the opening of a new scene.[19] The place name *Elon Moreh* ('the oak of Moreh', RSV), includes the root ירה (meaning 'to instruct, teach'), which belongs to the field of Education, close to the SF. At that location God is *seen* by Abraham and promises him the land where he is already situated (12.7a). Until this point, the routine of the movement of journey is achieved by the verbs 'Abram went' (v. 4), 'Lot went with him' (v. 4), 'departed from

17. Buber too, in his article 'Abraham the Seer', views these chapters as important landmarks in the history of Abraham.

18. The motif of seeing the Promised Land is also mentioned with reference to Moses in Deut. 34.1-5. According to Daube, the Abraham stories have influenced the stories about Moses in this issue (Daube, *Studies in Biblical Law*, pp. 28-30).

19. Amit, *Reading Biblical Stories*, p. 43.

Haran' (v. 4), 'set forth to go' (v. 5), 'they had come to the land' (v. 5), 'Abram passed through the land to the place' (v. 6). The verb of Sight in v. 7, 'Then Yhwh *appeared* (וירא) to Abram', breaks the dynamics of Abraham's movement. It creates a disturbance in the regularity achieved in the text up to that point, and thus sight becomes more noticeable. An additional pattern accentuates the seeing in these verses. The description of God's revelation opens with 'then Yhwh appeared (וירא) to Abram' (v. 7), and closes with 'to Yhwh, who had appeared (הנראה) to him' (v. 7). The opening and the ending which resemble each other, both being constructed from the verb ראה (see) in the niphal, to which is added the specification of who sees as indirect object (אל־אברם, אליו), highlight the matter of sight.

After the construction of the altar, additional journeys of Abraham are described in vv. 8-9. But, contrary to the travels described in the previous verses, there is no sign of visual perception in vv. 8-9. Moreover, both previously, in v. 7, and now, in v. 8, Abraham builds an altar, and the activity is described in an identical phrasing, ויבן שם מזבח (he built there an altar, vv. 7 and 8). However, in the second instance revelation is not mentioned. The appearance of God occurred in Elon Moreh, which is connected to the SF (§2.8.1.3). This pattern of the occurrence of a Sight-related term and its absence immediately afterwards in passages otherwise so similar to one another breaks into an automatic reading of the text and serves to emphasize the visual aspect.

3.2.2. *God's Promise and Covenant: Genesis 15*

The story of God's Promise and Covenant to Abraham in Genesis 15 opens as follows: 'After these things the word of Yhwh came to Abram in a vision (במחזה), "Fear not (אל־תירא), Abram, I am your shield; your reward shall be very great"' (15.1). The noun 'vision' (מחזה) and the verb 'fear not' (אל־תירא), which belong to the SF in different ways, appear in this strategic point of the opening.

Further on in the story of the covenant, we encounter a broad spectrum of words from the SF. Abram asks God for a son to be his heir, since, as he says, he remains childless (15.2). In response, God promises Abram a son to be his heir, and that promise is made during an act of seeing expressed thus: 'And he brought him outside and said, "*Look* (הבט) toward heaven, and number the *stars* (הכוכבים), if you are able to number them"'. Then he said to him, "So shall your descendants be"' (15.5). Opinion is divided as to whether or not Abram actually does go outside as part of the vision he sees, or if the vision has ended together with the blessing, in which case the request from God for Abram to come outside is made afterwards.[20] The

20. According to von Rad, the 'chief joint' in this text, which is filled with joints, occurs between v. 6 and v. 7 (von Rad, *Genesis*, pp. 179-81).

question also arises whether the dialogue that follows and the division of the animals are parts of the same vision, or whether they should be viewed as actions outside the vision (or form another vision). However that may be, for our purposes the important point is that the routine of the dialogue is broken by the divine request that Abram take some other action, that is, go out and look at the stars. The violation of routine emphasizes what is connected with Sight. The description of this stage of vision concludes with lexemes from the CPF in v. 6: 'And he *believed* (והאמן) Yhwh; and he *reckoned* (ויחשבה) it to him as righteousness' (see the discussion in §4.5, including n. 38).

The exchange of words continues in v. 7, in which 'Ur of the Chaldeans' is mentioned, at which 'Ur' belongs to the SF. In v. 8 Abraham makes things difficult and asks: 'O Yhwh God, how am I to *know* (אדע) that I shall possess it?' The verb 'know' is also linked to the SF since it belongs to the nearby CPF. As to the development of the theme of Sight, here Abraham's situation is one of not knowing at all.

In the story of the covenant, God's reaction to Abraham's query as to how he will know that he shall indeed possess the land has a symbolic character. God asks Abram to take a three-year-old heifer, a three-year-old she-goat, and a three-year-old ram, and also a turtledove and a young pigeon. Abram divides all these animals except for the birds, and waits. This period of uncertainty is accentuated by descriptions of defective visibility: as *the sun* (השמש) sets, and Abram falls into a *deep sleep* (תרדמה), and a 'dread and *great darkness* (חשכה) fell upon him' (15.12). Within this situation of extreme uncertainty, which, for Abraham, included conditions of dreadful darkness, God clarifies for Abram the future in store for him and his people: 'Then Yhwh said to Abram, "*Know of a surety* (ידע תדע) that your descendants will be sojourners in a land that is not theirs, and will be slaves there, and they will be oppressed for four hundred years"' (15.13-16). But afterwards the fourth generation shall come back to Canaan (v. 16). At the end of the divine words of God which continue for five verses, we return again to descriptions in which lexemes of Sight occur, but this time, elements of light penetrate the darkness as sudden fire passes among the pieces (15.17): 'When the *sun* (השמש) had gone down and it was *dark* (ועלטה), behold, a *smoking fire pot* (תנור) and a *flaming torch* (ולפיד אש) passed between these pieces'. The words 'sun' and 'dark' belong to the SF. The words 'fire pot' and 'flaming torch' join the periphery of the SF because of the feature 'light' in their semantic definitions.

Thus, in the story of God's Promise and Covenant, lexemes from the SF have been particularly emphasized, thanks to the structure of the text. In every instance, after a routine of dialogue between Abram and God, appear lexemes from the SF. Abram, who says of himself that he does not know, is immersed in darkness and gloom, and at a certain point is overcome by a deep sleep. God tries to bring him out of the darkness of his situation, both visual and cognitive, by informing Abram of his future, and by miraculously creating a situation of light by means of the fire pot and the flaming torch. And we need to recall that in the section under discussion, the visual means serve to accentuate the strategic importance of this event in Genesis, the event where God promises Abram that his seed shall inherit the Land that is given to him. As for levels of Sight, this event is characterized by God impelling Abram to look at the stars, and God himself begins to recognize Abram's faith (see further the discussion in §4.5).

3.2.3. *The Sacrifice of Isaac: Genesis 22*

The sacrifice of Isaac constitutes the climax of the Abraham narrative.[21] In this narrative God puts Abraham to the most difficult test, the sacrifice of his only son.[22] The plot of this narrative forms the pattern of the pediment.[23] The introduction is of a special kind since it contains a comment from the narrator, who reveals the objective of the narrative, or as Westermann puts it, offers a comment that summarizes the theme of the story, 'God tested Abraham' (Gen. 22.1).[24]

The flow of events begins only afterwards, in v. 1b, with a dialogue between God and Abraham, in which God commands Abraham to go to the land of *Moriah*. It is at this very point—when the command is given, that the complication begins. Abraham's equilibrium is disturbed by the divine command that he, the father of Isaac, sacrifice his son, a command that is almost impossible to carry out. The name of the place at which the sacrifice was to take place is connected to the SF (the land of Moriah; see §2.8.1.5).

Abraham, for his part, hastens to carry out the command, and the description mentions the time at which he begins: 'So Abraham rose early in the morning (בבקר), saddled his ass…' (22.3). This part of the day—'the morning'—belongs to the SF because it includes the semantic feature 'light' in its semantic definition. This indication of the morning hours could be viewed as an allusion that Abraham implements the command at a degree of increased awareness, that he does what follows with full awareness.

21. Wenham refers to Isaac's sacrifice as the aesthetic and theological climax of the entire section of the Abraham narrative (Wenham, *Genesis 1–15*, p. 99).

22. In the Midrash of the Sages the sacrificing of Isaac is the final of the ten trials which God placed before Abraham (*Pirke deRabbi Eliezer* 26). See also Buber, 'Abraham the Seer', pp. 22-43.

23. On this pattern, see Polak, *Biblical Narrative*, pp. 38-39.

24. Westermann, *Genesis 1–11*, p. 354. Amit observes that the exposition itself includes only four words: והאלהים נסה את־אברהם ('God tested Abraham', 22.1). The first part of the verse contains the words 'After these things', which were added by the editor in order to connect the story to its surrounding context (Amit, *Reading Biblical Stories*, p. 47).

A new stage in the complication is indicated by the solemn formula of seeing: 'On the third day Abraham lifted up his *eyes* and *saw* the place afar off' (22.4).[25] Indicating an act of seeing carried out by one of the main characters in a narrative sometimes serves to mark the beginning of a course of action.[26] Wenham points out that the use of the wording וישא את עיניו ('lifted up his eyes') prior to the act of seeing indicates that the object of vision is of special importance.[27] In this case the object of the gaze is the location where the sacrifice is supposed to take place.

The full implementation of the command does not occur immediately. The narrator delays the flow of events by inserting an exchange of words between Abraham and his servants and afterwards between Abraham and his son Isaac. First Abraham tells the servants to sit and wait with the ass, while he and Isaac continue along the way alone (22.5). Then the narrator increases the suspense by describing the list of items that those walking have taken with them: 'And Abraham took the wood of the burnt offering, and laid it on Isaac his son; and he took in his hand the *fire* (האשׁ) and the knife' (22.6). Among the items taken on the journey, 'fire' has a connection to light and thus indirectly to the SF, as a peripheral lexeme.

It is through the second exchange of words, a short dialogue between Isaac and Abraham, that the narrator creates another delay. The question comes from Isaac, walking beside his father: 'Behold, *the fire* and the wood; but where is the lamb for a burnt offering?' (22.7). Abraham's response to Isaac's question is of much significance so far as the SF is concerned: Abraham said, 'God will *provide* (יראה) himself the lamb for a burnt offering, my son' (22.8). This statement foreshadows what is to come, since God will in the end select an unexpected sacrifice, the ram. The narrator continues to describe in detail the actions of Abraham when they come to the

25. Auerbach explains that raising one's eyes is the only movement mentioned, and indeed the only thing that is told about the journey. This uniqueness of movement gives the 'impression of emptiness' of the journey. It is as if Abraham looked neither right nor left and suppressed any sign of life in himself or in those accompanying him. Auerbach calls it the march of silence (Erich Auerbach, *Mimesis: The Representation of Reality in Western Literature* [trans. W.R. Trask; Princeton, NJ; Princeton University Press, 1953], p. 7).

26. Westermann, *Genesis 1–11*, p. 339.

27. Wenham (*Genesis 1–15*, p. 107) cites more occurrences in Genesis. These include 18.2, where Abraham sees the three angels standing before him; 24.63, in which Isaac sees the camel caravan of Rebekah, and the following verse, which describes how she lifts her eyes, sees Isaac, and reacts by falling off her camel; 33.1, just before the meeting of conciliation between Jacob and Esau, Jacob lifts his eyes and sees Esau bringing four hundred men with him. Esau, for his part, lifts his eyes and sees the women and children accompanying Jacob, a sight that, in the end, apparently prevents him from attacking Jacob (33.5); Joseph lifts his eyes and sees Benjamin after many years of separation, when he is brought to Egypt by his brothers (43.29).

place of which God had spoken. Abraham builds an altar there, lays the wood in order, binds Isaac his son, and lays him on the altar, upon the wood (22.9). The complication reaches its climax in v. 10, which describes how Abraham 'put forth his hand, and took the knife to slay his son'.

The turning point occurs when the angel calls out to Abraham from the heavens, telling him not to touch the boy (22.11-12).[28] This reversal appears next to the unraveling that follows immediately in v. 13. The turning point contains an explicit expression of realization on the part of the angel, the representative of God: 'for now *I know* (ידעתי) that you *fear* God (ירא אלהים), seeing you have not withheld your son, your only son, from me' (22.12b). This verse is of special importance for the plot, since the cognitive change which God undergoes in regard to Abraham is described. This change is worded using language from the SF: 'I know' (ידעתי) and 'fear' (ירא).[29] Knowing belongs to the nearby CPF whereas 'fear' belongs to the field of Emotion, also close to visual perception. In addition, ירא includes sound resemblance to ראה ('see', §2.6.2.1), and thus the connection of the verb to the SF is strengthened. Not only in their content do these verses function as the turning point of the story, but also in their form. Moberly admits that fear is one of the key words in this story.[30] The words the angel speaks here stand out for their length compared to the other dialogues in this chapter (those between Abraham and his servants and between Abraham and Isaac).

Then, the solemn formula of seeing marks the beginning of the unravelling: 'And Abraham *lifted up his eyes and looked* (וישא אברהם את־עיניו וירא), and behold, behind him was a ram, caught in a thicket by his horns...' (22.13).

At the ending of the story of the sacrifice, at v. 14, Abraham calls the place of the revelation: ה' יראה. Abraham assigns a name to the place in order to commemorate the event that took place there.[31] In this case, the

28. Westermann too regards vv. 11-12 as the turning point in the narrative (Westermann, *Genesis 1–11*, pp. 360, 364).

29. In the words of Aristotle, we have before us a 'complex plot'. Aristotle categorizes stories according to the simplicity or complexity of their plots. A 'simple plot' is one in which the change that transpires within it occurs without peripety or recognition, whereas a 'complex plot' is one 'in which the shift of fortune is accomplished consecutively with recognition or peripety or both' (Aristotle, *Poet.* 52a.12-21). The term 'recognition' is important in the present context, because it denotes turning points involving a transition of the hero from a situation of uncertainty to certainty as happened to God's angel.

30. R.W.L. Moberly, 'The Earliest Commentary on the Akedah', *VT* 38 (1988), pp. 302-23 (304).

31. Gunkel defines this kind of story as a ceremonial legend, whose purpose was to explain the regulations of religious ceremonials in certain places. According to Gunkel, Gen. 22 is a legend about a primitive sanctuary of Israel at Jeruel (Gunkel changes the

name of the place, containing the root ראה (see), emphasizes the visual event that occurred there—God saw.

Yet the story has still not ended completely. The second call of the angel from heaven to Abraham, and the blessing accorded to him in vv. 15-18, still remain. This unit is perceived by scholars as a secondary unit within the story of the sacrifice.[32] However, according to Wenham and Polak, for example, the story cannot be considered complete without this declaration. Wenham argues that without it, there is no point in the trial which Abraham underwent successfully. Abraham deserves some kind of reward for his suffering.[33] Polak examines the web of events according to the basic patterns that shape the fable, using the approach of Dandes. He argues that Abraham, who obeys the divine command to sacrifice his son, has earned himself credit (v. 12), and as his reward, his seed is granted an eternal blessing (vv. 16-17). Only this element counterbalances the threat, since it is equal to the threat mentioned in the beginning and transforms the father from victim to beneficiary. In other words, this final unit should be seen as part of the unravelling and not necessarily as secondary to the story.[34]

As for the SF in this last scene, the word 'stars' (כוכבים) appears (22.17), as part of the divine promise to Abraham that his seed will be as numerous as the stars in the heavens. This lexeme is related to the SF in general and to the portrayal of Abraham's image in particular.[35]

Only after the blessing is conveyed does the narrative end on a note of tranquillity. Abraham returns to his young men, and they return to Beer-sheva (22.19). Amit classes this ending as circular, in that Abraham returns to the place from which he set out.[36]

SF lexemes appear at almost every stage of the plot. Local linguistic and literary phenomena serve to emphasize these lexemes, including topographic names that contain elements of seeing, temporal words from the SF, the use of a solemn formula of vision and wordings that create de-automatization (or estrangement, see §1.3.5, esp. n. 84). At one instance, the verb ראה (see) appears in its rare sense of 'to choose', and this semantic pattern also serves

Masoretic name to Jeruel, suggesting that this was the original name of the place of sacrifice; Herman Gunkel, *The Legends of Genesis: The Biblical Saga and History* [intro. by William F. Albright; trans. W.H. Carruth; New York: Schocken Books, 1964 [from the 1901 German edn], p. 32).

32. See, for example, Westermann, *Genesis 1–11*, pp. 355, 363; von Rad, *Genesis*, p. 237.

33. Wenham, *Genesis 1–15*, p. 111.

34. Polak, *Biblical Narrative*, pp. 132-33; Alan Dundes, *The Morphology of North American Indian Folk Tales* (Helsinki: Suomalainen Tiedeakatemia, 1980).

35. On the implications of Abraham observing the stars, see §4.5.

36. Amit, *Reading Biblical Stories*, p. 47.

to emphasize the SF. Abraham, as in the story of the covenant, is the subject who is brought to see, and it is God who is the motivating agent (who makes him see). In the end it is God (who speaks through his angel) who explicitly undergoes enlightenment in regard to Abraham's faith. In other words, Abraham at this point cannot be regarded as achieving a high level of sight since there is no declaration coming from his side about his own seeing and fearing God. Oddly, Abraham declares about God's sight. This conclusion matches Jonathan Jacobs's analysis of Abraham's character in Genesis 22, not as a one-dimensional figure eager to fulfil God's will, but rather as having inner doubts, as Jacobs focuses on the qualms that plague Abraham on his journey to Moriah.[37]

3.2.4. *Hagar's Flight: Genesis 16*

While it is customary to refer to the section at hand as the 'Abraham narrative', the analysis of the SF in the individual stories reveals that Hagar too has a central role.[38] The story of Hagar's flight in Genesis 16 is usually divided into three main scenes: vv. 1-6, 7-14, 15-16.[39] The first scene takes place in Abraham's home, the second includes a meeting between Hagar and the angel at the spring, and the third tells of the birth of Ishmael, with a concluding remark on Abraham's age.[40] Apart from the two concluding verses, SF lexemes appear throughout the narrative.

The exposition introduces the characters involved and the background for the events (v. 1), that is, Sarah's barrenness and the fact that she has a maidservant. Additional details conveyed by the narrator are the maidservant's place of origin, namely, Egypt, and that her name is Hagar.

The chain of events begins with an exchange of words between Sarah and Abraham, or more precisely, Sarah demands that Abraham have intercourse with her maidservant, and he assents to her request (v. 2). Performance of the deed is described immediately in v. 3; Sarah takes Hagar and gives her to Abraham as a wife (v. 3), and Hagar conceives (v. 4a). A new stage in the complication is marked by the act of sight ascribed to Hagar: 'and when she *saw* that she had conceived, she *looked* with contempt on her mistress' (v. 4b). The reader already knows that Hagar has conceived from what is

37. Jonathan Jacobs, 'Willing Obedience with Doubts: Abraham at the Binding of Isaac', *VT* 60 (2010), pp. 546-59.

38. Buber ('Abraham the Seer') discerned the centrality of the verb 'see' in the narratives concerning Abraham, including the narratives about Hagar.

39. See Skinner, *Genesis*, pp. 284-89; Westermann, *Genesis 12–36*, p. 235; Wenham, *Genesis 16–50*, pp. 3-4. Also see James C. Okoye, 'Sarah and Hagar: Genesis 16 and 21', *JSOT* 32 (2007), pp. 163-75.

40. A transition between scenes may entail a change in venue, or time, or the characters involved (Bar-Efrat, *Narrative Art in the Bible*, p. 102).

related in v. 4: ותהר. But it is Hagar's seeing that she has conceived that causes the complications in the plot: ותרא כי הרתה. Hagar sees and understands that she is pregnant; she comprehends her advantage over her mistress who has not succeeded in becoming pregnant, and from the moment of this understanding, she begins to look with contempt upon Sarah.[41]

Sarah speaks to Abraham and informs him of how matters have developed from her standpoint: 'May the wrong done to me be on you! I gave my maid to your embrace, and when *she saw* (ותרא) that she had conceived, she *looked* (בעיניה) on me with contempt' (v. 5). The clause ותרא כי הרתה ('she saw that she had conceived') is emphasized by its exact repetition, expressed both by the narrator (v. 4) and Sarah (v. 5).

The lexeme עין (eye) from the SF also stands out in these verses. The understanding 'she looked with contempt', which contains in Hebrew the lexeme 'eye' (ותקל גברתה בעיניה), is uttered by the narrator in v. 4, and again by Sarah in v. 5 (ואקל בעיניה). The eyes are also mentioned by Abraham, this time as part of the expression עשי־לה הטוב בעיניך ('do to her as you please', v. 6), and they are emphasized by virtue of the sound resemblance to ותענה ('dealt harshly with her') which follows immediately. The consonants נ and ע occur again in the root ענה which appears in the words of the angel in v. 9 (התעני), as well as in the commentary on the name Ishmael: 'because Yhwh has given heed to your affliction (ענ‍יך)' (v. 11).

The turning point is described in the following verse when the angel finds Hagar 'by a *spring* (עין) of water in the wilderness, *the spring* (עין) on the way to *Shur*' (v. 7). Along with other words from the SF, the word *eye* (עין) is again emphasized in additional appearances. After a short dialogue between Hagar and the angel (v. 8), we are led to a new stage in the plot. Step by step the narrator unties the knot that has been created thus far in the plot. Amit observes that this untying process presents the results of the change.[42] First, the angel commands Hagar to return to her mistress and submit to her (v. 9). Afterwards, he blesses her with descendants so numerous that they cannot be counted for multitude (v. 10), and he informs her that she is with child and that she will give birth to Ishmael (v. 11). Finally, he blesses Ishmael (v. 12).

41. Zucker and Colorado notice the recurrence of words of Sight and Hearing in the stories of Sarah and Hagar. They suggest that the repetition of these words is a purposeful literary device and connects Sarah to Hagar and both women to Abraham (David Jeremy Zucker and Aurora Colorado, 'Seeing and Hearing: The Interrelated Lives of Sarah and Hagar', *Women in Judaism* 7 [2010], < http://wjudaism.library.utoronto.ca/index.php/wjudaism/article/view/14663>).

42. Amit, *Reading Biblical Stories*, p. 55.

As in the narrative of the Akedah (ch. 22), the story reaches its end with a name explanation (though in Gen. 22 there is an additional ending). At the end of the narrative, there is usually a return to static data, a situation that is calm but that presents a reality of new habits.[43] Hagar refers to God, who speaks to her, as 'a God of *seeing*', for she said, 'Have I really *seen* God and remained alive after *seeing* him?' (Gen. 16.13). The narrator further comments that because of the revelation to Hagar, the well was called *Beer Lahai Roi* (16.14).[44] The explanations for these names, as in the narrative of the Akedah, are linked to the revelation described in the story, and they include words from the SF.

Again, we see that SF lexemes appear at key points in the story, in the names of places where events occur, and in their explanations. We have also seen how patterns of sound emphasize the appearance of lexemes from the SF (בעיניה, בעיניך, vv. 4, 5, 6; ותענה, v. 9; ענייך, v. 11). Thus, Hagar receives divine guidance, and feels God has seen her and keeps watch over her. Hagar's seeing in this place reaches a high level of Sight, since this is a situation in which God's angel reveals himself to a human character, and this character takes note of it in an explanation of names. Preceding this, the complication included Hagar's seeing at an intermediate level, when she realizes her pregnancy and understands the advantage of status it brings her in relation to Sarah.

3.2.5. *The Banishment of Hagar: Genesis 21*

The story of the banishment of Hagar in Genesis 21, her wandering in the desert and the angel of God rescuing her, very much resembles in its content and form the story of the Akedah. In the account of Isaac's sacrifice, Abraham's role is similar to that of Hagar in Genesis 21, and Isaac has a role reminiscent of that of Ishmael. Wenham describes the following parallels between the narratives:

In Gen. 21.12-13 God confirms the act of banishing Ishmael, and in 22.2 God commands Abraham to sacrifice his son.[45] In 21.14, food and water are

43. Amit, *Reading Biblical Stories*, p. 46.

44. In Gunkel's view the story originates with J, and according to that source, additional data are lacking at its conclusion. For example: How did Hagar remain beside the well? How did she give birth to Ishmael? And how did he grow up and become a great nation? According to Gunkel, vv. 15-16 originate in P. It is possible that the concluding verse of the story is Gen. 25.18, which tells of the dwelling place of Ishmael's offspring (Hermann Gunkel, *Genesis: übersetzt und erklärt* [Göttingen: Vandenhoeck & Ruprecht, 1966], p. 189).

45. Galpaz-Feller portrays Abraham's relations with Ishmael as 'the Akedah of Ishmael' (Pnina Galpaz-Feller, *Va' Yoled: Relations between Parents and Children in Biblical Stories and Laws* [Jerusalem: Carmel, 2006 (Hebrew)], pp. 23-29).

taken, and in 22.3, there is the taking of the lads and the wood for the offering. Genesis 21.14 describes the journey, as does 22.4-8. Both Ishmael and Isaac are about to die (21.16; 22.10). In both chapters the angel of God calls from the sky. In 21.17 the angel says to Hagar: '*Fear* not' (אל־תירא), and in ch. 22 there is a similar statement from the angel: 'for now I know that you *fear* (ירא) God' (22.12). In 21.19 we have 'Then God opened her *eyes*, and she *saw* a well of water', and in 22.13 'And Abraham *lifted up his eyes* and *looked*, and behold, behind him was a ram, caught in a thicket by his horns'. In 21.19 the child is saved when Hagar gives him water to drink, and in 22.14 the ram is sacrificed instead of the child.[46] In light of all these resemblances between the Akedah and the story of Hagar's banishment, it is no wonder that in both, the same semantic field is found, the SF, which contributes to the coherence of the section concerning Hagar.

Genesis 21.1-21 is a story about Abraham's house and his wives. These verses are commonly divided into two main episodes: vv. 1-7, which are concerned with the birth of Isaac, and vv. 8-21, telling of Isaac's weaning and the banishment of Hagar and Ishmael. However, according to the notion that the appearance of a new figure signifies a new scene, v. 8 as well is part of the exposition, and the plot actually begins in v. 9, where 'the son of Hagar, the Egyptian' appears for the first time in this chapter. Also, beginning with v. 9, the plot becomes more dynamic.[47]

Thus, the exposition of the story of Hagar's banishment would then include eight verses: vv. 1-8. The story opens with the statement that God *visited* (פקד) Sarah, and she conceived as he had promised (21.1-2). The form פקד (visited) is linked to the SF, because it is a lexeme from the nearby CPF (§2.6.1). Abraham calls the son who is born Isaac (v. 3), and he circumcises the child when he is eight days old, as God has commanded him to do (v. 4). Since in Gen. 17.11 circumcision is mentioned as a *sign* (אות) of the covenant between Abraham and his descendants and God, here too, although the lexeme *sign* is not explicitly mentioned, the circumcision is indirectly connected to the SF. The reader knows that this is an external mark visible on the body, and assumes the existence of an unspecified perceiver who sees the mark (see §2.3.5).

The exposition tells of the special relationship of the two parents towards Isaac. This is a son of their old age and he is the embodiment of God's promise that was made after long barrenness. A variety of means are used to describe the special love of the parents for this son of their old age. For example, the father, who is mentioned by name (Abraham), names his son

46. Wenham, *Genesis 16–50*, pp. 99-100.

47. Wenham sees v. 8 as exposition of the episode that continues until v. 21 (Wenham, *Genesis 16–50*, p. 78).

(v. 3),[48] the mother explicitly expresses her joy (v. 7), and a feast is held in honour of the child on the day he was weaned (v. 8).

This idyllic family picture is violated in v. 9, when the complication begins, as the verb of sight marks the beginning of a new phase in the plot: 'But Sarah *saw* (ותרא) the son of Hagar the Egyptian, whom she had borne to Abraham, playing with her son Isaac'.[49] Westermann attaches much importance to the two attributes joined to the name Hagar, the woman who is the object of Sarah's seeing: 'the Egyptian' and 'who bore Abraham'.[50] The first attribute emphasizes Hagar's Egyptian origin, and the second underscores the fact that Hagar has given birth to a child of Abraham. That is what Sarah sees, and that is the source of the confrontation between Hagar and Sarah, says Westermann.[51] Hence, this seeing incident is significant to the development of the plot.

Afterwards Sarah demands of Abraham that he banish the maidservant and her son, so that the child does not receive part of the inheritance together with her own son Isaac (21.10). Abraham's emotional response to this demand is presented. We are told that this was displeasing to him (בעיני אברהם, in *his eyes*) on account of his son (21.11). God intercedes, comforts Abraham, and tells him: 'Be not displeased (אל־ירע בעיניך) because of the lad and because of your slave woman'. God promises that his descendants shall be named after Isaac (21.12), and also that Ishmael is not in danger but rather will himself father a great nation (21.13).

The next stage of the complication is marked by the formula 'Abraham rose early in the *morning*' (21.14). This mention of the time of day, when conditions of visibility are good, may symbolize that Abraham is highly conscious and aware when giving Hagar bread and a skin of water and sending her and her son away. Hagar loses her way in the desert of Beer-sheba (21.14), and the situation becomes more complicated when she has no more water (21.15). Hagar throws down her son under one of the bushes

48. In various places the biblical narrator rather chooses the indefinite subject in the description of naming a child, for example in Gen. 2.23; 25.25, 26; 38.29. On naming children in the Hebrew Bible, see Yael Avrahami, 'Name Giving to the Newborn in the Hebrew Bible', *These Are the Names: Studies in Jewish Onomastics* 5 (2011), pp. 15-53.

49. According to Westermann (*Genesis 12–36*, p. 339), the opening of this scene with the phrase 'but Sarah saw' can be paralleled with similar openings that are found in the New Testament, for example in narratives of healing which open with such statements as 'and Jesus saw'. To this we can add that in comparison to Gen. 16, in which Hagar's sight leads her to disrespect Sarah, in the current narrative there is a reverse of roles of the two women; in ch. 21 Sarah is the one who sees, sight which leads her to act against Hagar.

50. This is my translation of the MT: אשר־ילדה לאברהם (Gen. 21.9).

51. Westermann, *Genesis 12–36*, p. 339.

and takes up a position from which she will be able to avoid *seeing* the death of the child (21.15-16). The scene peaks in the weeping of Hagar (21.16).[52]

The distress in which Hagar finds herself undergoes a reversal the moment God's angel calls to her from the sky, saying, 'What troubles you, Hagar? *Fear not* (אל־תיראי); for God has heard the voice of the lad where he is' (21.17).[53] In this way Hagar's immediate problem of the child's crying is resolved.

Afterwards, in the resolution, Hagar's remaining problems find their solutions, one after the other. The turnabout occurs at a single point, located in one verse only, whereas the resolution is complex and longer. One of the problems that is resolved is the lack of water, about which is written: 'Then God *opened her eyes, and she saw* a well of water; and she went, and filled the skin with water, and gave the lad a drink' (21.19). Lexemes from the SF are prominent here by virtue of their close appearance one after the other: 'eyes' and 'saw'.

To sum up, there is a large accumulation of Sight terms in this pericope, many of which belong to the nearby CPF. This accumulation strengthens cohesion and coherence between the first passage about the birth of Isaac, and the second which deals with Hagar's banishment. As to the meaning of the story in terms of the theme of Sight, once again an act of seeing triggers the development of events (Sarah's seeing causes Hagar's banishment). Also to be noted is that God makes Hagar open her eyes to see a well of water, and by this her life and Ishmael's are saved. Only here and in the story of the Garden of Eden are the eyes of humans opened, affording access to a new kind of reality.

3.2.6. *Abraham and Sarah Go Down to Egypt: Genesis 12.10-20*

In the first of the three wife–sister stories (Gen. 12.10-20; chs. 20; 26) Abraham and Sarah go down to Egypt because of the severe famine in the land of Canaan (Gen. 12.10). The chain of events begins with Abraham saying to Sarah: 'I *know* (ידעתי) that you are a woman *beautiful to behold* (יפת־מראה); and when the Egyptians *see* (יראו) you, they will say, "This is his wife"; then they will kill me, but they will let you live' (Gen. 12.11-12).

52. Skinner (*Genesis*, p. 323) and Westermann (*Genesis 12–36*, p. 337), based on the LXX, prefer to read וישׂא את־קולו ויבך ('the child lifted up his voice and wept'), rather than MT, ותשׂא את־קלה ותבך ('and she lifted up her voice and wept').

53. We should distinguish between the attitude of God towards Abraham and towards Hagar. In the turning point of Hagar's banishment, God says to Hagar 'Fear not; for God has heard…' (21.17), whereas, in the turning point in the Akedah, God says to Abraham 'for now I know that you fear God' (22.12). Attention to the use of the verb ירא (fear) in these two turning points informs us of the deep difference between these two characters, and in particular of the establishment of trust relationship between God and Abraham.

Sarah is described as being beautiful to behold, and the entire plot hinges upon this external feature of hers constituted of SF lexemes. Abraham's life is in danger because of her, and because of her, they are obliged to lie to the Egyptian king.

Verses 14 and 15 describe the arrival of Sarah and Abraham in Egypt and twice emphasize the matter of how Sarah is *seen* by the Egyptians; in v. 14 the Egyptians *see* (ויראו) that she is beautiful to behold, and in v. 15 Pharaoh's ministers *see* (ויראו) her, speak her praises to Pharaoh, and as a result she is taken into his house. Until this point, there is knowing, beauty, and seeing—all related to the SF. Because of the lie, Abraham receives property, and Pharaoh and his household are afflicted with adversity. From this point on lexemes of Oral Communication are dominant: '...because of Sarah' (על־דבר שרי), but literally 'because of Sarah's words/matter' (v. 17), 'So Pharaoh called' (ויקרא), 'and said' (ויאמר), 'Why did you not tell me' (לא־הגדת, v. 18), 'Why did you say' (אמרת, v. 19). And at the end, both Sight and Speech appear together—without lexemes from these fields, but by means of the presentative particle הנה (here, behold) and the imperative, v. 19: 'Now then, *here* (הנה) is your wife, take her, and be gone'.[54]

And at the end, again occurs a lexeme from the field of Oral Communication: 'And Pharaoh *gave* men *orders* concerning him' (ויצו, v. 20). Before v. 17 there are also lexemes from the field of Oral Communication: 'he said' (v. 11), 'they will say' (v. 12), 'Say' (the lie!, v. 13), 'they praised her to Pharaoh' (v. 15).

The story, then, concerns Oral Communication and Sight interwoven and appearing throughout the plot. Abraham asks Sarah to lie (= Oral Communication) in the matter of her connection to him because of her external beauty (= Sight). The SF and field of Oral Communication come together here, with the one serving to emphasize the other. Terms of Oral Communication highlight the lie that Abraham asks Sarah to tell Pharaoh, and the SF acts through the recurring motif of the beauty of the matriarch.

3.2.7. *The Destruction of Sodom and Gomorrah: Genesis 19*

The Sodom and Gomorrah narrative in Gen. 19.1-29 begins with what Lot saw in the evening: 'The two angels came to Sodom in the *evening* (בערב); and *Lot* was sitting in the gate of Sodom. When Lot *saw* them, he rose to meet them' (19.1), and it ends with what Abraham saw in the morning in vv. 27, 28: 'And Abraham went early in the *morning* (בבקר) to the place where he had stood before Yhwh; and *he looked* (וישקף) down toward Sodom and Gomorrah and toward all the land of the valley, and *beheld* (וירא), and lo, the smoke of the land went up like the smoke of a furnace'. This special

54. See Waltke and O'Connor, *Introduction*, §40.2.1. For a discussion on the uses of the word *hinneh*, see Berlin, *Poetics and Interpretation*, pp. 91-95.

structure of the characters' seeing at the beginning and at the end of the story emphasizes the dominant presence of the SF in the chapter.[55] Also, the evening, during which visibility is limited, is used here as a metaphor for partial consciousness connected with Lot, and an enlightened and clear awareness in connection with Abraham at this stage, since in the previous chapter (Gen. 18.1), the angels come to him 'in the heat of the day', when the sun is forcefully shining, and conditions of visibility are good.[56] To strengthen the tie between God and Abraham there is also the final half-verse which clarifies the situation more explicitly: 'God *remembered* (ויזכר) Abraham, and sent Lot out of the midst of the overthrow…' (19.29). I am taking 'remember' here as a term from the CPF and close to Sight.

Another special element in this narrative is the use of a wide spectrum of lexemes from the SF, while exploiting a wide range of their meanings. In this chapter cases of visual perception are mentioned, using the verbs ראה (vv. 1, 28), השקיף (v. 28), and הביט (v. 26), as well as the visual blindness that strikes the people of Sodom (סנורים, v. 11). The verb הביט (look) appears in Genesis only here and in the story of the Promise and Covenant (Gen. 15.5). The word סנורים is found only here, and outside Genesis it appears in 2 Kgs 6.18. The rare appearance of the form underscores its significance. The lexeme ידע (knew) belongs to the CPF, and occurs in vv. 5 and 8 in the sense of sexual intimacy. Immediately following this story, in the narrative about Lot's daughters, there is a repeated use of the verb ידע (knew), in the sense of a cognitive state, alongside the verb שכב (lay with), in the sense of sexual coupling—a fact that serves to emphasize the importance of ידע throughout the chapter.

In regard to the appearance of the lexemes at key points in the narrative, it may be observed that the people of Sodom are struck by *blindness* (סנורים) at the turning point, and another lexeme from the SF occurs nearby: 'they

55. Weston Fields sees the times of the day in this episode as a secondary motif, with special emphasis being placed on the night as the time of day presaging danger. The night, in which darkness prevails, is the time that symbolizes an uncertainty and a transition between two clear points of light. It can be compared to the physical passage during a journey between two geographical points, as is illustrated in the Bridegroom of Blood narrative (Exod. 4.24) and in the story of Jacob's Struggle with the Deity (Gen. 32.34). The night as a motif symbolizing danger is especially prominent in three episodes that Fields analyzes: the Sodom and Gomorrah narrative (Gen. 19), the Gibeah Outrage (Judg. 19–21), and the story of the arrival of the spies to Jericho (Josh. 2) (Weston Fields, *Sodom and Gomorrah: History and Motif in Biblical Narrative* [JSOTSup, 231; Sheffield: Sheffield Academic Press, 1997], pp. 103-15).

56. Though David Kimhi comments that this mention of Abraham sitting in the heat may hint that Abraham had experienced a direct revelation of God due to a slight dehydration and a rather unfocused state of mind, which was caused by the heating sun (*Rabbi David Kimhi's Commentary on Genesis*, in Menahem Cohen [ed.], *Mikra'ot Gedolot 'HaKeter'* [Ramath Gan: Bar-Ilan University Press, 1997 [Hebrew]).

wearied themselves *groping for* (למצא) the door' (19.11). This is a Story of Blindness—opposite to Narratives of Insight (see §1.4.3). While the blindness is physical, the degree of awareness of the people of Sodom is also expressed, since they are blind in the aspect of seeing God. In view of the disagreement between Abraham and God about the number of virtuous people in the city, it is clear that in God's view, the inhabitants of Sodom are not righteous.

Furthermore, the complication is involved with the SF, again from the negative standpoint, contrary to the act of seeing, by means of the verb ידע (know). The sin of the people of Sodom is in their desire *to know* (ונדעה) Lot's guests *at night* (בלילה, 19.5). Lot refuses to hand over his guests to them, and offers, in their stead, his two virgin daughters: 'who have *not known* (לא ידעו) a man' (19.8). He proposes to the inhabitants of Sodom that they should 'do to them *as you please*' (כטוב בעיניכם, 19.8). These verses emphasize the lowest possible level of vision. Lexemes of perception connected to the field signify concrete rather than abstract perception, expressing the desire of the men of Sodom for negative carnal knowledge under conditions of faulty visibility (it all happens at night).

Throughout this narrative there are a number of idioms that also contain lexemes from the SF: 'your servant has found favour *in your sight*' (מצא עבדך חן בעיניך, v. 19), 'Behold, I grant you (פניך, literally: your face) this favour also' (v. 21, פנים, 'face', a lexeme related peripherally to the SF), and '*as you please*' (כטוב בעיניכם, v. 8) previously mentioned above, '*he seemed* to his sons-in-law to be jesting (כמצחק בעיני)' (v. 14).

A relatively diverse group of lexemes in this story, which are related to visual perception, belong to the categories of time and conditions of visibility: 'in the evening' (v. 1), 'tonight' (v. 5), 'morning dawned' (v. 15), 'the sun' (v. 23), 'early in the morning' (v. 27). As a peripheral lexeme, the word 'fire' is also linked to the SF (v. 24), since its semantic definition contains the feature of 'light'. Finally, the name of the central character, Lot, is connected to the SF because it may refer to the sense 'veil', 'hide'.

Altogether, lexemes from the SF appear at key positions in the plots of the individual stories in the Abraham narrative, with various rhetorical devices from the planes of sound, semantics, and style enhancing their effect. We have seen that in the matter of the levels of sight, God comprehends that the main character, Abraham, believes in him. We have also seen God guiding Abraham and Hagar's seeing (ch. 21). In most cases this part does not include an explicit statement regarding the belief of Abraham and of Hagar in God; we usually become aware of the fact of their belief from God's recognition, not the characters'. Only in one story, at the conclusion of the account concerning Hagar's banishment, does the human character arrive at a high level of sight. This is understood from Hagar's own words: '"You are a *God of seeing*", for she said, "Have I really *seen* God and remained alive after *seeing* him?"' (16.13). Here we witness Hagar's clear recognition of having seen God or of her ability to still see after she has seen him. In any case, from what is said, we understand that she is aware that she has seen the angel of God, and recognizes his power. Other characters, such as the people of Sodom, and Lot's wife, are characterized by the lowest level of sight, even in its negative concrete, physical sense. Human beings behave cruelly towards each other, and the SF is drawn upon in order to emphasize this idea.

3.3. *The Jacob Narrative*[57]

This chapter presents a survey of lexemes in the SF in the principal episodes from Jacob's life.

3.3.1. *Deceiving Isaac: Genesis 27*

Jacob's impersonation of Esau is central to Genesis 27, in which Jacob deceives Isaac and steals Esau's blessing. The act of hiding an identity belongs to the spheres both of visual and cognitive perception. In this story, however, matters connected with other senses—speech and hearing, touch, and even taste and smell—are prominent.

Rebekah's plot is mentioned at the opening of the chapter: 'Now it came to pass, when Isaac was old and his *eyes were so dim that he could not see*' (27.1). This is not only a sight-connected rhetorical device that helps to create coherence between the episodes, but also a critical detail for the success of the deception described afterwards. Rebekah and Jacob succeed in their trickery because Isaac's sight was not as clear as before. In addition we encounter a state of lack of knowledge: 'Then he said, "Behold, I am old. I *do not know* (לא ידעתי) the day of my death"' (v. 2).

All the other senses mentioned repeatedly in the narrative seem to serve as if it were a compensation for Isaac's inability to see. Isaac sends Esau to prepare him savoury food, in Hebrew מטעמים, a lexeme based on the root טעם (taste, 27.4).[58] The tasty food is mentioned several times: when Rebekah tells Jacob what she has overheard (v. 7), when she orders Jacob to bring her two goodly kids to prepare savoury food for Isaac (v. 9), and also in vv. 14 and 17.

Rebekah tells Jacob to bring her a goat from the flock so she could prepare his father's favourite dish. She has overheard the conversation between Isaac and Esau and learned that Isaac is expecting Esau to bring

57. On the dominant semantic fields in the Jacob Narrative, see Talia Sutskover, 'Lexical Fields and Coherence in the Jacob Narrative', in Brenner and Polak (eds.), *Performing Memory*, pp. 126-39.

58. *HALOT*, p. 377.

him game, so that he would bless Esau before his death. Jacob twice shows his deep understanding of human nature: just as he knew that the red stew would tempt his brother, he now understands his father's nature. Jacob assumes that it would not be simple to carry off the scheme, since he suspects his father would probably want to feel him. Since Esau is hairy and he himself is smooth-skinned, he fears his father would know the difference. This is exactly what happens. Jacob is right. Isaac does ask to feel his son. The lexemes שׂעיר (hairy) and חלק (smooth, v. 11) belong both to the field of the sense of touch and to that of outward appearances, since both attributes relate to sense perception, that is to say, visibility and tactility. Verse 12 reads: 'Perhaps my father will *feel* me, and *I shall seem to be a deceiver to him*; and I shall bring a *curse* on myself and not a *blessing*'. Different fields—that of the sense of touch, the fields of Visual and Cognitive Perception, and the field of Oral Communication ('curse' and 'blessing')—are intermingled in this verse. These spheres come together again in vv. 22-25: 'So Jacob went near to Isaac his father, and he *felt* him and *said*, "The *voice* is Jacob's *voice*, but the *hands* are the *hands* of Esau". And he *did not recognize* (הכירו) him, because his *hands* were *hairy* like his brother Esau's *hands*; so he *blessed* him... He said, "I will *eat*...so that my soul may *bless* you...and he brought him *wine*, and he *drank*".'

Hereafter the sense of smell is intertwined with sight and speech: 'He said, "See, the smell of my son is like the smell of a field which Yhwh has blessed"' (v. 27).

While Isaac focuses on touch and taste, Rebekah's actions are dominated by lexemes from the field of Oral Communication. Rebekah 'overhears' (ורבקה שׁמעת בדבר יצחק) Isaac's request from Esau, and orders Jacob to 'obey my word as I command you' (שׁמע בקלי לאשׁר אני מצוה אתך, 27.8). When Jacob reveals his worry that his father will feel him and understand his deceit, she is willing to take the curse on her (27.13) and presses him to *listen* to her and *obey*.[59]

Apart from sight, all Isaac's other senses are highly alert, that is, he feels, touches, tastes, smells, and hears. When Jacob enters Isaac's room wearing the hairy mantle Rebekah has prepared for him, Isaac asks to feel him: גשׁה־נא ואמשׁך בני... (27.21). While feeling his son he declares: הקל קול יעקב והידים ידי עשׂו ('The voice is Jacob's voice, but the hands are the hands of Esau', 27.22). The voice is the instrument of speaking, and the hands the instrument of touching. Here the fields of Oral Communication and Touch intertwine at a high point of the plot, calling attention to the objects which

59. *Gen. R.* 65.15 tells that Jacob brought the two kids his mother had requested (Gen. 27.14) 'under constraint, bowed down, and weeping' (H. Freedman and Maurice Simon [trans. and ed.], *Midrash Rabbah* [London: Soncino Press, 1939]). Hence, the Midrash stresses Rebekah's commanding tone.

the characters focus on, and the way they perceive them. This leads to a better understanding of the characters' personality and motivations.[60]

Apart from taste and touch, Isaac's sense of smell is activated as well. After Isaac eats and drinks he asks Jacob to get closer to him, so that they can kiss (27.26-27). At this stage Isaac senses the smell of the field coming out of Jacob's garments, as prepared by his mother: וירח את־ריח בגדיו ויברכהו ויאמר ראה ריח בני כריח שדה... (27.27). Then Jacob receives Esau's blessing.

In keeping with Isaac's failing eyesight, his perceptive abilities are described as negative. In the beginning of the episode Isaac does not know the day of his death (לא ידעתי, 27.2), and as the story unfolds he does not recognize Jacob (ולא הכירו, 27.23). In this description of Isaac in his old age, neither visual nor mental perception is as sharp and effective as his other senses. This will stand in opposition to Jacob's developing sense of sight in the broader sense, but at this stage of the plot the son is still not active in this area. At the end of this scene Rebekah orders Jacob to run away from Esau and go to her brother Laban in Haran (27.42-43). The personal name Laban resembles the Hebrew designation for the colour white. If metaphorically interpreted, the colour 'white' often represents a pure and sinless state in the Hebrew Bible (Isa. 1.18; Ps. 51.9; Job 9.30); hence an allusion may be made to the Hebrew sense of the name 'Laban' as 'white' in this context.[61] This interpretation could be connected with the notion that Jacob is sent to Laban to repent and purify himself of his sins.

3.3.2. *The Dream of the Ladder: Genesis 28.10-22*

The story of Jacob's dream[62] is delimited by details concerning place and time of day, and these are meaningful for the Sight factor. The lexemes 'stayed for the night' (וילן) and 'sun' (שמש; 28.11) are meaningful for our field since 'light' (or lack of it, in the case of וילן), the necessary condition

60. Polak analyzes the contrastive semantic fields of motion-towards and motion-away-from and revelation via vision vs. auditory revelation in the Narrative of the Burning Bush (Exod. 3.1-6). Polak concludes that this intertwining of semantic fields in a narrative calls the attention of the reader to their contrastive meanings and roles (Polak, *Biblical Narrative*, pp. 102-104).

61. Heard also makes this connection when titling his discussion about Laban 'White Lies', and about Esau 'Seeing Red' (Christopher R. Heard, *Dynamics of Diselection: Ambiguity in Genesis 12–36 and Ethnic Boundaries in Post-Exilic Judah* [Atlanta: Society of Biblical Literature, 2001]).

62. Many commentators opine that the story of Jacob's dream extends from v. 10 to v. 22 (Skinner, *Genesis*, p. 375; von Rad, *Genesis*, p. 277; Wenham, *Genesis*, p. 217). Wenham claims that the story begins in v. 10, in which succinct details of Jacob's journey are given. The function of this verse is also to connect the story with matters which appear before and after it: ch. 27, which deals with the theft of the blessing and Jacob's necessity to flee to Haran; and ch. 29, which describes the meeting with Rachel in the land of the sons of Kedem.

for sight, is a constituent in their basic meaning. According to Fokkelman, this nocturnal episode is part of a general motif of nocturnal revelations which characterizes the Jacob stories: the revelation described here, in Bethel, marks Jacob's flight, whereas the nocturnal revelation in Penuel marks his return.[63] 'Then he dreamed, and behold…' (v. 12) comes immediately after the indication of time. As noted in the Introduction, the lexeme ויחלם ('dream'), which describes the channel through which God reveals himself to Jacob, belongs to the SF, thus connecting the episode to the overall sight theme. Also, this is the first explicit information about Jacob's engagement in the act of seeing, which is positioned, as we can see, at the moment of his leaving home. The scene continues to describe how Jacob dreams about a ladder set on earth with its top reaching to the sky and God's messengers ascending and descending it, while God himself stands above the ladder and blesses Jacob (28.12-15).

When Jacob wakes from his dream he understands something which he had not understood previously. The narrator expresses his new-found insight in lexemes from the SF: 'Then Jacob awoke (וייקץ) from his sleep (משנתו) and said, "Surely Yhwh is in this place, and I did not know it (ידעתי)"'. And he was afraid (ויירא) and said, "How awesome (נורא) is this place! This is none other than the house of God, and this is the gate of heaven!"' (vv. 16, 17). According to Fokkelman, the narrator is describing a psychological insight; as he knows that people often attain significant insights when they awaken from sleep.[64] From our point of view this is the turning-point of the plot, which tells of Jacob's cognizance of the fear of God. Like the stories of the Garden of Eden, the sacrifice of Isaac, and perhaps also the stories of Hagar, we may speak of a Narrative of Insight (see §1.4.3).

After this comes the denouement, in the course of which Jacob takes the stone on which he had laid his head, pours oil on it, changes the name of the place from Luz to Bethel, and makes a vow (vv. 18-20). All this is done in the morning as Jacob awakes (v. 18). 'Morning' and 'awakening' are SF terms.

The SF in this story explicitly shows Jacob's cognizance of God. Jacob sees God in a dream and acknowledges his presence when he wakes up, therefore he may be said to experience a high level of sight. From this point onwards Jacob fears God. Hence, Jacob has come to a very close relationship with God, but has yet to develop his ability to perceive visually and cognitively in the human sphere, that is, with his family members.

63. Fokkelman, *Narrative Art in Genesis*, p. 48.

64. Fokkelman, *Narrative Art in Genesis*, p. 62. Fokkelman believes that the themes of place and time unite Genesis as a whole. He claims that the motif of place is specially emphasized in this story. Jacob's dream appears in the opening with the seemingly neutral word 'place' (28.11), but as the narrative develops the place turns out to be 'the gate to Heaven' (v. 17), which is later called Bethel (the house of God; v. 19).

3.3.3. *Mahanaim: Genesis 32.2-3*

The story of Jacob's encounter with the angels of God in Gen. 32.2-3 is particularly short. Though it consists of only two verses it still includes a verb of Sight. The verb ראם (he saw them) occurs in v. 3, and the sound plays of the verse emphasize this occurrence: ויאמר יעקב כאשׁר רָאָם מחנה אלהים זה ויקרא שׁם־המקום ההוא מחנים ('When Jacob saw them, he said, "This is God's army". So he called the name of that place Mahanaim'). In this clause the letters *resh* and *mem*, which are also the constituents of ראם, are frequently repeated. If the story begins in the previous verse, at 31.55, the sounds of the *mem* in the word למקמו (to his place), and the word בבקר (in the morning), which belongs to the SF and in which the letter *resh* appears, strengthen our analysis of a prominent occurrence of the verb of sight.

Thus, though this might look like an insignificant side happening, it is not in fact so. The stylistic design de-familiarizes the verb of sight, and thereby Jacob's seeing the camp of God is emphasized, and his awareness proclaimed. The reader is called to attribute special significance to this event in the framework of the general development of the theme of sight in this section; thus we have to acknowledge that Jacob experiences a high level of sight, which is in other words seeing God and admitting it.

3.3.4. *Jacob's Encounter with the Divine Being at Penuel: Genesis 32.22-32*

Jacob gets up in the *night*, pulls his wives, maidservants and sons together, and takes them across the ford of Jabbok (32.22-23). After he has taken them all across he is left alone, and at the stage of the complication there is a description of how a 'man' comes to wrestle with him until *daybreak* (32.25). In this important incident in Jacob's life, in which his name is changed, the senses are again commingled, just as they were in the narrative of Isaac's deception in Genesis 27. At the turning-point we are told that the man of God *sees* (וירא) that he cannot prevail against Jacob (32.25), and injures Jacob's thigh by touching it. Sight is combined with touch.

Their wrestling takes place at *night*, the time when there is no light, when conditions for seeing are poor, and continues until daybreak (עד עלות השׁחר, 32.24, 26). Jacob names the place of the wrestling Peniel, explaining: 'For I have *seen* God *face to face*, and yet my life is preserved' (32.30). Jacob admits that he has seen God. In this instance God's face is mentioned, whereas previously it was the sight of Laban's face (31.1); and later, the sight of his son Joseph's face will be mentioned several times (e.g. 46.30; 48.11).[65]

65. On the phrase 'to see the face', see further discussion in §4.7.

Moreover, this episode opens at *night*, and closes with sunrise (32.31). The lexeme שמש (sun) belongs to the SF, and so does the name of the place: Penuel (v. 31). Hence, conditions for sight, depicted by SF words, define this tale's boundaries, and the place name explained by SF lexemes underlines the theme of the unit—Jacob's recognition of having seen God face to face. In this episode Jacob attains a high level of seeing—the sight of God and the recognition of it—and he is unharmed.

3.3.5. *List of the Descendants of Ishmael: Genesis 25*

The genealogy in Genesis 25 is not without lexemes from the SF. Verse 9 tells that Abraham was buried 'before Mamre', and v. 11 that after his death Isaac lived in Beer Lahai Roi (באר לחי ראי), which is related to the SF since it contains the verb 'see'. At the end of the genealogy of the sons of Ishmael it is said that they dwelt 'from Havilah to Shur, which is opposite Egypt in the direction of Assyria, he settled over against all his people' (25.18). The place name Shur belongs to the SF, and the name Ashur is linked to it by assonance. Thus, these genealogies have points of contact with the SF, and they are linked to the overall theme of sight by means of cohesive elements.

3.4. *The Joseph Narrative*

In many of the individual stories which compose the Joseph Narrative, lexemes from the SF are consistently intertwined at key points with lexemes from the field of Oral Communication, and together they function to stress the deep meaning of the narrative. The recurrence of dreams has been noted as a central motif in this narrative, and its contribution to the construction of the main theme has been discussed.[66] Significantly, 'dream' is also a term from the SF (§§2.3.1.3-4). The following discussion focuses on four chapters in the Joseph Narrative, which were chosen because of their key positions in the macro-plot of the Joseph Narrative as a whole, or because of an interesting deployment of SF terms in them. In each of these chapters terms from the SF alone, or together with terms from the field of Oral Communion, consistently appear at turning points. These chapters are (1) ch. 37, which is the opening of the Joseph Narrative; (2) the story of Judah and Tamar (ch. 38), which is sometimes regarded as secondary in the Joseph Narrative; (3) the story of Joseph and Potiphar's wife (ch. 39); (4) and the climactic point of the renewed encounter between Joseph and his brothers (ch. 45). Other key episodes in this narrative are discussed in §4.8, which deals with the coherence of the Joseph Narrative as a whole.

66. See, for instance, D.B. Redford, *A Study of the Biblical Story of Joseph* (VTSup, 20; Leiden: E.J. Brill, 1970), pp. 89-91.

3.4.1. *The Selling of Joseph: Genesis 37*

As will be shown, key points of the plot of Genesis 37 are consistently constructed with the use of lexemes from the semantic fields of Sight and Oral Communication.[67] To begin with, the complication of the plot of ch. 37, that is, the growing hatred of Joseph's brothers toward him, starts off with an issue from the field of Oral Communication. The first reason for their hatred is that Joseph brings unfavourable *reports* about them to their father, in Hebrew: ויבא יוסף את־דבתם רעה אל־אביהם (37.2). But it was not enough that Joseph maligned his brothers. Another problem was that Jacob loved Joseph, and gave him a robe (כתנת פסים, 37.3). The robe itself, which is mentioned several times in this story and which is perceived by some commentators as one of the main motifs in it,[68] is related to the SF, since it functions as a visual identifier of its owner, Joseph (see §2.5.5).[69] Moreover, identification is an act of mental perception, which is part of the SF in the broad sense.

The narrator continues, 37.4: 'But when his brothers *saw* (ויראו) that their father loved him more than all his brothers, they hated him, and could not *speak* peaceably to him (ולא יכלו דברו)'. What we have here is the narrator's evaluation of the brothers' hatred for Joseph, that is, the strategic point of the marking of the main problem in the narrative, expressed in terms of Sight and Oral Communication.[70]

Shortly after this comment, the narrator describes Joseph dreaming the two symbolic dreams of the ears and the luminaries (§2.8.3). Joseph's dreams, which predict that in the future he will be elevated above his brothers and parents, are an important element in the life of Joseph and the development of the plot of his story.[71] Both the verb 'to dream' (חלם) and

67. T. Sutskover, 'The Semantic Fields of Seeing and Oral Communication in the Joseph Narrative', *JNSL* 33.2 (2007), pp. 33-50.

68. Westermann, *Genesis 37–50*, pp. 66-67; Matthews, 'The Anthropology of Clothing', pp. 28-31.

69. Matthews notes: 'on the symbolic level, clothing always serves as a means of visual communication' (Matthews, 'The Anthropology of Clothing', p. 25).

70. White remarks: 'With this the narrator points to the central problem with which the narrative will be occupied until it is initially resolved..., i.e., the problem of communication between Joseph and his brothers'. When White cites v. 4 he stresses the verb 'saw'. Thus, he recognizes its importance but does not include sight as part of the overall theme of the story (H.C. White, 'Reuben and Judah: Duplicates or Complements?', in J.T. Butler, E.W. Conrad and B.C. Ollenburger (eds.), *Understanding the Word: Essays in Honor of Bernhard W. Anderson* [JSOTSup, 37; Sheffield: JSOT Press, 1985], pp. 73-97 [86]).

71. Amit speaks of the paired dreams in the Joseph Narrative—the two dreams of Joseph, of Pharaoh and of Pharaoh's servants—as part of a more general poetic principle. The narrator of the Joseph Narrative has made frequent use of repeated events, such are the paired dreams, two attempts of two brothers to save him instead of the original plan to

the noun 'dream' (חלום), which appear frequently in this chapter, are included in the SF, since the perception of images by the brain is involved in the act of dreaming. But it is not only these lexemes which are prominent here; both the contents of the dreams and the way Joseph acts after dreaming them are of great importance, from the point of view of the intertwining of the two fields under discussion.

Joseph *tells* his brothers about the dreams, an act which deepens their hatred toward him (v. 5). The recounting of the dreams to the brothers opens with Joseph's own words, which are connected to the fields of Sight and Oral communication: 'He *said* to them, "*Hear* this *dream* which I have *dreamed*"' (v. 6). Moreover, these dreams also include symbols that echo both fields in question. In each of these two verses (vv. 5, 6) the root חלם (to dream) occurs twice, and in each of them it is said that he *told* his dreams to his brothers.

In the first dream Joseph pictures his sheaf rising and standing upright. The brothers' sheaves gather around Joseph's and bow down to it. The Hebrew word for 'sheaf' is אלומה, but the root אלם has another meaning as well—dumbness (*HALOT*, p. 57); thus it may be considered to belong to the field of Oral Communication, or at least evoking it. This meaning is illustrated by other verses in which the root אלם appears, such as in Isa. 53.7: 'He was oppressed, and he was afflicted, yet he did not open his mouth; like a lamb that is led to the slaughter, and like a sheep that before its shearers is silent (נאלמה), so he did not open his mouth'; and Ezek. 3.26: 'And I will make your tongue cling to the roof of your mouth, so that you shall be dumb (ונאלמת) and unable to reprove them; for they are a rebellious house'. It is striking to note the irony of Joseph alluding to himself as a sheaf when these passages show that the root אלם can also be used in reference to a dumb lamb led to slaughter.

The first dream concludes with the following statement by the narrator, which explicitly connects seeing and speaking as reasons for the brothers' hatred: 'So they hated him yet more for his *dreams* and for his *words*' (37.8). This verse and v. 6 mentioned above are clear illustrations for the close combination of two different semantic fields.

Joseph's second dream, like the first one, is introduced by the statement that he had dreamed a dream and recounted it to his brothers (v. 9, which is similar to v. 5). The pattern of the double occurrence of the root חלם is repeated, this time as a verb and a noun, 'And he *dreamed* yet another *dream*' (v. 9), when the problem is Joseph's words, 'And he *told* it to his

kill him, two selling occasions of Joseph, two journeys of the brothers to Egypt (Yairah Amit, 'Repeated Situation—A Poetic Principle in the Modeling of the Joseph Narrative', in *In Praise of Editing in the Hebrew Bible: Collected Essays in Retrospect* [trans. Betty Sigler Rozen; Sheffield: Sheffield Phoenix Press, 2012], pp. 70-83).

brothers', and again חלם twice: 'Look, I have *dreamed* another *dream*. And this time, the *sun*, the *moon*, and the eleven *stars* bowed down to me' (v. 9).[72] The semantic definition of these heavenly bodies includes the feature 'light', and since light is a necessary condition for seeing, they are also included in the SF as indicators of time. Again we can see how the symbols that appear in the dreams are connected to the fields of Sight and Oral Communication.

Jacob reacts to these dreams in a verbal response, in which the idea of verbal discourse is prominent: 'So he *told* (ויספר) it to his father and his brothers; and his father *rebuked* (ויגער) him and *said* (ויאמר) to him, "What is this *dream* (החלום) that you have *dreamed* (חלמת)? Shall your mother and I...indeed come (הבוא נבוא)..."' (v. 10). The root חלם again appears twice, in Jacob's reply as well. The fact that בוא also appears twice, together with the special construct of an infinite absolute and the imperfect, highlights the entire saying.

In the opening of the next scene (vv. 12-17) Jacob sends Joseph to inquire after his brothers using lexemes from the fields of Sight and Oral Communication: 'Go now, *see* (ראה) if it is well with your brothers and well with the flock; and bring me *word* again (והשׁבני דבר)' (v. 14). A man finds Joseph wandering in the field and asks him: 'What are you *seeking*'? (v. 15). The Hebrew verb used to express the idea of seeking is תבקשׁ, which makes another contribution to the variety of terms of sight.[73] This verb is repeated in Joseph's answer, in addition to another verb of Oral Communication, הגידה־נא (tell me, 37.16). In this short interlude of vv. 12-17 Sight and Oral Communication continue to exert their influence on the level of verbal texture and on the level of plot-development.

The brothers see Joseph from afar, and call him, among themselves, 'this *dreamer*' (v. 19). The brothers want to kill him, to throw him into a pit and lie about it: 'We shall *say*, "Some wild beast has devoured him". We shall *see* what will become of his *dreams*!' (v. 20). Speech in this verse means deception, and in any case the fields of Oral Communication and Sight meet here. The brothers take Joseph's tunic off (ויפשׁיטו את־יוסף את־כתנתו את כתנת הפסים אשׁר עליו, v. 23) and throw him into the pit (v. 24). Sight is emphasized in the formulaic phrase: 'Then they *lifted their eyes and looked*, and there was a company of Ishmaelites' (v. 25).

Genesis 37.18-30 mentions a few proper names that consist of terms from the semantic fields of Sight and Oral Communication. The occurrence of

72. On repetitions in the Joseph Narrative, see Amit 'Repeated Situation'.

73. The Hebrew term תבקשׁ may also connect to the field of Oral Communication, since in some places it has the meaning of 'to demand', and in others 'to require' or 'to request' (*HALOT*, p. 152). This could be a special case in which the SF and the field of Oral Communication intersect in one and the same lexeme.

words of the dominant semantic fields as constituents in names of characters is a special phenomenon that serves to highlight the role of these fields in the text. The name of the eldest brother, Reuben, includes the verb ראה (see) and thus relates to the SF. Reuben tries to prevent the conniving plan of the brothers to murder Joseph, suggesting that they throw him into a pit without killing him first, so that he (Reuben) could later save him and return him to their father: וישמע ראובן ויצלהו מידם... (vv. 21-22). Thus, Reuben's role must not be minimized; it is Reuben who saves Joseph.[74] In the following verses, Judah indeed makes the suggestion to refrain from killing Joseph and, instead, to sell him to the Ishmaelites. A close reading shows that he makes this proposal when he *sees* the caravan approaching, and after Reuben has already been assured that the lad has been put in the pit without first having been killed by his brothers. The name Judah can be related to the field of Oral Communication, since it has graphic and sound resemblances to the root ידה (give thanks, praise; see also 49.8). The contrasting roles of these two brothers in the episode of vv. 18-30 are part and parcel of the framework of the narrative, which stresses Sight, Insight and Oral Communication throughout. Details, such as these roles, which were often thought to be duplications and contradictions, may also be considered as integral parts of the plot.[75] In my view, and along with such scholars as Wenham, White, and Longacre,[76] the role of these two figures may be explained in terms other than those of source criticism, and may be seen as part of a coherent, unified discourse. Hence, the proper names Judah and Reuben stress the presence of the fields of Sight and Oral Communication in the text, and draw attention to the thematic meaning connected to them. Metaphorically speaking, we may conclude that, as regards Reuben, Sight and Speech are used positively, but with respect to Judah and the other brothers, oral communication and visual perception are both used in a negative manner.

By the same token, the names of the peoples involved in the two acts of selling Joseph to Egypt should be noted—Ishmaelites and Midianites. These names, as stated by Redford,[77] were used for generations to demonstrate the validity of source criticism. It may be suggested, however, that these names fit the paradigm of the dominant semantic fields in the following manner: the

74. R. Pirson, *The Lord of the Dreams: A Semantic and Literary Analysis of Genesis 37–50* (JSOTSup, 355; London: Sheffield Academic Press, 2002), p. 62. But compare J.P. Fokkelman, 'Genesis 37 and 38 at the Interface of Structural Analysis and Hermeneutic', in L.J. de Regt *et al.* (eds.), *Literary Structure and Rhetorical Strategies in the Hebrew Bible* (Assen: Van Gorcum, 1996), pp. 152-87 (161).

75. Skinner, *Genesis*, pp. 446-47; S.E. Loewenstamm, 'Reuben and Judah in the Cycle of Joseph-Stories', in Loewenstamm, *From Babylon to Canaan: Studies in the Bible and Its Oriental Background* (Jerusalem: Magnes Press, 1992), pp. 35-41.

76. Wenham, *Genesis 16–50*, p. 350; White, 'Reuben and Judah'; Longacre, *Joseph*.

77. Redford, *A Study of the Biblical Story of Joseph*, p. 145.

designation 'Ishmaelites' is connected to the Hebrew verb שׁמע (hear), and 'Midianites' (v. 28) to the Hebrew verb דין (contention). Judah's words '*Let us conceal* (וכסינו) his blood' (v. 26) contain a lexeme from the SF (v. 26). The brothers *hear* (וישׁמעו) Judah's words (v. 27, 'And his brothers heeded him').

The variety of proper names connected to Sight and Oral Communication in this episode stresses the centrality of these fields to understanding the main theme. Now that Joseph is sold to Egypt he is out of sight, and there is no oral communication between him and his brothers. The divine aspect should also be noted: God is not mentioned anywhere in this scene and therefore he may be considered as being absent from the characters' cognition.

The first chapter of the Joseph story ends with Jacob staring at the blood-stained robe, recognizing it as belonging to Joseph, and at the end refusing to stop mourning for his son (vv. 31-35). This scene is constructed by recurring lexemes connected to the SF: the robe, which is mentioned five times, and the recognizing of the robe, which is mentioned twice (הכר־נא, ויכירה).[78] The verb 'to find' (זאת מצאנו), which involves seeing and thus belongs to the SF, is mentioned once, in v. 32. Jacob mourns for his son, and his children rise up to *comfort* him (vv. 34, 35). Jacob *weeps* (ויבך) for Joseph (v. 35). The story ends with these lexemes from the field of Oral Communication.

The concluding verse (v. 36) is particularly significant, since the Midianites are mentioned again, but with a small variation in spelling: *Medanim* (מדנים) instead of *Midianim* (מדינים). This spelling emphasizes the sense of dispute, since *madon* means 'contention, strife', as shown by the phrase ריב ומדון, which appears in Jer. 15.10 and Hab. 1.3. This underscores the idea that the main problem presented in this chapter is a dispute in the family caused by Joseph's sight, that is, his dreams, and his talk about them to the brothers. As regards the field of Oral Communication, the brothers are accused of not speaking peaceably to him and plotting his murder. This negative talk eventually turns to years of complete silence between the parties. From the aspect of Sight, they are accused of putting him in the pit, and thus, by implication, causing his disappearance.

Another word concerning the classic view of Genesis 37, that is, its division into sources, is needed. Many scholars consider the story of Joseph to be derived from two sources—a Judaean source, and an Israelite source which is expressed in the allusions to the figure of Reuben.[79] In the analysis

78. According to Malul, Jacob is legally obliged to say that he recognizes the robe (Exod. 22.9-12); in other words, the verb הכיר (recognize) is legally binding (Malul, 'Law in the Narratives,' pp. 23-36).

79. According to Loewenstamm, there was an ancient tradition of the story in which only Reuben was mentioned. This old tradition was later dominated by the Judaean

presented here, however, the characters of Reuben and Judah are not derived from different sources, but represent the literary dialogue between two semantic fields: Reuben represents the field of Sight, and Judah the field of Oral Communication.

3.4.2. *The Story of Judah and Tamar: Genesis 38*

The Story of Judah and Tamar emphasizes that aspect of the SF that deals with cognitive perception. Faber and Wallhead, in their analysis of the Vision field in Fowles's novel *The French Lieutenant's Woman*, express the opinion that one of the functions of the field in this novel is a result of the focusing on one aspect in this field, in what they call: 'the VISION-Intellect metaphor, SEEING IS UNDERSTANDING'.[80] They claim that in this novel characters who see, understand, and have self-knowledge are the ones who command the twentieth-century reader's admiration, in contrast to those characters who have a distorted view of themselves or who are slaves to appearances. I think that the SF in the Judah and Tamar narrative (Gen. 38) acts in a similar way. The narrative of Judah and Tamar has often been analyzed as a secondary unit inserted into the Joseph Narrative,[81] but Clifford presents a different approach, perceiving it as an integral element of the surrounding narrative.[82] Clifford sums up many of the thematic and linguistic connections between Genesis 38 and the Joseph Narrative. For example, both Joseph and Judah 'went down' (ירד) from their brothers (38.1; 39.1), married foreign women, and played a role in deceptions involving a kid from the flock and an item of clothing (37.31-33; 38.15). Also, there is a verbal parallel, הכר־נא (recognize), which is in one case used by Tamar referring to Judah (38.25-26), and in another is used by the brothers addressing Jacob (37.32-33). Clifford suggests that this connects the two narratives, and, as I shall show below, it is also related to the theme of ch. 38 and the presentation of Judah's character. The notion of a persistent dominant presence of lexemes of the SF in key positions of this plot too may be considered as an additional argument in support of the literary approach already suggested by others.[83] I will now allude to some of the

tradition (Loewenstamm, 'Reuben and Judah', pp. 35-41). The current form of the story could also be explained as a result of the intervention of an implicit editor (Amit, 'The Repeated Situation', pp. 70-83). This implicit editor could have combined the two sources, and used the poetics of the semantic field to create a coherent text.

80. Faber and Wallhead, 'The Lexical Field of Visual Perception', pp. 127-44 (the capital letters appear in the original article).

81. Skinner, *Genesis*, p. 450; von Rad, *Genesis*, p. 351-52; Speiser, *Genesis*, p. 299.

82. R.J. Clifford, 'Genesis 38: Its Contribution to the Jacob Story', *CBQ* 66 (2004), pp. 519-32 (519).

83. Clifford, 'Genesis 38: Its Contribution to the Jacob Story'; U. Cassuto, 'The Story of Tamar and Judah', in Cassuto, *Biblical and Oriental Studies*. I. *Bible* (trans.

lexemes of the SF and CPF appearing at key positions and constructing the central theme of the story.

After a short exposition the story opens with Judah physically *seeing* (וירא) Shua's daughter (38.2), an act which leads to him marrying her. Judah's first son was called Er (ער), which is connected to the SF from the angle of the CPF, because the name can be interpreted as referring to a cognitive state of awakeness. Judah takes a wife, Tamar, for his first-born son, Er (38.6). Er does evil in the eyes of God and dies, and Judah gives his second son, Onan, to Tamar. Onan spills his semen on the ground, and God kills him, too. Now Judah is afraid that if he gives his daughter-in-law to his third son he, too, will die, so he sends her to her father's home. Much time passes, Judah's wife dies, and one day Judah goes up to Timnah with his friend (רעהו). A notable sound-play is the use of the phonemes *ayin* and *resh*. The sound-play emphasizes the states of cognition: Er (ער) was evil (רע) *in the eyes* (בעיני) of God (38.7). Onan did evil (וירע) *in the eyes* of God (38.10), and Judah went to Timnah with his friend (רעהו, 38.12). By not giving his third son to Tamar, Judah is infringing the law of levirate marriage.

Tamar disguises herself by putting on a veil and wrapping herself up (38.14), so that Judah would not recognize her. The veil (צעיף) and the covering up (ותכס) are connected to the SF, since the covering and the hiding stand in opposition to the act of exposing or creating conditions for seeing.[84] Tamar sits and waits for Judah at the entrance of Enaim, which can be either translated as 'eyes' or 'springs of water'. Stendebach asserts that עין in the sense of 'eye' has expanded its meaning to denote 'spring of water' due to the metaphorical resemblance between the spring on the face of the earth and the eye's location in the human face.[85] In Akkadian, as in Biblical Hebrew, the one and the same word, *īnu(m)*, denotes both of these meanings.[86] Thus, the covering, the scarf, the clothes, and the name Petah Enaim all belong to the SF.

The SF also appears in the episode of Judah having intercourse with Tamar, 'for he *did not know* (לא ידע) that she was his daughter-in-law' (v. 16). Eventually, Tamar's identity is made known to Judah as a result of his own identifying objects, which belong to the SF: 'Mark (הכר נא), I pray

I. Abrahams; Jerusalem: The Magnes Press, 1973 [first published in Hebrew in 1929]), pp. 29-40; R. Alter, *The Art of Biblical Narrative* (New York: Basic Books, 1981), pp. 5-12; Wenham, *Genesis 16–50*, pp. 363-64.

84. Balentine treats the semantic field of hiding separately (Balentine, *The Hidden God*). Another lexeme from the SF in v. 14 is 'for she saw (ראתה) that Shelah was grown up'.

85. F.J. Stendebach, 'עין', *TDOT*, XI, p. 44.

86. *CAD*, I–J, p. 153.

you, whose these are, the *signet* (החתמת) and the *cord* (והפתילים) and the *staff*' (והמטה, v. 25).

The turning point of the story comes after Tamar succeeds in her plot to conceive Judah's child without him being aware of her identity, at the moment when Judah realizes the truth: 'Then Judah *acknowledged* (RSV, ויכר, "recognized") them and said, "She is more righteous than I, inasmuch as I did not give her to my son Shelah". And he did not lie with her again (לדעתה)' (v. 26). This realization on the part of Judah comes after the narrator explicitly mentions his unawareness of what is done to him by Tamar (vv. 15, 16). Terms from the SF point to a theme, which is concerned with the cognitive state of the main character, Judah. Judah, who at first lacked insight, finally realizes that he was wrong in not giving his third son to Tamar. Thus, the phrase הכר־נא, also mentioned in the final episode of ch. 37 (37.32, see also the same root in 37.33), is an element in the SF which creates lexical cohesion between chs. 37 and 38 and at the same time is related to the central theme of the story of Judah and Tamar—as summarized in Pirson's words: 'the story shows how Tamar opens Judah's eyes and teaches him to take responsibility and secure his family's future'.[87]

The end of the last unit of the story is the emergence of the second infant from Tamar's womb—the infant who is called Zerah (זרח, stemming from the Hebrew root זרח, 'to shine'). This name can be thought of as symbolizing of the father's cognitive state: a state of lucidity and awareness.

Until this point we have seen the profusion of lexemes from the SF at critical points in the story of Judah and Tamar—at the beginning, at the turning-point, at the conclusion, and also in other parts of the plot. There are character names which are also connected with the SF: Er and Zerah, and, indirectly, Tamar, and perhaps also the place-name Timnah (see the discussion below). All these allude to Judah's cognitive state, which changes from ignorance and non-recognition to a state of understanding of his sin. The veil Tamar covers herself with as she dresses as a prostitute can also be interpreted as a metaphorical expression of Judah's cognitive state. Tamar's body is covered, and so is Judah's ability to perceive clearly. Words from the SF function on the symbolic level, or as Hasan put it, the words have a double function of significance—both at the straightforward level of meaning, and at the symbolic level (§1.3.2). Thus, when Tamar removes the concealing veil (v. 14), this hints at the turning point and the beginning of the process which will bring about Judah's moral awakening.[88]

87. Pirson, *The Lord of the Dreams*, p. 85

88. Clifford ('Genesis 38: Its Contribution to the Jacob Story') also points out the change in Judah's cognitive state, a change which enables him to behave morally towards Joseph in Egypt later on.

In relation to the cognitive states of the characters, it should be noted that the first two letters in the name Tamar (תמר)—*tav* and *mem*—can denote a cognitive state of perfection and pure intentions (תָם, תֹם). It is not insignificant that Judah was sent to a place called Timnah (תמנה), the first two consonants of which make up the word תֹם (innocence). This hints at the central theme of the story, having to do with the cognitive state of the main characters, especially that of Judah. Judah's cognitive state is about to change. And again, among his personal possessions, through which his identity is revealed, there is a seal (חותמת); in this word, too, the letters *tav* and *mem* appear.

Thus, in this story an assortment of SF lexemes occurs at strategic points. Many commentators, as mentioned above, consider this chapter as a secondary unit in its surroundings, since it interrupts the continuity of the account of Joseph's descent to Egypt, with Genesis 39 continuing the history of Joseph from ch. 37. This raises a question: How is it that, although the story is thought of having different origins, SF lexemes which it contains are uniquely distributed in it and contribute to its theme, as they do in its surroundings? In this case we may say that the author of this text unit or the implicit editor[89] of the story of Joseph used the poetics of the SF in order to adapt Genesis 38 to the Joseph Narrative as a whole, and to create by means of the SF, cohesion and coherence between this story and its surroundings. The deployment of the SF in this story, turns it into a unified whole with the rest of the Joseph Narratives, even though it is Judah rather than Joseph who takes the centre stage. Nonetheless, it is impossible to suggest a comprehensive rule that would explain whether a certain semantic field is introduced into the story by the author, or rather by the editor. Whether the lexemes of a certain semantic field belong to the stage of authorship or the editorial stage, or perhaps the combination of both, is a question to be considered *ad hoc*.[90]

89. Amit writes: 'The implied editor is thus the sum of the authors-editors and redactors of the work who were guided by the central unifying principle or who, despite their involvement, did not distort its sections or remove it from the guiding editing line which gives integrity to its various portions' (Yairah Amit, *The Book of Judges: The Art of Editing* [trans. Jonathan Chipman; Leiden: Brill, 1999], p. 16).

90. On this aspect we may draw conclusions about the semantic field from research about the leading word. On the appearance of the leading word in different stories, Buber says: 'But the correspondences are so exact, and fit so perfectly into the situation as a whole, that we have to accept the idea: that the roots of the "secret meaning" reach deep into the earlier layers of the tradition' (Buber, 'The Style of the Leading Word', p. 120). As a development of his work on the leading word, Amit broadens the discussion on the integration of a leading word in a literary work, and considers whether it is the work of an author or an editor. She distinguishes between the function of a 'key word', a term taken from literary criticism, and that of the leading word. When the leading word

3.4.3. *Joseph in Potiphar's House: Genesis 39*

The episodes of ch. 39 open with the narrator's statements of sight and insight; Joseph's success in Potiphar's house is introduced by the verb 'to see'. Genesis 39.3 reads, 'His master *saw* that Yhwh was with him', and v. 4 has, 'So Joseph found favour in his *sight*' (וימצא יוסף חן בעיניו).

The story of Joseph and Potiphar's wife also opens with SF terms. Joseph's external characteristics are described; he is said to be '*handsome and good-looking*' (יפה־תאר ויפה מראה, 39.6). These visual traits led Potiphar's wife to *cast* her *eyes* (ותשא... את־עיניה) on him, and ask him to lie with her (39.7). Her persistent and ongoing talk to Joseph is described in v. 10: 'And although she *spoke* to Joseph day after day, he would not *listen* to her...' The wife kept his *garment* (בגדו), an identifying sign (39.12-13), and relied on this evidence when she falsely accused Joseph of attempting to lie with her. The clothing motif appears here once again with its connection to the SF since it discloses the identity of its owner, as it does in the preceding scenes of Genesis 37 and 38.

The rest of this episode is very much connected to Oral Communication, since it is about the different versions of Potiphar's wife regarding the alleged attempt to rape her. In the account she gives to the servants of the house and to her husband she lies about her crying out for help (39.14, 18). When Potiphar himself *hears* (כשמע) from his wife about the incident, he puts Joseph in prison (39.19). The story ends with an act of seeing (or not seeing) on the part of the keeper of the prison. 'The keeper of the prison paid no heed (literally: "did not *see*", אין שר בית־הסהר ראה) to anything that was in Joseph's care, because Yhwh was with him' (39.23).

To conclude, this narrative includes lexemes of the SF and Oral Communication field at key points. This special deployment enhances the connection of the unit to the Joseph Narrative as a whole. As to the levels of Sight, we may say that Potiphar's wife is engaged in low-level sight since she sees Joseph in the physical sense. The keeper of the prison is also engaged in seeing what Joseph does in the more concrete sense. Moreover, paying attention to the fields under discussion leads to the understanding that this is the third narrative in succession in which certain characters behave violently towards others, including lying and deceiving. Joseph's brothers cannot speak peacefully to him, after he reveals his dreams. They

appears as a tool for connecting texts she calls this a connective-leading function, which may have originated with an author, a later adaptor, or an editor. When the leading word is found in a unit in which the interpretative tradition has not discovered levels of editing, it functions as a leading word. Here the author introduces words not only in order to strengthen the connections between the parts of the plot, but also in order to hint at a particular meaning. The word becomes a tool through which the reader discovers this meaning (Amit, 'The Multi-purpose "Leading Word"').

also plot to murder and sell him (ch. 37). Tamar dresses as a prostitute and deceives Judah, while Judah announces that Tamar should be taken out and burnt (ch. 38). Lastly, Potiphar's wife lies to Potiphar and to his servants about Joseph trying to rape her (ch. 39).

3.4.4. *Joseph's Reacquaintance with his Brothers: Genesis 45*

The story of Joseph reaches its solution when Joseph *makes himself known* (בהתודע) to his brothers (Gen. 45.1). At this climactic point, as at the beginning of the Joseph Narrative, the field of Oral Communication appears together with the SF. First Joseph weeps aloud, and all the Egyptians and the house of Pharaoh hear him. After this, in 45.12, he reveals himself, continuing to use terms from the SF combined with the field of Oral Communication: 'And now your *eyes see*, and the *eyes* (עיניכם ראות ועיני) of my brother Benjamin see, that it is my *mouth* that *speaks* (פי המדבר) to you'. 45.13 continues: 'You must tell (והגדתם) my father of all my splendour in Egypt, and of all that you have *seen* (ראיתם). Make haste and bring my father down here'.[91]

This chapter concludes with the brothers returning to their father in Canaan, and reporting on all that has happened to them. The narrator adds that Jacob *sees* the wagons full of the gifts which Joseph has sent with his brothers (45.27). Jacob's last request also uses the SF: 'And Israel *said*, "It is enough; Joseph my son is still alive; I will go and *see* (אראנו) him before I die"' (45.28).

From the point of view of the levels of sight, both this episode and other chapters in the Joseph Narrative are characterized by a human performance of visual perception. The turning point of the story centres on visual perception—the encounter in which the brothers see Joseph and he sees them. None of the characters sees God, but God is mentioned several times in Joseph's speech as working behind the scenes—for example in 45.5, 'for God sent me before you to preserve life', and similarly in vv. 7, 8, 9. As to Oral Communication, Joseph's crying aloud ends years of silence between Joseph and his brothers (excluding dialogues between the parties taking place when the brothers did not recognize him).

3.5. *Conclusion*

Up to this point I have examined the SF in individual stories. In some pericopes, such as that of the Joseph Narrative, the field of Oral Communication was also taken into account, because of its dominant role. The next

91. For Polliack's discussion on the reacquaintance between Joseph and his brothers, see §4.8 n. 67.

step will be to assemble key points from various stories in which the SF is prominent, link them together, and examine the overall pattern of the theme of sight in Genesis. My point of view will be more distant, that of the macro-plot of Genesis as a whole.

Chapter 4

THE THEME OF SIGHT UNIFIES THE SECTIONS OF GENESIS

In the previous chapter I showed how lexemes from the SF are distributed in key positions in selected individual narratives in Genesis, and how they are sometimes accompanied by patterns of sound plays which emphasize their presence. Similarly, I began to present a general description of how different levels of sight are expressed in these individual stories, and in two central contexts—divine sight and human sight.

The aim of this chapter is to show how the theme of sight contributes to the unity of Genesis as a whole. In some pericopes the SF is intertwined with the semantic field of Oral Communication, and they both play a significant role in the design of the central theme. Now I shall track the occurrences of lexemes from the SF at strategic points, from the perspective of the macro-plot of Genesis. The SF is now examined in its contribution not only to the inner coherence of the individual story, but also to the coherence of the book as a large entirety. Previously, in the analysis of the individual stories, it was shown that Genesis opens with God's seeing the world and his creatures, and that he aimed his sight on human behaviour. On the other hand, the story of Joseph, which comes at the end of Genesis, makes no mention of God's direct sight, but rather of divine activity behind the scenes. In the following sections I shall discuss the intermediate stages in this process of the reduction of God's explicit involvement in seeing humans, and shall examine how human sight develops.

Before discussing the theme of sight which contributes to the coherence of the book, I shall present a brief outline of modern interpretations which is divided into two main schools: those commentators who focus on dividing Genesis into its components, and those who emphasize its unitary aspects, and consider it to be a cohesive and coherent literary composition.

4.1. *Diachronic Aspects of Genesis: The Division of the Book into its Parts*

The beginning of modern critical research of Genesis, and of the Pentateuch in general, dates from the late nineteenth century.[1] Following Wellhausen's

1. Since this is not the main subject of the present book, I shall mention here only a few well-known diachronic analyses of the Pentateuch. For elaborations on this issue see,

work on the sources and components of the Pentateuch, source criticism enjoyed a consensual status for some time.[2] According to Wellhausen, Genesis consists of three main written sources: the earliest is the Jahwist source (J), followed by the Elohist (E) and then by the Priestly source (P).[3] Wenham gives a clear summary of five primary criteria for this division of sources: the different names of God (Yahweh in J, and Elohim in E); duplicate stories (for instance, Gen. 1–2.3 and 2.4–3.24); differences in vocabulary; different styles (the Yahwist and Elohist sources include narratives described vividly, whereas P has a more lacklustre style expressed in the tendency for repetitions, and in its many genealogies); and their theologies are different (according to the Priestly source, God is transcendental, whereas in the Yahwist and Elohist sources he is anthropomorphic).[4]

To this discussion Gunkel added the pre-literary stage, and distinguished between the written stage of the documents and their earlier oral stage, when they were circulated orally.[5] The motives for the stories were varied: some consisted of the aetiology of the growth of cultic spaces, the growth of tribes, or explanations of natural phenomena. It should be pointed out that Gunkel considered the classical sources to be a collection of stories compiled by J and E as editors.

Von Rad, who developed the classic form of the Documentary Hypothesis, acknowledges that the written documents were based on traditions of their own, that the different documents were not homogeneous—some early, others later—and that it is harder to date the traditions from which they are

among others, Joseph Blenkinsopp, *The Pentateuch: An Introduction to the First Five Books of the Bible* (New York: Doubleday, 1992), and 'The Pentateuch', in John Barton (ed.), *The Cambridge Companion to Biblical Interpretation* (Cambridge: Cambridge University Press, 1998), pp. 181-97; Joel S. Baden, *The Composition of the Pentateuch: Renewing the Documentary Hypothesis* (New Haven: Yale University Press, 2012); Thomas B. Dozeman, Konrad Schmid and Baruch J. Schwartz, *The Pentateuch: International Perspectives on Current Research* (Tübingen: Mohr Siebeck, 2011); David McLain Carr, *The Formation of the Hebrew Bible: A New Reconstruction* (New York: Oxford University Press, 2011); T.C. Vriezen and A.S. van der Woude, *Ancient Israelite and Early Jewish Literature* (trans. Brian Doyle; Leiden: Brill, 2005); Thomas B. Dozeman, and Konrad Schmid (eds.), *A Farewell to the Yahwist? The Composition of the Pentateuch in Recent European Interpretation* (Atlanta: Society of Biblical Literature, 2006); James Mckeown, *Genesis* (Two Horizons Old Testament Commentary; Grand Rapids: Eerdmans, 2008).

2. J. Wellhausen, *Die Composition des Hexateuchs und der historischen Bücher des Alten Testaments* (Berlin: W. de Gruyter, 1963 [repr. 3rd edn 1899]).

3. Although this is controversial, there is an additional editorial layer, known as JE. Also, the main sources are frequently divided into sub-sources (e.g. Skinner, *Genesis*, pp. liv-lviii).

4. Wenham, *Genesis 1–15*, p. 26.

5. Gunkel, *The Legends of Genesis*.

compiled.[6] Von Rad goes further in that he believes that there was already a continuity of stories at the stage when the traditions took shape. In his view, two central continuous historical narratives can be discerned in Genesis: the Primeval History, and the sacred history. The first treats the period from before the patriarchs, and the latter begins with the patriarchal period, which starts at Genesis 12, and deals with God's salvation of Israel. Von Rad considers that Genesis is based on these documents, but he lays special emphasis on the unifying redaction done by the Yahwist and the last scribe/editor of the Pentateuch. For this reason, von Rad will also be mentioned in the following discussion of synchronic approaches.

Many scholars have challenged the consensus regarding the dates of composition of the documents, as well as the nature of their authors and the texts which they comprise. Van Seters, for instance, relying on literary and archaeological arguments, dates the composition of J approximately in the sixth century BCE.[7] According to Westermann, Genesis is based only on J and P, and he denies the existence of the Elohist source.[8] Another variation is the historical approach to the traditions. According to Rendtorff the stories of the Pentateuch developed by being told and retold. He doubts the existence of any documents in Genesis or in other parts of the Pentateuch. Since the material attributed to J is heterogeneous, he believes that it cannot have been arranged by a single hand.[9] In his discussion of the stories of the patriarchs, Rendtorff speaks of the crystallization of individual traditions into larger units, which led to the creation of a continuous group of stories of the patriarchs. He considers that this was a gradual process, and distinguishes late and early elements in the promises to the patriarchs, and the way in which they were integrated into the text by the Deuteronomistic redaction. Since Rendtorff discusses points of coherence in the Pentateuch, he is also mentioned in the following discussion concerning synchronous approaches to Genesis.

6. G. von Rad, *Old Testament Theology*. I. *The Theology of Israel's Historical Traditions* (trans. D.M.G. Stalker; Edinburgh: Oliver & Boyd, 1962), and *Genesis: A Commentary* (Old Testament Library; trans. J.H. Marks; London: SCM Press, 1963).

7. John Van Seters, *Abraham in History and Tradition* (New Haven: Yale University Press, 1975), and *The Pentateuch: A Social-Science Commentary* (Sheffield: Sheffield Academic Press, 1999). Von Rad has dated the Yahwist to the tenth century BCE, the 'enlightenment' period of Solomon. The Elohist he dates one or two centuries later, and the Priestly document is the latest, taking its final form after the Babylonian exile (von Rad, *Genesis: A Commentary*, pp. 23-27). For a different approach and a later date of the composition of Genesis, see Heard, *Dynamics of Diselection*.

8. Westermann, *Genesis 12–36*, pp. 31-35.

9. Rolf Rendtorff, *The Problem of the Process of Transmission in the Pentateuch* (JSOTSup, 89; trans. J.J. Scullion; Sheffield: JSOT Press, 1990).

But I stop this basic survey here, because a historical analysis is not the main issue in this work.[10]

4.2. *Synchronous Aspects in the Book of Genesis: Discerning Coherence*

Along with diachronous methods such as the Documentary Hypothesis, form criticism (Gunkel), and tradition history criticism (von Rad), a school of interpretation has evolved which aims at considering the text as it is. According to this approach to the text, phenomena such as repetition, duplication of narratives, different names for God, and other changes in the vocabulary are not viewed as indications of different documents, or traditions, but are rather considered as changes in the author's style and technique, put to use for thematic, or literary reasons, or in order to attract the attention of the readers.[11] This literary method of analysis does not necessarily replace the Documentary Hypothesis, but commentators who apply it choose to emphasize synchronic research of the text rather than diachronic research and historical questions.

In his essay 'Abraham the Seer', Buber considers the stories of Abraham as a homogeneous composition, in which the leading word ראה (see) is prominent. Despite the great number of authors and editors of the Hebrew Bible and the differences between their styles, he nonetheless emphasizes their 'common spiritual atmosphere':

> And yet this story has an amazingly homogeneous character, although the homogeneity did not exist from the beginning, but developed in time. For all the chroniclers, i.e., all the custodians of the tradition, regardless of any particular tendencies or peculiarities of each individual, inhabit a common spiritual atmosphere which I would like to designate as the proto-biblical, that is, the biblical atmosphere that existed before the Bible. All who contributed something to history of beginnings—the beginning of the world, of the human race, of Israel—were ultimately concerned, each in his own way, with one thing: to show the people how their God prepared the goal and the road for them, even before they were yet a people.[12]

Wenham and Turner explicitly state that their aim is to read Genesis in its present form, though neither of them denies the stages of its historical development.[13] They prefer to explore the text in its final form, and apply a

10. For further reading on this topic see n. 1 above.
11. Wenham, *Genesis 1–15*, p. 36.
12. Buber, 'Abraham the Seer', p. 24.
13. Wenham, *Genesis 1–15*, p. 36; Laurence A. Turner, *Announcements of Plot in Genesis* (JSOTSup, 96; Sheffield: JSOT Press, 1990).

literary approach in their analyses. They start by relating to Genesis as a whole, with certain themes they find throughout it, or at least throughout considerable parts of it.

Von Rad, besides his historical approach, also speaks of a leading ideological approach in the books from Genesis to Joshua, which is mostly the work of the Yahwist author/editor.[14] With regard to the patriarchal narratives in Genesis, he claims that the varied material on which they are based, which he refers to as 'a varied mosaic', has been harnessed to the concept of the promises to the patriarchs: in particular, the promise of the Land, but also the promise of an abundant posterity. Von Rad claims that the unifying concept of Primeval History (Gen. 1–11) is that the sins of humankind are the source of the negative events in the world. Moreover, the stories show a growing distance between God and humanity, and an increase of God's power. In his view the idea of divine salvation is also a unifying factor; the stories of the expulsion from the Garden of Eden, Cain and Abel, and the Flood display redemption by a merciful and compassionate God. Only in the narrative of the Tower of Babel, when the unity of humanity is brought to an end, does it seem that God's judgment is irreversible. According to von Rad the Yahwist is concerned with God's approach to foreign nations, and from this point on the question of God's relation to foreign nations arises. The history of primeval times does not give a sufficient answer to this question. The answer is given in Gen. 12.1-3, where God's plan is that Abraham will be a blessing to all the families of the earth. In these verses the universal goal to which God wishes to bring history is mentioned, and this is the point of contact between the Primeval History and the history of the salvation of the people of Israel. The salvation history must be understood in the context of the unsolved problem of God's relationship with foreign nations. When Israel and the significance of its being a chosen people are spoken of, the Primeval History has to be considered as one of the important elements in the theological aetiology of Israel.

In addition to his diachronic analysis of the book, Van Seters discusses the entire work of the Yahwist, joining up the small units discussed by Gunkel to a whole.[15] In his view, most of the work of collecting the materials and combining them in Genesis was done by the Yahwist. However, the structural arrangement, the chronology of the genealogies, and a unifying ideological theme which seems to emerge, show, according to Van Seters, that the work of the Yahwist was much more than simply collecting traditions. Van Seters, like von Rad, considers that throughout the whole history of primeval times at Genesis 1–11 there runs a single theological concept, of sin and punishment; or, more accurately, the concept of human sin and

14. Von Rad, *Old Testament Theology*, I, and *Genesis: A Commentary*.

15. Van Seters, *The Pentateuch: A Social Science Commentary*.

God's judgment broadens out here to the universal sphere in which God acts in the Yahwistic history. Here, there is no longer a code acting at the level of the nation, as depicted by the Deuteronomist, but a code of moral behaviour which is applied throughout Genesis. God is both the creator and the judge of humankind. Van Seters explicitly rejects the contention that the Primeval History is an independent unit which is not part of the work of the Yahwist, and has no connection with the subsequent patriarchal narratives. He denies the supposed linguistic and ideological differences between these two units. In his view, the traditions which compose the first section of Genesis, were edited so as to fit the genealogical chronology. Since the chronological lists appear throughout Genesis, this is, he believes, yet another indication of the connection between this section and the rest of Genesis, and of the continuity of the Yahwist's work. The many promises of the inheritance of the Land and Israel's becoming a great nation function as a unifying factor between the traditions of Abraham and Jacob. Isaac, on the one hand, was added as a link between these two; on the other hand, the influence of the Abraham stories on those of Isaac and Jacob is clearly noted.

Clines, Goldingay, and Turner also focus on the promises to the patriarchs in Genesis.[16] According to Clines, the central subject of the whole of the Pentateuch is the partial fulfilment of the promises of blessing which were given to the patriarchs, and the hope that these promises will be carried out fully. Goldingay holds that what unifies the patriarchal narratives is the concept of the promise, and, as against this, the obstacles which delay its fulfilment. Among other obstacles, for instance, Goldingay mentions the barrenness of the matriarchs. Turner, who analyzes only Genesis, divides it into four main parts: the Primeval History, the Abraham narratives, the Jacob Narrative, and the narrative of Jacob's family. He examines the 'announcements of plot' in the book, which are in fact the divine promises. Turner describes how some of the principal divine promises which are situated at the beginning of the four parts of Genesis are fulfilled and others not fulfilled as the plot develops. Rendtorff discusses the way in which the central traditions of the Pentateuch coalesce from small units to larger ones. He maintains that the promises given to the patriarchs, and in particular the promise of divine guidance and the promise to be a blessing to the other peoples, unify the traditions of the patriarchs and contribute to their coherence.[17]

16. D.J.A. Clines, *The Theme of the Pentateuch* (JSOTSup, 10; Sheffield: JSOT Press, 1997); J. Goldingay, 'The Patriarchs in Scripture and History', in A.R. Millard and D.J. Wiseman (eds.), *Essays on the Patriarchal Narratives* (Winona Lake, IN: Eisenbrauns, 1983), pp. 1-34; Turner, *Announcements of Plot*.

17. Rendtorff, *The Problem of the Process of Transmission in the Pentateuch*.

Not only divine promises have been held to be a unifying factor of the Genesis narratives. Westermann, who remains faithful to his own version of source criticism (the lack of E), also views the text synchronically. Westermann speaks of an ideological conception of family relationships, which runs through the patriarchal narratives: in the Abraham narrative (Gen. 12–25) the relationship of parents and children is emphasized, and, thereafter, in the Jacob and Esau narrative (chs. 25–36), attention is diverted to relationships between siblings; in the story of Joseph (chs. 37–50) the relations between several members of the same family are emphasized. In fact, Westermann also connects the stories of the primeval period with the patriarchal narratives: the former deal with basic elements of the world and humanity, whereas the patriarchal narratives deal with basic elements of the community.[18]

Alter, who does acknowledge the unity of Genesis, nevertheless argues that it was composed by a 'collage technique'. According to his view the author allowed himself to use different materials, such as an etiological legend and a genealogy, or to compose such materials and present them side by side.[19] Alter, too, divides Genesis into two sections between which there are many differences: the section dealing with the Primeval History (chs. 1–11), and the section of stories of the patriarchs (chs. 12–50). The first eleven chapters of Genesis deal with the past, and not the future, while the stories of the patriarchs deal with the future: for instance, God promises Abraham descendants in the future, and Jacob's blessing will be fulfilled in the future—'in days to come' (Gen. 49.1). There is also a stylistic difference between the two sections: in the first section characters are described at a distance, as generalized types, not as individuals with a personal history, as in the patriarchal narratives. Moreover, in the section of early stories there are few dialogues, whereas in the patriarchal narratives there are many dialogues, which display the complexity of emotions and relationships. Despite these and other differences between the sections, Alter claims that there is a general line of observation in both sections, and an overall theme which connects the two. The history of the family which will become the people of Israel is seen as part of a broader universal history. The family's travels to and fro between Mesopotamia and Canaan, and the descent to Egypt, show that the region includes not only the Promised Land of Canaan, but also a wider sphere of other cultures. Also, national existence is conceived of as an effort to renew the act of creation: the story of creation repeatedly emphasizes the precept to be fruitful and multiply, whereas the stories of the patriarchs, through the very process of the linguistic echo of

18. Westermann, *Genesis 12–36: A Commentary*, pp. 23-24.

19. Alter, *Genesis*, pp. xlii-xlvii.

fertility from the opening chapters of the book, make it clear that the creation of descendants is very far from being an automatic biological process, since it involves danger, and is unceasingly threatened with extinction. According to Alter, although Genesis looks forward to the book which follows it, it stands independently and demands our attention when we consider the legend from its beginning to its end.

I shall conclude by describing Fokkelman's approach.[20] He considers Genesis to be part of a macro-structure which unites the Pentateuch with Joshua, Judges, Samuel and Kings to form a single work with a line of development from the creation, through the choice of the people of Israel and its settlement in Canaan until the Babylonian exile. Genesis furnishes two building blocks for this macro-plot: the Primeval History (chs. 1–11), and the history of God's covenant with Israel. Fokkelman gives the term תולדות (generations/history) the status of a leading term in Genesis. The root ילד (to give birth) appears frequently, and birth constitutes a general framework emphasizing the different parts of the book. The word תולדות appears at strategic locations: for example, at the beginning of the genealogical lists which conclude two scenes (chs. 1–4, 6–9), and two cycles (of the stories of Abraham and of Jacob). Again and again, claims Fokkelman, we see that fertility, in various forms, and survival by means of progeny are the prime concern of Genesis. The theme of the book is constituted by words from the field of Birth and Fertility, which are expressed by God, and these recur throughout the book. This is connected with the fact that God promises the patriarchs many descendants, and the Land of Canaan as a permanent place for them to dwell in. Thus, space and time are bound up together in the framework of a single theme in Genesis: seed and the descendants represent time, and the Land of Canaan the space. The two parts of the promise are inseparable and interdependent; there can be no progeny without a place to settle in, and there can be no land without somebody to settle in it. In Genesis, space is divided, organized and hallowed by the divine promise, and it also becomes a theme, connected with the origin, and wanderings of the patriarchs. Time, too, is organized in a certain order, and because of the promise it is characterized by expectation and fulfilment.

According to Fokkelman, the theme of space and time influences our view of Genesis as a whole. The differences and contradictions which arise from the texts of which the book is composed become integrated, from many aspects, into a level of conformity:

20. J.P. Fokkelman, 'Genesis', in R. Alter and F. Kermode (eds.), *The Literary Guide to the Bible* (Cambridge, MA: Belknap Press, 1987), pp. 36-55.

> The differences and shifts in language and in types of text which we noted at the outset and which seemed so disturbing now fade... We are now in a position to reevaluate them as dynamic contrasts. The better we realize that time and space, theme and plot merge to create a synthesis of the heterogeneous, the easier it becomes to enjoy the intended play of differences and oppositions. The more we know our reading to be based on centripetal forces, the easier it is to surrender to the centrifugal movements and explore them as a system of counterpoise.[21]

All these studies, like that of Fokkelman, maintain that a level of conformity in Genesis is created by literary and stylistic elements. The present work leans on the point of view shaped in the studies mentioned above regarding coherence in Genesis, but considers the SF as a central aspect of the thematics which unify the book.

Moreover, when studying the deployment of the SF in Genesis I have come to recognize that the instances of seeing practiced by the characters can be grouped into four main categories, which I organize in a hierarchical fashion. The hierarchy is based on the semantic development from concrete to abstract; this is what generally distinguishes between the first two levels of sight. However, since God plays a central role in the entire Bible, the divine factor is added into my hierarchical considerations. When human sight is involved it is significant whether humans visually perceive God or perceive him in a more abstract way. God as the object of sight is what differs between the first two levels of sight and the third and fourth levels. Interestingly, when Faber and Wallhead analyze the field of Vision in John Fowles's *The French Lieutenant's Woman*, they, too, discern a scale of levels of sight.[22] Of course, God is not included as a factor in this scale, and there is no division into a divine sphere and a human sphere as is required in the analysis of religious scriptures. Lastly, although I consider in my analysis characters that practice sight, I do not consider this an analysis of the focal points in the narrative.[23] This is because focalization takes into account not only who sees but the point from which the events are told, seen or thought. Though my analysis of the SF in Genesis does have points of contact with the notion of focalization, the method and the general interest of my discussion are different.

21. Fokkelman, 'Genesis', p. 44.

22. Faber and Wallhead, 'The Lexical Field of Visual Perception', p. 132; see also the Introduction §1, n. 5.

23. According to Bal, the speech act of narrating is actually separated from the vision, the memories and thoughts that are being recounted. She is interested not only in who sees, but also who is telling about the act of sight, and who is reporting about other actions occurring in the narrative (Bal, *Narratology*, pp. 142-74).

4.3. *Levels of Sight*

In general, we may distinguish in Genesis two spheres in which the act of sight occurs: divine sight, when God practices sight; and human sight, when humans practice sight. The levels of sight in the framework of these spheres are based on the proximity between the SF and the CPF, and on the fact that verbs of Sight sometimes mark cognitive perception, and not only sensory visual perception (see §1.1.2).

It appears, then, that the theme of sight relates not only to the character that sees, but also the object perceived: whether it is an object in the world (level a), or God himself (levels c and d). From the literary point of view, I have found that seeing is divided into four main levels, which are based on the nature of the act of seeing itself (visual or cognitive perception), and, as mentioned, on the nature of the perceived object.

a. Low-level sight is sensory-visual, and is performed by the character in the context of tangible objects in the world seen through the eyes. This type of sight is exemplified when the Egyptians see Sarah: 'And when the princes of Pharaoh *saw* her' (Gen. 12.15). Similarly, in the contexts of Lot and Abimelech: 'And Lot *lifted up his eyes* and *saw* that the Jordan valley…' (13.10), and 'Abimelech king of the Philistines *looked out of* a window and *saw* Isaac fondling Rebekah his wife' (26.8). The character sees the object through his/her eyes: the Egyptians see Sarah, Lot sees the plain of Jordan, Abimelech sees Isaac and Rebekah. At the lowest level of sight there is also the knowledge about physical aspects in the world, including carnal knowledge.
b. Intermediate-level sight is cognitive sight, expressed by a verb of sight, which marks the occurrence of a cognitive act together with sensory-visual seeing or without it. The phrase 'When Rachel *saw* that she bore Jacob no children, she envied her sister' (30.1) refers to Rachel's understanding that she cannot bear children. The verb ראה (see) here indicates a cognitive process which the character practices. It is, however, not always possible to distinguish between low-level and intermediate-level seeing: it is not always certain whether sensory visual perception or cognitive perception is being described. This is the case with the passage immediately after the opening of Genesis, after the creation of light, when God's seeing is mentioned: 'And God *saw* that the *light* was good' (1.4), or 'And God *saw* that it was good' (1.10). It is hard to know whether God thinks that his creations are good, whether 'saw' in these places means 'thought' or 'understood', and the sight referred to is sensory-visual, or whether it is a combination of both.

c. High-level sight occurs when the character that practices sight perceives God in some sensory-visual way, and the character explicitly mentions seeing in this way. At this high level of sight, the sight of God is included in a visual medium, seeing him in a dream, or when he appears in human shape, and so on. In order to reach the high-level sight, however, we need to look for the character's explicit acknowledgment that he/she recognizes that he/she has seen God. This is what happens when Jacob awakes from his dream in Bethel, and says: '"Surely Yhwh is in this place, and I *did not know* it". And *he was afraid* (ויירא) and said, "How *awesome* (נורא) is this place! This is none other than the house of God, and this is the gate of heaven!"' (28.16-17). On the other hand, when the angels of Yhwh appear in Sarah's tent she does not declare that she recognizes God and fears him. On the contrary, her lack of faith leads her to laugh inwardly when she hears the prophesy concerning the birth of her son (18.12). Thus, we cannot say that Sarah experiences sight at the high level.

d. Highest-level sight is when humans perceive God in an abstract fashion, and it is not connected with the sense of vision. Seeing at its highest level is realized in the belief in God when he is not revealed in any sort of visual communication. Although the theme which marks the deepest meaning is generally expressed in lexemes from the SF, it is sometimes expressed in rather different terms. When the highest level of seeing is in question, we seek verbal expression on the part of the character of the fact that he/she believes in the actions of God which take place in the world, but without God being revealed to him/her.

All four levels of sight occur when analyzing the human sphere throughout Genesis. As for the divine sphere, God may be involved in concrete visual perception (level a) or in cognitive perception (level b). Levels c. and d. are irrelevant for God. Also, the chosen designations 'Low', 'Intermediate', 'High', and 'Highest' predominantly allude to the development of sight in the human sphere. Nevertheless, as shall be shown further on, divine and human sight interrelate in a special manner. So, in the following discussion I address the levels of sight in both spheres, but I also continue to speak of Sight terms at key points. This time the key points are not only of the individual narratives, but of the macro-plot of the sections of Genesis, thus they contribute to the coherence of the book as a whole.

4.4. *The Primeval History*

The first section of Genesis begins at ch. 1, v. 1, and ends at the end of ch. 11. The SF, which is deployed at key points in this section, emphasizes the process of seeing practiced by God and humans. Instances of seeing in this section show that very often it is God that tries to see, and thereby to learn (also see Licht below). In these instances God tries to learn how the cosmos, which he has created, and the creatures within it behave; God inspects the nature of the earth, and how the forces of nature behave. As the reading of this section proceeds, God's sight becomes clearer, in that he understands that he must guide his creatures and rule over them. Although he himself created them, a close examination of the words of the SF shows that he looks at the behaviour of his creatures in order to learn about them.

Licht, who discusses the term ניסיון (trial/test) in biblical texts, among them the story of the Akedah, argues that God's knowledge of his creatures is limited. According to Licht, God subjects humans to various trials in order to find out how they will behave: 'So it appears that God, who commits strange and terrible acts in order to know, does not know everything'.[24]

The view that God has been looking down on his creatures and observing them ever since the creation of the world is expressed in *Gen. R.* 3.8:

> R. Jannai said: From the very beginning of the world's creation the Holy One, blessed be He, foresaw the deeds of the righteous and the deeds of the wicked. 'And the earth was desolate' alludes to the deeds of the wicked. 'And God said Let there be light', to those of the righteous. 'And God saw the light, that it was good', to the deeds of the righteous. 'And God made a division between the light and the darkness'—between the deeds of the righteous and those of the wicked.[25]

At the beginning of Genesis, in ch. 1, sight and insight are achieved only by God. This is expressed in the phrase so frequently repeated at the end of most of the stages of creation, 'And God saw that it was good'. The fact that this SF formula is repeated so often makes it a key expression, of special importance in the narrative. Nahmanides, in a comment on Gen. 1.4, claims that God himself was not aware in advance of the nature of his creation: 'As in a matter of a man who did not know the nature of a thing until it existed'.

Genesis 3 describes the expulsion of mankind from the Garden of Eden. The climax of the narrative comes when Adam and Eve's eyes are opened: 'Then the *eyes* of both were *opened*, and they *knew* that they were *naked*' (3.7). This verse describes the turning-point within the Adam and Eve

24. Jacob Licht, *Testing: In the Hebrew Scriptures and in Post-Biblical Judaism* (Jerusalem: Magnes Press, 1973 [Hebrew]), p. 25.

25. Freedman and Simon (trans. and eds.), *Midrash Rabbah*.

narrative, by describing an extreme change in their behaviour. Now they, as human beings, no longer feel at ease when they are naked. Nonetheless, Adam and Eve are still at a low level of sight, in that they understand only that they are physically naked. The consequences of sight here apply only to the body, and not to the sight of God; I therefore call this low to intermediate sight on the graduated scale of seeing. Thus, human sight at this point is still sensory-visual, even though it also contains understanding of their situation. On this insight of Adam and Eve, Polak comments: 'Hence the bitter irony in the recognition of the man and his wife "that they were naked". All of their wisdom is concentrated in this pitiful recognition.'[26] It may be that this seeing involves more abstract implications, and that at this point humans had discovered their sexuality; but this, I think, is still on the level of the sensory and physical, of seeing which has no connection with matters of spirit and belief on an even more abstract plane.

After the story of the Garden of Eden the relationship between Cain and Abel, the children of Adam and Eve, is described. Seeing is a crucial factor in the complication and development of the plot: 'And Yhwh had regard for Abel (וישׁע) and his offering, but for Cain and his offering he had no regard (לא שׁעה). So Cain was very angry, and his countenance fell' (Gen. 4.4-5). The lexeme שׁעה, which means 'to gaze, look at' (*HALOT*), belongs to the SF, and the circumstances related in these words serve as a reason for the sequence of events up to the murder. The climax of the story is the short description of the murder of Cain by Abel, defined by Longacre as 'an action peak'. After this there is another peak, this time a complex 'didactic peak',[27] which comes to a head with the marking of Cain: 'And Yhwh put a mark (אות) on Cain, lest any who came upon (מצאו) him should kill him' (4.15). At the didactic peak the word 'mark' is connected with the SF, since it functions by being seen. The mark must be a sign shown clearly on Cain's body. Thus, it is shown how the complex narrative about murder and punishment is made coherent by means of the SF.

The genealogy of the first man continues beyond Cain and Abel, and it is connected to the environment of Sight by means of a number of lexemes which belong to the field: וידע (and he knew, 4.25);[28] בדמות (in the likeness of, 5.1); בדמותו כצלמו (in his own likeness, after his image, 5.3). In 5.1, it is said that humans were created *in the likeness* of God (5.1), and that Adam begat Seth *in his own likeness, after his image* (5.3). Thereafter the names of

26. Polak, *Biblical Narrative*, p. 102.

27. On peaks which are actions, as against peaks expressing morals ('didactic peak'), see Longacre, *The Grammar of Discourse*, p. 37.

28. The lexeme ידע (to know) in Gen. 4.1, 17, 25 refers to carnal knowledge, though in 4.9 it means intellectual perception.

the ancestral lines of Seth and Enosh are enumerated. Hence, these genealogies are connected with the SF by means of the lexemes from the field which appear at their commencement of vv. 5.1-5.

Between the end of these genealogies and the Flood story comes 6.1-4, which describes the daughters of men who are taken by the sons of God, and the 'mighty men' who were born as a result of this coupling. The reasons for the taking of the daughters of men by the sons of God are formulated in terms of the root ראה (to see), with a subordinate accusative clause, describing the fairness of the daughters of men (כי טבת הנה): 'the sons of God saw that the daughters of men were fair; and they took to wife such of them as they chose' (6.2). Opposed to this is God's sight, accompanied by a subordinate clause, which also opens with the particle כי (that), and tells of the wickedness of the sons of man: 'Yhwh *saw* (וירא) that the wickedness of man was great in the earth, and that every imagination of the thoughts of his heart was only evil continually' (6.5). Immediately following Noah's selection, the representative of humankind, who survives the Flood, is described by Sight terms: 'But Noah *found favor in the eyes* (מצא חן בעיני) of Yhwh' (6.8). Two more indicators of sight from the point of view of God are mentioned: 'And God *saw* (וירא) the earth, and behold, it was corrupt; for all flesh had corrupted their way upon the earth' (6.12), and 'for I have *seen* (ראיתי) that you are righteous before me in this generation' (7.1).

It should be pointed out that the formulae of sight in 6.5, 12 are reminiscent of the recurring formulae of sight in the Creation narrative of Genesis 1. In Genesis 1, as mentioned above, the formula 'and God saw that it was good' is repeated after the different stages of the Creation. Here, however, the formulae of sight serve as a prelude to God's destruction of the world by means of the Flood. The formula '*Yhwh saw* (וירא) that the wickedness of man was great in the earth' (6.5), stands as a contrastive parallel to 'and God *saw* that it was good'. The concluding statement, 'And *God saw* the earth, and *behold* it was corrupt' (6.12), corresponds, by contrastive relations, to the concluding statement in the creation story: 'And God *saw* everything that he had made, and behold, it was very good' (1.31).

The formulae of sight at 6.5 and 6.12, encapsulate the process of God's observation of the behaviour of his creations up to this point. So far, he has witnessed the infringement of the prohibition which he laid down in the Garden of Eden, a case of fratricide, and the generally corrupt behaviour of humankind.

All these indicators of sight constitute part of the complication, and lead to the narrative of the Flood itself, in which there is a concrete description of the activity of the forces of nature, conveyed through words from the SF: for instance, the *fountains* (מעינֹת) of the deep burst forth (7.11); the mountains were *covered* (ויכֻסו) with water (7.19, 20), and *seen* (נראו) again at the end of the Flood (8.5), after the *fountains* were stopped (8.2). The flood abated, the dove was sent out to *see* (לראות) if the waters were abated off the face of the earth (8.8). When the dove returns with an olive leaf in her mouth, Noah knows (וידע) that the waters had subsided from the earth (8.11). After Noah removes the *covering* (מכסה) of the ark, he *sees* (וירא) that the face of the ground is dry (8.13). The flood ends with God's promise not to curse the earth again, and he promises humankind 'The *fear* of you (ומוראכם)and the dread of you shall be upon every beast of the earth' (9.2). From that moment it is forbidden to shed blood, 'for God made man in his own image (בצלם)' (9.6 [RSV translation]). This conclusion is accompanied by a didactic peak in which God gives humans the sign (אות, 9.12, 13) of the covenant between him and humankind, the rainbow in the clouds: 'I will *look upon* (וראיתיה) it, and *remember* (לזכר) the everlasting covenant between God and every living creature of all flesh that is upon the earth' (9.16).

The act of sight triggers the effect of the rainbow. According to 9.14, the rainbow will be *seen* without describing who will see it. But God's explicit purpose in creating the rainbow, as expressed in vv. 9, 15, 16, is that he himself will *remember* the covenant between him and every living creature; the rainbow must first of all prompt the act of memory within him himself, and this happens as a result of his *seeing* the rainbow (9.16). If he does not look at the rainbow, he will not remember. This may be compared with the fringes which Israel are commanded to put on the edges of their garments: 'And it shall be to you a tassel to look upon and remember all the commandments of Yhwh... So you shall remember and do all my commandments' (Num. 15.39-40). The sign on the fringe of the garment is meant to be *seen* by Israel. In the case of the rainbow, the sign must be seen by God, so that he may remember his covenant and not cause another Flood (Gen. 9.14-16). The lexemes of sight, as we have seen, are connected with God, and appear at key points in various stories. These lexemes emphasize the processes of seeing experienced by God, and the notion that he learns about human behavioural patterns. Human sight, however, is still limited to the physical-sensory area of the SF.

At 8.1, the appearance of the rainbow is preceded by the description of the turning-point of the Flood narrative: the moment when God decides to stop flooding the world with water: 'But God *remembered* (ויזכר) Noah and all the beasts and all the cattle'. The form ויזכר, from the CPF which is linked to the SF (§1.2.5.2), again reinforces the general conception that it is mostly God who experiences cognitive seeing in the first section of Genesis, seeing which is focused on understanding the behaviour of humans.

The Flood narrative is followed by the story of Noah's drunkenness. The turning-point describes the process which Noah undergoes: 'When Noah *awoke* (וייקץ) from his wine and *knew* (וידע) what his youngest son had done to him' (9.24). Noah's insight is about the understanding of what happened to him when he was drunk. This understanding is not connected with

God but with the relationship between Noah and his sons. Through this story we learn about the dangers inherent in relationships between human beings, and of forbidden deeds.[29] Thus, the reader discovers more about the way in which humans behave.

In the narrative of the Tower of Babel (Gen. 11.1-9), lexemes from the field of Oral Communication are prominent, but the narrative is divided at its midpoint by the central verb of the SF—לראות (to see, at 11.5)—which occurs here only once. This verb appears after the description of the human plan to build a city and a tower, and before the description of God's reaction to this plot: 'And Yhwh came down *to see* the city and the tower' (11.5). It is precisely the unexpected and peculiar occurrence of the verb of sight, single and in the middle of surroundings of Oral Communication, that highlights the difference between God and his creatures in the process of seeing. He sees them, but they do not see him, yet.

Hence, a general look at this section shows that God creates his world, sees it, and learns it. As to the divine sphere, God sees his creations and discovers their character. As to the human sphere, the sight of human characters in the first section of Genesis is generally limited to the sensory aspect, and the insights which they achieve are connected only with themselves, and not with God. The insights of human beings in Genesis 1–11 are personal or have to do with humans, not yet involving the sight and insight of God: Adam and Eve realize they are naked, the first man knows his wife bodily, the first city is built, instruments are played, iron is smelted, and cattle are grazed. In the story of the Tower of Babel, humans talk to each other in order to accomplish their common objective of building a city with a tower reaching up to the heavens. In this section, humans generally deal with themselves or each other, and are not interested in seeing God or learning his ways. God, on the other hand, is busy learning the behaviour of the world and his creatures, animals and human beings, attempting to

29. Though I am interested in terms of Sight in this narrative, some words are called for concerning the interpretation of Ham's seeing the nakedness of his father (Gen. 9.22). Several problems are raised while reading this pericope. One such problem has to do with the fact that though Ham sees the nakedness of his father, Ham's son, Canaan, is cursed by Noah (v. 25). Another difficulty is the understanding of what exactly Ham has done wrong. Bergsma and Hahn suggest that Ham has perpetrated an act of maternal incest (John Bergsma and Scott Hahn, 'Noah's Nakedness and the Curse on Canaan', *JBL* 124 [2005], pp. 25-40). See also F.W. Basset, 'Noah's Nakedness and the Curse of Canaan: A Case of Incest?', *VT* 21 (1971), pp. 232-37. Recently, Embry has summarized the different solutions given to these difficulties, such as maternal and paternal incest between Ham and his mother or his father, but suggests that the problem of the narrative is rather the voyeurism of Noah, that nakedness is a problem in the prehistory, also to be found in the Fall account, in Gen. 1–3 (Brad Embry, 'The "Naked Narrative" from Noah to Leviticus: Reassessing Voyeurism in the Account of Noah's Nakedness in Genesis 9.22-24', *JSOT* 35 [2011], pp. 417-33).

impose certain rules on their lives, and trying to understand how to control their behaviour. He aims to establish a covenant between himself and humankind, a mutual covenant involving commitments both on his part and on the part of humankind to a particular regularization of the relationships between them. The Midrash, too, discerned this overall programme of God to establish a covenant with humans, which already guided him at the stage of the Creation:

> R. Samuel b. Ammi said: From the beginning of the world's creation the Holy One, blessed be He, longed to enter into partnership with the mortals.[30]

4.5. *The Abraham Narrative*

The discussion concerning the Abraham narrative (Gen. 12–25) will be divided in accordance with the key stations in Abraham's life and his relationship with God; thereafter I shall discuss the secondary characters and their connection with the theme of sight. From his observation of human behaviour in the previous section, God realized that 'the imagination of man's heart is evil from his youth' (Gen. 8.21). Since the behaviour of humans as a whole is not suitable for the establishment of a covenant, God had to choose one representative who would be worthy of it. At the beginning of the Abraham narrative God chooses Abraham as the representative of humankind with whom he can establish a covenant, and throughout the section he observes his behaviour and tests him. The rabbinical concept of the ten trials which Abraham underwent reinforces this theme:

> With ten trials our father Abraham was tried, and he stood firm in them all, to make known how great was the love of our father Abraham.[31]

The section opens with the divine command to Abraham: 'Go…to the land that I *will show* (אראך) you' (12.1). From this saying onwards, the promise of the Land is connected with the sight of the Land.[32] God wants to send

30. *Ber. R.* 3.9 (Freedman and Simon, *Midrash Rabbah*).

31. *Abot* 5.4. This Midrash may be interpreted in two different ways. It may be that Abraham's success in his trials shows how great his love of God was; or that his success shows how greatly God loved him (Rabbi Morris Schatz, *Ethics of the Father in the Light of Jewish History* [New York: Bloch, 1970], pp. 207-208).

32. This motif—the connection between sight and the promise of the Land—appears also in the life of Moses, and this is evidence of its importance. For instance, God tells Moses to encourage and strengthen Joshua, because he is the next leader of Israel after Moses: 'and he shall cause them to inherit the land which *you will see* (תראה)' (Deut. 3.28). Further on, God shows Moses the Land, but does not allow him to enter it (Deut. 34.1-5). Daube discusses the motif of the sight of the Land appearing in the history of Moses, and claims that it is based on its occurrence in the stories of Abraham (Daube, *Studies in Biblical Law*, pp. 28-30).

Abraham to a certain land, a land which he will *show* him. In this same chapter God shows himself to Abraham: 'Then Yhwh *appeared* (וירא) to Abram and said, "To your descendants I will give this land". So he built there an altar to Yhwh, who had *appeared* (הנראה) to him' (12.7). These verses show that up to this point God is the active party in seeing, and causes Abraham to see him and to see the Land.

In Genesis 15 Abraham and God are again central characters, demonstrating a development in the relationship between them as they establish a joint covenant. The promise of the Land is no longer given in the *yiqtol*, meaning the future, as in 12.7 or in 13.15, rather it is formulated, for the first time, with the use of the *qatal* (נתתי, 'I have given'). The qatal expresses the idea of a gesture that is performed at the time of speaking as if it had already been done: 'To your descendants I give this land' (RSV, 15.18, but KJV, JPS: 'have I given').[33] Also, the importance of the promise of Gen. 15.18 is greater, since it contains the beginning of the fulfilment of the promise.

The Abraham section opens, then, with the divine command to Abraham to go to the land which God will show him. This command is the beginning of the relationships between God and Abraham; the next turning-point is the establishment of the covenant at ch. 15. In what follows I shall discuss the episodes in between these two high points. Yet the Hebrew Bible is silent as to what happened before the command given to Abraham to leave his family and kindred (12.1), and does not give any details of the circumstances connected with the beginning of the relationship between God and Abraham. The Midrash casts light on this point, which is not mentioned by the biblical narrator, and is expressed on the level of the SF. In *Jubilees*, which is representative of the apocryphal writings, the beginning of Abraham's faith is connected with the performance of sight:

> And in the sixth week, in the fifth year thereof, Abram sat up throughout the night on the new moon of the seventh month to observe the stars from the evening to the morning, in order to see what would be the character of the year with regard to the rains, and he was alone as he sat and observed.
>
> And a word came into his heart and he said: 'All the signs of the stars, and the signs of the moon and of the sun are all in the hand of the Lord. Why do I search (them) out? If He desires, He causes it to rain, morning and evening; And if He desires, He withholds it, And all things are in his hand.' And he prayed that night and said, 'My God, God Most High, Thou alone art my God, And Thee and Thy dominion have I chosen. And Thou hast created all things, And all things that are the work of thy hands' (*Jub.* 12.16-19).[34]

33. Driver speaks of performative forms which indicate the immediate past, a time which, in his words, we call the present (S.R. Driver, *A Treatise on the Use of the Tenses in Hebrew and Some Other Syntactical Questions* [Oxford: Clarendon Press, 3rd edn, 1969 (first published 1882)], p. 15).

34. Translation taken from R.H. Charles (ed.), *The Apocrypha and Pseudepigrapha of the Old Testament* (Berkeley, CA: Apocryphile Press, 2004).

Thus, *Jubilees* continues the poetics of the SF: Abraham's first observation of the skies does not occur during the story of the Promise and Covenant, as in the Masoretic text, but earlier. Abraham's observation of the skies is linked in *Jubilees* to the beginning of his faith in God. According to this source, the turning point, which was the beginning of Abraham's monotheistic path, is also marked by the notion of sight, Abraham's observation of the heavens.

Kasher writes of the conception that looking at the heavenly bodies is a way of knowing God. She quotes various statements found in the Midrash which deal with the beginning of Abraham's path of faith, and concludes: 'Abraham, who neither inherited his faith from his father nor absorbed it from his geographical surroundings, is presented as one who acquired the knowledge of him who sits in heaven through his own observation'.[35]

In the Babylonian Talmud the concept of Abraham's ability to read the stars seems to be well known: 'Abraham our forefather was so well versed in astrology (איצטגנינות), that all the kings of the east and west would arrive early at his door to seek advice' (*b. Bat.* 16b).[36] The Midrash *Genesis Rabbah*, too, attributes to Abraham skill in the field of observation of the heavenly bodies:

> He lifted him up above the vault of heaven; hence He says to him, 'Look (הבט) now toward heaven' הבט signifying to look down from above. The Rabbis said: 'You are a prophet, not an astrologer'... In the days of Jeremiah the Israelites wished to entertain this belief [in astrology], but the Holy One, blessed be He, would not permit them. Thus it is written: 'Thus saith the Lord: Learn not the way of the nations, and be not dismayed at the signs of heaven, etc.' your ancestor Abraham wished to entertain this belief long ago, but I would not permit him. (*Gen. R.* 44.12)

It seems, then, that God's request of Abraham to look at the skies and count the stars at Genesis 15 is one of the echoes of a more general tradition regarding Abraham's sight abilities. This tradition is hinted at in the Hebrew Bible, in *Jubilees*, and in the rabbinical literature. It may be, therefore, that this is an example of a certain pre-biblical tradition which left traces in both earlier and later sources.[37] It must, however, be remembered that the Bible

35. Hannah Kasher *et al.* (eds)., *Abraham, Father of Believers* (Ramath Gan: Bar-Ilan University Press, 2002 [Hebrew]), p. 331.

36. Y.S. Schorr and C. Malinowitz (gen. eds.), *Talmud Bavli: The Gemara: The Classic Vilna Edition, with an Annotated, Interpretive Elucidation, as an Aid to Talmud Study* (elucidated by Gedaliah Zlotowitz; Brooklyn, NY: Mesorah Publications, 2000).

37. This example is parallel to that of Loewenstamm with regard to the tradition of the death of Moses. He maintains that it may be surmised that a tradition of Moses' ascent to heaven had taken shape as early as biblical times. It was rejected by the Pentateuch, but is reflected in the words of Josephus (*Ant.* 4.8, 48), and also in the story of

itself does not discuss these powers; on the contrary, the biblical narrator is silent regarding the question of Abraham's ability to interpret the heavenly bodies, just as he is when he describes the beginning of Abraham's faith in God, and he certainly makes no connection between the starting point of his faith and his experience of looking at the skies. Abraham's first act of communication with God is rather linked with the sight of the Promised Land, not the skies.

As for the development of the theme of sight in Genesis, the Abraham narrative shows that it is God rather than Abraham who is the active party in the processes of sight, and this hints at the type of relations between them.[38] It is God who shows Abraham the Land, it is he who sends him to look at the heavens and see the stars, and the flaming torch which appears in the story of the Promise and Covenant is a symbol of God's presence.

In 15.6 it is said of Abraham: 'And he *believed* in Yhwh' (והאמן ביהוה), and that God, for his part '*reckoned* (ויחשבה) it to him as righteousness'. These words relate to a specific promise given to Abraham at that place (God promises him a son who will succeed him, and many descendants: 15.4-5). At the same place, Abraham also expresses his doubts, asking 'How am I to *know* (אדע) that I shall possess it?' (15.8). Since the statement about Abraham's belief in God is concerned with a specific context, and since it is followed by Abraham's expression of doubt in God's doings, I do not consider this place as a demonstration of a high level of Sight on the part of Abraham.[39] There is no explicit declaration coming from Abraham about his fear of God. Therefore, God continues to reveal himself to Abraham in order to know whether he is in absolute fear of him. On this, the Midrash comments:

> A potter does not examine defective vessels, because he cannot give them a single blow without breaking them. What then does he examine? Only the sound vessels, for he will not break them even with many blows. Similarly, the Holy One, blessed be He, tests not the wicked but the righteous.[40]

Elijah's ascent to heaven (1 Kgs 2.11) (S.L. Loewenstamm, 'The Death of Moses' [Hebrew], *Tarbiẓ* 27 [1958], pp. 142-57 [148-49]).

38. Polak remarks that God here is an active subject, as against Abraham, who is a passive object (Frank Polak, 'לא כקורא תגר: A Structural and Thematic Analysis of the Covenant among the Divided Parts [Genesis 15.1-21]' [Hebrew], in Y. Avishur and J. Blau [eds.], *Mehqarim Bamikrah Uvamizrah Haqadum* [Jerusalem: Rubinstein, 1978], pp. 319-27 [321]).

39. On the dispute regarding Gen. 15.6, see, for instance, Bertil Alberktson, 'A Disputed Sense in a Covenant Context: On the Interpretation of Genesis 15:6', in *Covenant as Context: Essays in Honour of E.W. Nicholson* (New York: Oxford University Press, 2003), pp. 1-9; Daniel Klein, 'Who Counted Righteousness to Whom? Two Clashing Views by Shadal on Genesis 15:6', *Jewish Bible Quarterly* 36 (2008), pp. 28-32.

40. *Gen. R.* 55.2 (Freedman and Simon, *Midrash Rabbah*).

The next episode in which God and Abraham are the central figures is the story of the circumcision at ch. 17. This chapter opens with a mention of Abraham's age, and says that God *appeared* (וַיֵּרָא) to him (17.1). In the course of this revelation God promises Abraham an abundant posterity, and that the covenant between them will continue to be valid between himself and Abraham's descendants; he then promises the land of Canaan to Abraham and his descendants (17.6-8). God demands of Abraham and his descendants that they circumcise their foreskins: 'And it shall be a *sign* (אות) of the covenant between me and you' (17.11). The lexeme אות (sign) is included in the category of lexemes that are connected by the schema: 'objects which fulfil their function by being seen'. This event of circumcision, as can be seen, is deployed by terms of Sight. Abraham and his descendants are thus connected to the SF by these Sight terms, and play a part in the general theme of sight. The injunction to carry out circumcision is another significant underpinning to the covenant between Abraham and God, and the role of humans in this act is prominent.

In 18.1-15 Abraham and Sarah are told that a son will be born to them. As the opening—'And Yhwh *appeared* (וַיֵּרָא) to him by the *oaks of Mamre* (באלני ממרא)' (18.1)—suggests, the events which take place in ch. 18 unfold against the background of God's appearance, in a place whose name is also connected with the SF. The story closes with Sarah's words, 'But Sarah denied, saying, "I did not laugh"; for she was *afraid* (יראה). He said, "No, but you did laugh"' (18.15). The narrator says that Sarah was afraid, and he uses the lexeme ירא, linked to the SF, due to its role in the nearby field of Emotion. Its link to the SF is also enhanced since it bears sound resemblance with the verb of sight ראה ('see', see §2.6.2.1). Though ירא means fear, and also specifically the fear of God, it does not indicate that Sarah, Abraham's wife, experienced sight at the highest level. The narrator refers only to Sarah's human fears. Here the narrator adduces no specific evidence of Sarah's faith, or that she understands that she is close to God. He speaks only of her laughter at the prophecy that she will give birth (18.12).

In the following episode God involves Abraham in his doubts as to whether to destroy Sodom and Gomorrah, in words taken from the SF: 'Shall I *hide* (המכסה) from Abraham what I am about to do?' (18.17). The bargaining between God and Abraham about the number of righteous men in Sodom and Gomorrah is discussed in terms which repeat the verb מצא (find), which belongs to the SF. God is the active party in the finding process—'If I *find*' (אם־אמצא, 18.28, 30)—as he is when the verb appears in the passive with no specific subject in Abraham's statement: 'Suppose…are *found* (אולי ימצאון)' (18.29, 30, 31, 32), possibly because of Abraham's reverence for God.

The three angels[41] who came to visit Abraham at the beginning of the story now rise from the place where he has camped, and *look* (וישקפו) towards Sodom (18.16): that is to say, God's attitude, represented here by the angels, is still that of testing his creatures. Abraham accompanies them, and on his way receives a promise from God that he will multiply and become a great people: 'No, for I have chosen him (כי ידעתיו), that he may charge his children and his household after him to keep the way of Yhwh by doing righteousness and justice; so that Yhwh may bring to Abraham what he has promised him' (18.19). The narrator uses here the verb ידע to express the idea of choosing Abraham, a verb which more often means 'to know'. Whether its significance is the choice of Abraham or whether it is recognition of the fact that Abraham believes in God, the knowledge is attributed here to God and not to Abraham. Immediately after this God decides to descend and *see* (ואראה) whether the people of Sodom and Gomorra have sinned 'and if not, I *will know* (אדעה)' (18.21). Here again, it is God who sees and knows. Together, Sight and Insight construct the theme of the unit.

In Genesis 19 which describes the destruction of Sodom and Gomorrah, Lot, rather than Abraham, is the central figure. But the story of the destruction ends with the following words: 'God *remembered* (ויזכר) Abraham, and sent Lot out of the midst of the overthrow' (19.29). The word ויזכר (he remembered) belongs to the CPF, which is close to that of Sight. Here again, divine activity on the cognitive level is emphasized, and the insights are attributed to God, and not to the man he has chosen.

As for sight on the human level, it appears that humans in this episode are involved in carnal knowledge (19.5, 33, 35), and their seeing or blindness are sensory-visual, both in the case of Lot (19.1), of his wife (19.26), and even of Abraham (19.28). Abraham *looks* towards Sodom and Gomorrah, and *sees* the ruins and the smoke rising from the land (19.28), for all of which God was responsible, but the higher conceptual process in the story takes place in the divine sphere (19.29). Human beings are still limited to the lower level of seeing, and in the case of the Sodomites and Lot's daughters, to carnal sight and knowledge.

41. The dispute as to the identity of Abraham's three visitors is well attested in biblical commentaries. The problem is that in some instances they are referred to in the plural (18.2, 4, 5, 8, 9), whereas in others they are referred to in the singular (vv. 3, 10). According to Skinner, one possibility is that the visitors were Yahweh accompanied by two angels. Skinner thinks that it is more probable that to the original Yahwist the men were representatives of Yahweh, who was not visibly present (Skinner, *Genesis*, p. 299). According to von Rad, 'one is therefore rather inclined to think that Yahweh appeared in all three…for Yahweh is one in spite of this form of his appearing' (von Rad, *Genesis*, p. 199). Also see Benjamin D. Sommer, *The Bodies of God and the World of Ancient Israel* (New York: Cambridge University Press, 2009).

In the story of the Akedah, which constitutes a climax in the section of the Abraham narratives, a high point in Abraham's relationship with God is described. It finds its expression when God admits: 'For now I know (ידעתי) that you fear (ירא) God, seeing you have not withheld your son, your only son, from me' (22.12). Thus, tracing the SF leads to the conclusion that in the second section of Genesis God tries to see whether his chosen one was chosen rightly and fears him absolutely. This question is answered positively in the story of the Akedah.

In addition to the main circle of the theme of sight in the Abraham narratives, which involves Abraham and God, there are secondary plots, relating to the lives of the characters close to Abraham; they, too, may contribute to the theme of sight which I have presented. Apart from the story discussed above in which Sarah is involved (Gen. 12.10-20, see §3.2.6), there are stories about his other wife, Hagar. Consideration of the SF in the narratives concerning Hagar shows that she undergoes an experience of sight at the highest level. After the angel has appeared to her and promises her a son, she gives God a name connected with sight: 'You are the God who sees me' (אתה אל ראי), for she said, 'I have now seen the One who sees me' (16.13, NIB translation). This declaration by Hagar constitutes explicit recognition that she appreciates the importance of the divine presence, thus reaching a high level of Sight (§3.2.4). It also demonstrates that the theme of sight indeed goes beyond Abraham's figure. Next I shall consider how the theme of sight functions in the history of Lot the son of Haran, Abraham's brother.

When Abraham parted from Lot, at Genesis 13, Lot *lifted up his eyes and saw* the whole plain of Jordan, which was well watered everywhere, before God devastated the region (13.10). This description parallels the description of the promise of the Land to Abraham. Just as in the framework of the command 'Go from your country' God commands Abraham to look upon the Land (12.1; 13.15), so Lot's eyes are raised and he *sees* the land which he chooses. But it becomes clear that the results of seeing are opposite in each of the two cases. Abraham receives the Promised Land, which will flourish in the future, whereas Lot chooses the land of the plain, which is doomed to destruction. Moreover, the negative aspect of sight in Lot's life is also to be found in the narrative of Sodom and Gomorrah, at the beginning of ch. 19. In the narrative of the destruction of Sodom and Gomorrah, Lot's wife *looks* backwards at the city as it is being overthrown, despite the divine injunction not to do so. She is punished by being turned into a pillar of salt (19.17, 26). The men of Sodom are stricken with *blindness* (סנורים, 19.11): whether a strong blinding light or night blindness is meant, the result is their inability to see.

To sum up, the study of the Abraham narrative from the point of view of the SF, enables the reader to grasp the section as an entirety. Many texts within it are now consolidated under the aegis of the theme of sight. The words of the SF turn the individual stories of Abraham into a unified whole. They join the parts of the plot to each other within the stories and across them, and create a developing theme concerned with divine sight and human sight. In the divine sphere, God tests his elected one, and also the people close to him: Abraham's two wives, and his nephew, Lot. The recognition of the functioning of the SF in the cycle of the Abraham stories shows that the whole history of Abraham is formed in a way leading to the climactic point—the binding of Isaac—in which God acknowledges that Abraham does indeed fear him.

As for the secondary characters, their sight completes the picture of the sight of Abraham. Sarah is beautiful, but God does not believe that she fears him sufficiently ('No, but you did laugh', 18.15). Lot and his wife are characterized by negative sight, but in the case of Hagar we see a high level of sight.

The section of the Abraham narratives concludes at 25.11, and immediately after it begins the history of Ishmael, which separates it from the subsequent section—the Jacob Narrative. Genesis 25.8-10 tells of the episode of Abraham's death and burial in the cave of Machpelah, which is situated in the field of Ephron the Hittite '*before Mamre*' (על־פני ממרא, 25.9). As shown previously (§2.8.1.4), ממרא derives from the root ירא (fear), which belongs to the field of Emotion, close to the SF (§2.6.2.1).

In 25.11 the reader is informed that God blessed Isaac after the death of Abraham, and that Isaac dwelt by *Beer Lahai Roi* (באר לחי ראי). The names of *Mamre* and *Beer Lahai Roi* are both connected to the SF, and bind the characters of Abraham and Isaac to the overall theme of sight. The genealogy of Ishmael, which is recorded immediately thereafter, at 25.12–18, concludes with an account of the death of Ishmael and with the observation that his descendants 'dwelt from Havilah to *Shur* (שׁור), which is opposite Egypt in the direction of Assyria (אשׁורה)'[42] (25.18). Here again, the name of *Shur*, a place connected with the SF, is mentioned, and thus connects Ishmael to Abraham and Isaac. The use of these place-names adds to the coherence between the Abraham narratives and the following section of Jacob from the point of view of the theme of sight, which continues to develop across them.

4.6. *The Jacob Narrative*

The first episode in the Jacob Narrative is the conception and birth of the two twin brothers, Jacob and Esau (25.19-26). This episode involves more Oral Communication than Sight on the part of the parents and God. Isaac

42. The sound resemblance between Shur (שׁור) and Assyria (אשׁורה, 25.18), especially felt in Hebrew, stresses the presence of the SF term (also see §2.8.1.7).

entreats God to put an end to his wife's barrenness, and God grants his request (25.21). Rebekah feels the struggling children within her and says, 'If it is to be this way, why do I live?', then she goes to inquire of God (25.22). The divine blessing for the children (25.23) is another act in the field of Oral Communication. Thus the scene of the birth of the sons is characterized by verbal communication between Isaac, Rebekah, and God. However, the theme of sight does not give way entirely to the field of Oral Communication.

The description of Esau in his birth tale includes the lexeme 'red', from the Colour field, which is linked to the SF as a peripheral category (§2.7.6), 'The first came forth *red*,[43] all his body like a hairy mantle' (אדמוני כלו כאדרת שׂער, 25.25). Visible colouring, Brenner explains, is the phenomenon whereby 'Energy distribution reaches the eye of the observer, is then transmitted through the observer's vision and interpreted and turned into a sensation'.[44] Since colours are visually accessible through the eyes they are connected to the SF.

The red colour follows Esau further on when he craves to eat from the red stew that Jacob prepares for him, causing him to give up his birthright (25.30). The narrator explains that Esau was named 'Edom' because of his request of the red stew, highlighting the sound resemblance between Edom and the Hebrew word אדם (red). Hence, the colour 'red' is connected with Esau's hairiness (25.25) and his strong drive to satisfy his hunger. In other words, not only sight, but also touch and taste senses, are closely linked in the description of Esau's character.

Although Jacob is not mentioned throughout Genesis 26, the chapter continues with the display of many SF lexemes at key points. God *appears* (וירא) to Isaac (26.2) and promises him the Land and an abundant progeny (26.3-4), as he promised his father. But the phrasing is slightly different from that of the promise to Abraham: God said to Isaac 'dwell in the land of which I shall tell (אמר) you' (26.2), whereas with Abraham, the Land is connected with sight as God sends him 'to a land that I will *show* (אראך) you' (12.1). The giving of the Land to Isaac is explained later: 'because Abraham obeyed my voice and kept my charge, my commandments, my statutes, *and my laws* (תורתי)' (26.5). The laws or instructions are connected to the SF, since they are included in the field of Education, close to the SF

43. It should, however, be noted that according to Brenner's findings the colour term אָדֹם, usually translated as 'red' in the Hebrew Bible, may also carry the value of orange, yellowish orange, or yellowish brown (Brenner, *Colour Terms in the Old Testament*, p. 61). Nevertheless, in this work I translate the term אָדֹם as 'red' in order to maintain consistency with the translations.

44. Brenner, *Colour Terms in the Old Testament*, p. 3. This has also been cited in §1.2.6.5. See also the discussion in Sutskover, 'Lexical Fields'.

(§2.6.3.1). At this point God begins his educational activity. He attempts to teach Isaac that the covenant between them obliges him to execute certain actions, and to adopt a way of life founded on faith.

Meanwhile the men of Gerar show interest in Rebekah, since she is beautiful. Her external attributes are depicted by lexemes from the SF, כי־טובת מראה היא (26.7). Additional SF lexemes occur as the narrative continues. Abimelech happened to *look out* (וישקף) of the window and *saw* (וירא) Isaac fondling his wife (26.8).

Verses 12-22 describe the digging of Abraham's wells, filled with earth by the Philistines. The Hebrew verb מצא (to find) is mentioned twice (vv. 12, 19); it links with the SF since the act of finding presupposes the act of looking for, or the process of seeing something and recognizing it.

The theme of sight progresses in this episode about Isaac to a higher developmental level than that observed in the Abraham cycle. God appears (וירא) before Isaac once again (v. 24) at *night*, asks him not to fear (אל־תירא), and blesses him. In reply, Isaac builds an altar at the place where God appeared to him, calls upon the name of the Lord, and even pitches his tent there (26.25). Isaac does not declare that he believes in God, but the Philistines acknowledge him. In a discussion between Isaac and Abimelech and his advisors, the latter tell Isaac that they *see* (ראו ראינו) that God is with him (v. 28), and wish to make a covenant with him. When morning comes the parties take an oath with one another, and on that same day Isaac's servants tell him about the well they had dug and in which water was *found* (v. 32, cf. vv. 12, 19). This statement concerning the acknowledgment of God's involvement in the life of humans comes from foreign peoples, not from the chosen ancestor.

Hence, although ch. 26 seemingly deviates from the main storyline, which is mostly concerned with Jacob, it contains the recurrence of SF lexemes (see, look out, find, beautiful) at plot key points, thus connecting it to the overarching theme of sight.

Thereafter, ch. 27 describes the deception practiced by Rebekah and Jacob—the theft of the birthright of the oldest son. The cycle of rivalry between Jacob and Esau develops apace, and this can take place only on the background of Isaac's weak eyesight (27.1). Although Isaac's eyesight is failing, he is sensitive and alert as regards the senses of hearing, touch, taste and smell. Jacob's visual perceptions are still to be developed further. Jacob is sent to Haran, to the house of Laban, whose name may also refer to the colour 'white' in Hebrew. This may hint at the idea that Jacob's vocation in Haran was to repent and purify himself of his previous sins.[45]

45. Brenner notes that לָבָן and אָדֹם are applied in descriptions of sins and of garments (Brenner, *Colour Terms in the Old Testament*, p. 53).

Chapter 28 is particularly important from the aspect of the theme of sight, since the relationship between God and his elected one—Jacob—evolves here. On this occasion God is not revealed directly to Isaac's son; he appears to him in a dream. From the moment of Jacob's awakening, God begins to act towards the patriarchs less and less openly. In his dream, Jacob sees a ladder whose top reaches the heavens, and the angels of God ascending and descending it. God is also standing above the ladder or beside Jacob[46] and promises him great progeny and the gift of the Land. When Jacob awakes from his dream he acknowledges that God was in the place where he himself is, 'and I *did not know* it' (לא ידעתי, 28.16).[47] In addition, this is the first time that a descendant of Abraham experiences fear at the appearance of God: 'And he was *afraid* (ויירא) and said, "How *awesome* (נורא) is this place!"' (28.17). He calls the place where God was revealed in his sleep Bethel—meaning 'the house of God'. Jacob's knowledge when he wakes up from his dream, and his fear, constitute a turning-point in the relationship between God and man. This is a sign of sight at its highest level (the fourth level), that is, seeing in the sense of fear of God. Sight of the third level is also involved (high level sight), since the actual seeing of God was involved and accompanied by an explicit declaration about this matter by the human character. From now on the open interference of God in the lives of humans decreases.

From the point of view of the relationship between the two brothers, reminiscence of their continued rivalry is expressed here by the use of the verb ראה (see): 'Esau *saw* (וירא) that Isaac had blessed Jacob and sent him away to Paddanaram to take a wife from there' (28.6). Esau understands that their father Isaac wants the best possible for his brother, while he himself is not enjoined to avoid taking a wife from among the Canaanite women. It appears that, for the sake of emphasis, the narrator takes care to state explicitly that Esau *sees* that the Canaanite women are bad in his father's eyes. Here, sight is accompanied by an act of understanding, and the drawing of conclusions: 'So when Esau *saw* (וירא) that the Canaanite women did not please Isaac his father' (28.8, literally, 'the Canaanite women were bad *in the eyes* [בעיני] of Isaac'). From the SF perspective, a development in Esau's personality is observed, since here for the first time the narrator

46. See these differences of interpretation, for example, in the translations of RSV, 'And behold, the LORD stood above it', as opposed to JPS, 'And, behold, the LORD stood beside him' (Gen. 28.13).

47. As noted when discussing the individual narrative of Gen. 28, Fokkelman maintains that Jacob had a psychological insight as a result of his waking from his dream. He claims that people often have insights of this type when they wake up from sleep (J.P. Fokkelman, *Narrative Art in Genesis: Specimens of Structural and Stylistic Analysis* [Assen: Van Gorcum, 1975], p. 62).

explicitly notes Esau's insight, using terms from the SF. It is important enough to mention that Esau cognitively understands his father's view on the subject of Canaanite women. He achieves sight at the intermediate level, seeing in the sense of understanding another human being. As for Jacob, he has come to a very close relationship with God, but has yet to develop his relationship with other human beings.

From ch. 29 on, seeing between human beings is emphasized. To interpret the development of personalities, it is essential to compare the levels of sight each individual—Jacob, Leah, Rachel and Laban—achieves in this text unit. Significantly, the setting of this episode is Laban's household, and the symbolic meaning of Laban's name ('white'), as representing a state of purity from sins, should be taken into account. It is the house in which Jacob will have to atone for his wrongdoings to his brother, and generally turn into a better man with regard to his relations with other people.

Once again the scene opens with a statement regarding sight of the main character, this time with the use of a few fixed formulas:[48] וישׂא יעקב רגליו וילך... וירא והנה... ('Then Jacob went on his journey, and came... As he looked, he saw...', 29.1-2). This instance illustrates the consistency of the appearance of SF lexemes at key points. Further on Jacob *sees* Rachel, and immediately rolls the stone from the well (29.10). Both Leah and Rachel are depicted in SF terms: 'Leah's *eyes* were weak' (ועיני לאה רכות),[49] while Rachel 'was *beautiful and lovely*' (יפת־תאר ויפת מראה, 29.17). With her first son as a mediator, Leah develops a relationship with God. God *sees* that she is unloved and opens her womb (29.31). Leah, in return, calls her first child *Reuben* ('*See*! A son!'), thanking God for *seeing* her distress (29.32). Further on, Rachel *sees* that she is barren and envies her sister (30.1). The tense relationship between the two sisters is also expressed by the interpretation of the name Naphtali, the second son of Rachel's maid, Bilhah. When giving an explanation for his name Rachel alludes to her wrestling with her sister as 'a mighty wrestling' (נפתולי אלהים) in which she had prevailed (30.8).[50] Immediately after this we are informed of Leah's perception as she *sees* she has stopped bearing children (30.9). The two continue in their dispute, this time over the mandrakes Reuben *found* (וימצא, 30.14) in the field. We can

48. On fixed formulas in the Hebrew Bible and their development from the oral tradition, see Polak, 'Linguistic and Stylistic Aspects of Epic Formulae'.

49. Here I follow the RSV translation, though the Hebrew clause describing Leah's eyes has been widely debated, starting with early translations, through Hebrew traditional exegesis, and onto modern contemporary commentators.

50. The reader senses the analogy between Jacob's wrestling with the man of God and prevailing in ch. 32, and Rachel's wrestling with Leah and prevailing. Gunkel, however, omits עם אחתי ('with my sister') of 30.8, thus strengthening the analogy further (Gunkel, *Genesis übersetzt und erklärt*, p. 334).

see, then, that the SF continues to create cohesion between the different plots. As to the development of the theme of sight in relation to Leah and Rachel, we learn that the sight of both sisters is directed at each other and involves cognitive perception. Both sisters attain the same intermediate level of sight that Esau reaches.

Right after Rachel gives birth to Joseph, Jacob approaches Laban and demands to take all his belongings and return to Canaan (30.25-26). Using their sense of sight Jacob manipulates the flock, encouraging them to mate and multiply by gazing at the *white* streaks he peels in fresh rods of poplar, almond and plane trees, then places them in front of the flock coming to drink at the watering troughs.

The lexemes used to describe the appearances of the flock in this unit—'striped', 'speckled', and 'spotted'—are also connected to the SF since, like the phenomenon of colour, they too depend on energy distribution that reaches the observer's eye. The colours 'white' and 'brown' (חום),[51] for example in vv. 32, 37, 40, are peripheral constituents of the SF. The lexeme 'eye', a primary term from the SF, is also mentioned when describing Jacob setting the rods before the eyes (לעיני) of the flock (30.41).

Up to this point Jacob has seen God, explicitly acknowledged his presence, and also shown sensitivity and understanding of the visual perception of his flock. However, he has yet to develop his sight in the human sphere. Jacob now proceeds to use his own perception in order to understand his relationship with his family members: 'And Jacob *saw* that Laban did not regard him with favour as before' (31.2). As if he has noticed the positive development in Jacob's attitude toward his family members, God immediately responds by giving Jacob specific guidance, commanding him to go back to Canaan, and promising protection (31.3).

Jacob shows sensitivity to and consideration for his wives when he assembles them to announce what he has *seen* in their father's face. ראה אנכי את פני אביכן... (31.5). He tells them of his *dream*, in which a divine messenger appears and promises him success with the breeding of his flock. Here Jacob quotes the messenger's words: 'for *I have seen* all that Laban is doing to you' (31.12). Thus, an additional instance of sight in the divine sphere is displayed: the messenger, God's representative, *sees* Jacob.

Another *dream*, this time seen by Laban, connects the next paragraph too to the theme of sight. Laban pursues Jacob, who has taken advantage of Laban's absence to run away, taking all his belongings—women, children,

51. Brenner states חום may be considered a dialectal colour term restricted to the sphere of sheep husbandry and the technical language spoken by shepherds. Within the scope of the Hebrew Bible, she concludes, חום is underdeveloped and structurally a subordinate within the sector governed by שָׁחֹר (Brenner, *Colour Terms in the Old Testament*, p. 123).

and property. God comes to Laban in a *dream* at *night* and tells him to be careful and say nothing to Jacob, either good or bad (31.24). We might say that Laban achieves sight at a high level (the third level of sight),[52] but not the highest level. Laban acknowledges the appearance of God in his dream, but does not admit having faith in him. God is referred to by Laban as the God of Jacob's fathers (v. 29). There is no recognition of divine providence on Laban's part at this stage of the story, thus he does not yet reach the fourth and highest level of sight.

Next, Laban starts searching Jacob's tent and the tents of his daughters and their maids to find the *teraphim* Rachel has taken from him. The lexeme מצא (to find), an SF constituent, occurs in vv. 32, 33, 34, 35 and 37. Another constituent, חפש (to look for), occurs in v. 35. Hence, this episode is also connected to its surrounding by SF terms.

Jacob confronts Laban (31.36-42), mentioning God's *seeing* his misery the night before, probably referring to Laban's dream (31.42). Laban answers that everything Jacob *sees* in front of him actually belongs to him, to Laban (וכל אשר־אתה ראה לי־הוא, 31.43). However, he offers to make a covenant with Jacob. The pile of stones gathered by Jacob's kinsmen is called 'Galed', but also 'Mizpah' (Watchtower), with the explanation given by Laban '*Yhwh* watch (יצף) between you and me, when we are absent one from the other (כי נסתר איש מרעהו)' (31.49). Although Laban does recognize God's providence, he still does not trust Jacob. Hence, Laban's character does not develop as regard to his relations with other human being.

And so the Laban–Jacob connection ends here, with the covenant between the two parties, both admitting God's crucial role in preserving the peace between them, while the name of the place where the covenant is made contains a SF lexeme. Metaphorically speaking, Jacob is now 'white', that is, he has made amends for all his sins in the human sphere. This accords with Polak's description of Jacob as a developing character. According to this view, Jacob starts on his way in the world by deceiving, but gradually learns to attain his goals through hard work and diplomacy.[53]

In ch. 32, Jacob and God again play the leading roles, while chs. 28–32 tell of Jacob's years with Laban. Chapter 32, then, opens with a short scene telling that Jacob *sees* the camp of God (*Maḥanaim*). There is visual communication between God, or, more exactly, between the 'camp of God', and Jacob. Later in the chapter comes a description of Jacob's struggle with the man who, as it appears, is an angel of God, or God himself. As mentioned above (§3.3.4), this episode opens at night, and closes with sunrise (32.31).

52. Though the text does not explicitly say that Laban sees God in a dream, it is said that God came to Laban at night in his dream and talked to him. I refer to this coming and talking to Laban, as a meeting between the two.

53. Polak, *Biblical Narrative*, p. 292.

Conditions for sight, depicted by SF words, define its boundaries, and the place name, Peniel (/Penuel), explained by SF lexemes underlines the theme of the unit, Jacob's recognition of his ability to see God *face to face*.

The next episode opens with the mention of Jacob *lifting up his eyes* and *seeing* Esau approaching, escorted by four hundred men (33.1), another instance in Genesis in which an episode opens by mentioning the sight of the main character. When the brothers finally meet, Esau lifts up his eyes and notices Jacob's women and children (33.5). Jacob compares the meeting between them to seeing the face of God, 33.10: 'Just *to see your face* is like *seeing the face* of God', he says. In my opinion, this is the most significant point in the development of Jacob's character, as depicted in SF terms. At this stage Jacob compares the sight of his brother to the sight of God, as if from now on giving God and family the same amount of respect.

Up to this point we have learned about Jacob's special ability to see and understand human and divine nature. Analyzed from the angle of seeing, the variety of topics treated in the different scenes of this cycle has been shown to display a certain narrative unity.

Now that the main issues concerning the Jacob–Esau and the Jacob–Laban relationships have been resolved, the question as to whether the SF continues to prevail in the remaining text units of chs. 34, 35, and 36 still remains.

In ch. 34, it is immediately apparent that the act of sight triggers the entire episode: 'Now Dinah the daughter of Leah, whom she had borne to Jacob, went out to visit the women of the land (34.1). The Hebrew has the verb לראות, literally 'to see', although it is translated as 'to visit' (RSV). Then Shechem the son of Hamor the Hivite, *saw* her (וירא אתה...) seized her, and lay with her by force (34.2). In the eyes of some Masoretic exegetes Dinah has probably done wrong when going out, 'to see' the women of the land, since the consequences of this seeing were that Shechem set his eyes on her, and then raped her.[54] Sight, in ch. 34, once again appears at a key position.

Chapter 35 opens with God's command to Jacob to go to Bethel, dwell there, and make an altar to the God who *appeared* to him (לאל הנראה אליך, 35.1). The condensed scene is brought to a conclusion by another mention of God's sight: '...and there he built an altar, and called the place El-bethel, because there God had *revealed* (נגלו) himself to him...' (35.7). God reveals himself to Jacob again at the beginning of the next scene, in 35.9.

In addition, each time Edom is mentioned in the genealogies of ch. 36 the SF is echoed (e.g. 36.9, 21, 31; see the beginning of this discussion §4.6). The appearance of SF lexemes in chs. 35–36 seems to combine into creating an overall lexical cohesion with the preceding narrative units.

54. *Qoh. R.* 10, *Tanḥ.* (Buber), *Parashat Wayishlah* 19.

4.7. *'Seeing the Face': A Unifying Phrase in the Jacob and Joseph Narratives*

The phrase ראה פנים (saw the face) has a special importance among the terms of sight in the narratives of Jacob and Joseph. This phrase includes two SF terms and does not occur in Genesis before 31.2, and from this point onwards it appears at key points up to the end of the book.[55]

Our phrase is found for the first time in the Jacob Narrative at the moment when he *sees* the *face* of Laban and notices that 'it was not towards him as before' (31.2). There follows the divine commandment to Jacob to return to the land of his fathers (31.3), and from that moment Jacob takes steps to leave Laban's house. As mentioned above, Jacob calls Rachel and Leah, and explains what he has seen in their father's face, repeating the matter of seeing the face: 'I *see* that your father does not regard me with favour as he did before (ראה אנכי את־פני אביכן, literally: I see the face of your father). But the God of my father has been with me' (31.5). This propinquity between Jacob's sight of Laban's face and the divine command to go back to Canaan (31.2, 3) may hint at a divine intervention, that God himself influenced Laban's expression, and thereby signalled to Jacob to take steps and leave.

In fact, Jacob leaves Laban, and eventually makes an agreement with him, and they part peacefully. As I have shown above, this agreement is also connected with words from the SF (such words as Mizpah ['Watchtower'], יצף ['watch'], and נסתר ['hide'], 31.49). The phrase 'to see the face' is found again just before Jacob's reunion with Esau. Jacob sends a gift in advance of the meeting between the brothers, and says, 'I may appease (אכפרה פניו) him with the present that goes before me, and afterwards I shall *see his face* (אראה פניו); perhaps he will accept me (literally: "my face", פני). So the present passed on before him; and he himself lodged that *night* in the camp' (32.20-21). The gift was intended to prepare the ground for the meeting with Esau.[56] In the same night the struggle between Jacob and the man takes place; at its conclusion Jacob declared that he had *seen* God *face to face*, and his life was preserved (32.30). Further on, in the course of the meeting between the brothers, there is a reference to the struggle between Jacob and the man, 'for truly *to see your face* is like *seeing the face* of God, with such favour have you received me' (33.10). Jacob compares the two incidents, and it appears that the meeting with the man of

55. It is not unusual for a particular phrase which is part of a semantic field and bears important meanings connected with that field to recur frequently. Balentine's discussion of the field of Hiding leads him to focus on the phrase הסתר פנים (hide one's face) in the divine context. The hiding of God's face is central to his thematic discussion (Balentine, *The Hidden God*).

56. There is a similar root in Akkadian, *kapāru(m)*, one of whose meanings is 'to spread' or 'to oil' (*CAD*, K, pp. 178-79).

God constituted a sort of psychological preparation for the real meeting between the two brothers. Jacob refers to the meeting with Esau as though he had seen God's face, and God wanted him.

In the story of Judah and Tamar the SF appears, as we have seen above. Although the combination 'to see the face' is not found there, its opposite, to hide the face (כסה פנים), does appear. Tamar waits for Judah in the entrance to Enaim on the way to Timnah with her face covered (38.15). Her stratagem succeeds as a result of her covering her face, which is an act of deception.

The phrase 'to see the face' leads directly to the very centre of the Joseph Narrative, and connects the history of Jacob with that of Joseph. In order to complete the picture, I shall continue to follow the occurrences of the phrase in the Joseph Narrative, even though I have not yet discussed the narrative itself in terms of the overall theme of sight. When Joseph first meets his brothers he abuses them, and does not expose his identity immediately nor after a while.[57] He keeps Simeon with him as a hostage, and the dialogue between the SF and that of Oral Communication (of which hearing is part) is continued in this section.[58] Joseph makes the release of Simeon conditional on his brothers' returning to Egypt and showing him their young brother Benjamin. When Judah tells his father Jacob of this condition, his words contain the phrase 'see the face': 'But Judah said to him, "The man solemnly warned us, saying, 'You shall not *see my face*, unless your brother is with you"' (43.3, see also v. 5).

When the brothers meet Joseph for the second time, he threatens that this time he will keep Benjamin with him. Judah begs that their young brother be not left with Joseph. In his speech Judah reminds Joseph of his earlier demand, repeating the phrase: 'Then you said to your servants, "Unless your youngest brother comes down with you, you shall *see my face* (לראות פני) no more"' (44.23). Judah tells Joseph that they have passed this demand on to their father, 'for we may not *see* (לראות פני) the man's *face* unless our youngest brother is with us' (44.26).

At 46.30 Jacob declares that, for him, seeing his lost son's face closes the circle of mourning: 'Now let me die, since I have *seen* your *face* (ראותי את־פניך), and know you are still alive'. After Jacob has blessed his son Joseph, he again speaks of the sight of Joseph's face as the essence of his

57. Polliack explains Joseph's sardonic accusation of the brothers (42.9) as a manifestation of his being in a state of 'altered consciousness', which is characteristic of post-trauma (Meira Polliack, 'Joseph's Trauma: Memory and Resolution', in Brenner and Polak [eds.], *Performing Memory*, pp. 72-105 [79]).

58. Here I am referring to the connection between the name Simeon שמעון and the verb שמע (to hear), from which it derives (see the discussion §3.4.1 in which שמע as a constituent in the name Ishmaelites is connected to the field of Oral Communication).

life: 'And Israel said to Joseph, "I had not thought *to see your face* (ראה פניך); and lo, God has let me see (הראה) your children also"' (48.11).

An examination of the verses in which the phrase ראה פנים (to see the face) occurs shows that in most cases there are differences in status between him who sees and him whose face is seen. In general the status of the one whose face is seen is the higher. None can actually see the face of God and survive. This can also be seen in places where this phrase occurs outside Genesis. In Exod. 33.20 God says to Moses, 'You cannot *see my face* (לראת את־פני); for man shall not see me, and live'. We also find, 'Then I will take away my hand, and you shall see my back; but my *face shall not be seen* (ופני לא יראו)' (Exod. 33.23). Moreover, God demands that when Israel will come to him on the three major festivals their hands shall not be empty: 'none shall *appear before me* (literally: "my face shall not be seen") empty handed' (Exod. 23.15).

Apart from 'seeing the face' alluding to God, it is generally the king whose face may be seen. At Exod. 10.28 Pharaoh says to Moses, 'Get away from me; take heed to yourself; never *see my face* again (אל־תסף ראות פני); for in the day you *see my face* (ראתך פני) you shall die'. To which Moses replies, 'I will not *see your face* (ראות פניך) again' (Exod. 10.29). The brothers' seeing the face of Joseph is another example of this type of sight. And, similarly, David says to Abner: 'You shall not *see my face* unless you first bring Michal, Saul's daughter, when you come to *see my face*' (2 Sam. 3.13).

From the occurrence of this phrase in Jeremiah it appears that a special function in the king's court was reserved for men called 'those who see the king's face': 'And from the city he took an officer who had been in command of the men of war, and seven men of the king's council (literally: "men who see the king's face" [מראי פני־המלך]), who were found in the city; and the secretary of the commander of the army who mustered the people of the land…' (Jer. 52.25). It may be noted that the office-holders, among whom were those 'who see the king's face', are distinguished from the 'sixty men of the people of the land who were found in the midst of the city', mentioned at the end of the same verse.

In short, the phrase ראה פנים, to see the face, generally appears in a context in which lower-class persons see the face of a member of a higher class: more exactly—subjects can see the face of the king. God sets himself apart in that he does not allow mortals to see him and survive (Exod. 33.20, 23). God allots the seeing of the face to the relationships between humans and kings, while he himself is characterized by the hiding of his face.[59] This

59. Balentine (*The Hidden God*, 1983) discusses the hiding of the face of God in the different genres of the Hebrew Bible. His discussion contains an extensive consideration of the phrase הסתר + פנים (hide + face) in the divine context.

process begins in Genesis, and concludes with the divine pronouncement on this matter in Exodus 33. It may be added that in Akkadian the phrase *pān(ī) dagālu(m)* (to see the face) is interpreted in certain contexts as 'to obey'.[60]

As for the texts in which the status of neither the one seeing nor the one seen is mentioned, we may argue from the general to the particular. When the biblical narrator writes 'Jacob saw the face of Laban' (my translation, Gen. 31.2), it may be inferred that on this occasion Jacob's status is lower, and during his stay in Laban's house Laban did not relate to him as an equal. And indeed, when they meet after Jacob has left Laban's house, Laban emphasizes his superiority, saying: 'It is in my power to do you harm' (31.29; cf. v. 43).

Jacob's status is also lower than that of Esau when they meet. Jacob, as we have seen above, is the one who *sees* his brother's face (32.10), rather than the opposite. As for the relations between Joseph and his brothers, we may note that Joseph himself does not use the phrase 'to see the face', though Judah does so in his speech (44.23-24). This may hint at the brothers' feelings of inferiority to Joseph the high official.

Finally, as we have seen, Jacob's life is focused on his last sight of the face of his son. In this final father–son scene, we may say that Jacob is the inferior party, since he is described as the one who *sees the face* of his son (46.30; 48.11). This accords with the interpretation of Joseph's dream of greatness at the beginning of his narrative, in which he sees the sun, the moon, and eleven stars bowing down to him (37.9-10). Thus, in the final meeting between Jacob and Joseph, Joseph's dreams come true, and the use of the phrase 'to see the face' reveals the difference in status between the two.

4.7.1. *Concluding the Jacob Narrative*

Summing up the events of the Jacob Narrative from the viewpoint of the sight theme, we can firstly say that a significant turning point in the plot involves the chief character making an explicit declaration of his fear of and belief in God; this is expressed after Jacob wakes from his sleep in ch. 28, and in the calling of the place 'Bethel'. From that moment onwards, God appears not in a direct revelation but through dreams, in night visions, through a camp (32.2-3), and as an anonymous man (Penuel, ch. 32). This is, therefore, a turning-point not only in the Jacob Narrative but also in the book of Genesis. From this point on God gradually adopts hidden operations, until, in the story of Joseph, he is present by the sending of symbolic dreams. Since God's actions take place according to his own plan, and he retreats gradually behind the scenes, the SF is expressed mainly in the

60. *CAD*, D, pp. 23-24.

context of human relationships. From here onwards lexemes of sight express visual contacts between human beings—Jacob and Esau, Jacob and Laban, Laban in the search for his *teraphim*, Leah and Rachel.

The diverse and consistent usage of Sight lexemes at key points in the individual episodes creates a coherent network that covers the entire Jacob Narrative, thus contributing to the description of the gradual development in Jacob's personality, as well as to the development detected in the surrounding characters. The overarching theme of the Jacob Narrative is how Jacob and the other characters develop their ability to see and perceive each other and God. Surprisingly, Jacob and Laban are the only characters in this narrative cycle who achieve a high level of sight, that is, God reveals himself to both, and both eventually admit of his providence. However, while Laban lacks the sensitivity to see and perceive his family members, Jacob gradually develops his ability to see in the human sphere. Jacob starts off with no sign of sight directed toward God or his brother,[61] but as the narrative unfolds he shows awareness of God, continues to develop the sensitivity to observe and perceive his wives, his flock, Laban, and finally his brother—in that order. Nevertheless, we may argue whether Jacob's developing sensitivity toward his family members is maintained in the story of Dinah and when sending young Joseph to his brothers after he told them about his dreams.

This ability to see the Other is not always developed by the other characters who surround Jacob. Rebekah is strictly characterized by a speech style, that is, the SF does not dominate in her story. Isaac's sight dims in his old age, which gives space for the senses of touch, taste, smell, and some hearing to take place.

Esau's sight is directed towards his father; although at the end he sees Jacob's women and children, and hugs and kisses his brother; yet, there is no sign of Esau reaching a high level of sight. This is also true of Leah and Rachel, who direct their sight almost exclusively toward each other; of Reuben, who finds the mandrakes, which leads to sexual relations between his mother and Jacob; and of Dinah, who goes to *see* the women of the Land, sight which ended with her rape.

In short, in the Jacob Narrative Jacob himself attains sight at its highest level; this is the turning-point in the narrative and in the book of Genesis. Jacob also experiences sight in the human sphere. Uniquely, he succeeds in combining the two sight modes when, upon uniting with Esau, he sees the face of God in the face of his brother. By contrast, most of the characters

61. Note that in ch. 31 Laban seeks the *teraphim* without success: he is looking for a material symbol of the divine, and this is the opposite of the fourth and highest level of sight.

round him enact lower-level types of seeing, which are not connected with the sight of God. This does not include Laban, who does acknowledge God, but fails to see and understand his close family members.

4.8. *The Joseph Narrative*

In the Joseph Narrative (Gen. 37–50) we see a further distancing of divine activity from human life. In this section God works behind the scenes until he is revealed only in Joseph's explicit declarations, or in a number of observations by the narrator. However, not only the semantic field of Sight is prominent in the Joseph Narrative, but rather Sight and Oral Communication reappear at key points and contribute to the overall theme of the narrative.[62]

Chapter 37, which is the beginning of the Joseph Narrative, tells of the friction between Joseph and his brothers, which leads the brothers to leave him in the pit and sell him to the Ishmaelites. This chapter has been analyzed in detail in §3.4.1 and I shall therefore summarize some of the points essential for the general discussion. The beginning of the narrative describes Jacob's special love for Joseph, the child of his old age. The brothers' jealousy is aroused when their father makes a *long-sleeved tunic* (כתנת פסים), and the bothers *see* in the sensory-visual sense that their father prefers him to them (37.4). The lexeme 'tunic', which belongs to the SF, is considered by many scholars to be a central motif connecting between the different individual stories of the Joseph Narrative.[63]

The brothers' hatred for Joseph grows stronger as a result of the content of Joseph's dreams, and of the fact that he told them about the dreams. The dreaming of the dreams and the discussion about them have aroused hatred toward him. The sound resemblance between אלומה (sheave), the symbol in Joseph's second dream, and the verb אלם (to be silent), which is constructed of the same consonants as 'sheave', connects between the SF and the field of Oral Communication. I have also shown how the ideas of sight and speech are echoed in the names of Judah, Reuben, the Ishmaelites and the Midianites.

Matters connected with identification, concealment and revelation of identity constitute an aspect of the SF which returns often in the story of Joseph, first appearing in ch. 37. After Joseph has been sold to the Ishmaelites the brothers dip his robe in the blood of a kid which they have killed, and ask their father to *recognize* it, that is, to identify it as Joseph's: 'and

62. The discussion here is based on my earlier study, 'Semantic Fields'.

63. See Matthews, 'The Anthropology of Clothing', pp. 25-36, and J.R. Huddlestun, 'Divestiture, Deception, and Demotion: The Garment Motif in Genesis 37–39', *JSOT* 98 (2002), pp. 47-62.

they sent the *long robe* with sleeves (כתנת הפסים) and brought it to their father, and said, '"This we have found; see now whether it is your son's robe or not". And he *recognized* (ויכירה) it, and said, "It is my son's robe (כתנת)"' (37.32-33). As regards the field of Oral Communication, the brothers are accused of not speaking peaceably to Joseph and plotting his murder. From that point until the reunion between Joseph and the brothers there is no oral communication or visual contact between the parties.

Matters of recognition and identification, which are linked to the SF, are also specially emphasized in the incident following that of the sale of Joseph, the story of Judah and Tamar (Gen. 38; see §3.4.2). In this narrative Judah, one of the main characters, undergoes a process of awakening, and his personal belongings, which identified him, serve to expedite this process.

The plot of the following story, that of Joseph and Potiphar's wife (Gen. 39) is furthered by means of the background details which tell in words of sight that Joseph's master *saw* that God was with him (39.3), that Joseph *found favour in the sight* of his master (39.4). I have shown that Joseph's external characteristics (39.6) led Potiphar's wife to *cast longing eyes* on him, and ask him to lie with her (39.7). Joseph's *garment* (also connected to the SF), which she kept, served as her evidence when she falsely accused Joseph of attempting to lie with her. She tells her side of the story to the guards and to her husband, and in these paragraphs the field of Oral Communication is stressed.

Hence, the fields of Sight and Oral Communication connect the individual stories of the Joseph Narrative. As for the theme of Sight, it is shown to operate between humans, whose sight is at a low level. God is not an explicit visual presence. God protects Joseph, but this is not yet explicitly acknowledged by the human participants.

The scenes described in chs. 40 and 41 are also connected to the theme of sight. In ch. 40 Joseph explains the *dreams* of Pharaoh's servants and in ch. 41 he interprets those of Pharaoh himself. In these chapters we witness Joseph's developing character in terms of insight and oral communication. His experience as a prisoner teaches him that God is responsible for his dreams and their solutions (41.28): 'It is as I *told* (דברתי) Pharaoh, God has *shown* (הראה) to Pharaoh what he is about to do' (also 40.8; 41.16, 25). Once again Oral Communication and Visual Perception act together at a critical juncture in the narrative. Joseph talks about what God has shown him, and understands that God appears in the world in an implicit manner, through symbolic dreams.

In ch. 42, the scene shifts back to Canaan and to Jacob's house. The narrative starts with the Hebrew verb of seeing, ראה, denoting here abstract vision, and is translated as follows: 'When Jacob *learned* (וַיַּרְא) that there was grain in Egypt, he said to his sons, "Why do you keep *looking at one another* (תתראו)?"' (42.1). The use of the verb ראה in the hithpael form is unusual and appears only here, and in 2 Kgs 14.8, 11 (= 2 Chron. 25.17, 21). In the latter verses it is a constituent in the idiom נתראה + פנים, denoting aggressive intentions. The use of an unusual form (תתראו) of this common verb in Gen. 42.1 stresses the special function of the SF in the narrative.

The narrator is not satisfied with reporting that Jacob saw that there was grain in Egypt (42.1); this is repeated by Jacob in the succeeding verse: '"I have *heard*", he *said*, "that there is grain in Egypt; go down and buy grain for us there, that we may live and not die"' (42.2). Seeing and hearing are mentioned here side by side, at the strategic point of the opening of the episode: Sight and Speech continue to predominate throughout the history of Joseph's family.[64]

Next, ten of Joseph's brothers go down to Egypt to get food for the starving family (42.4). When the brothers stand in front of Joseph, now an Egyptian governor, they bow before him with their face to the ground. The text tells that Joseph *sees* them, and *recognizes* them, but decides to act as a stranger (42.7). This verse makes use of no fewer than three Sight terms: וַיַּרְא (he saw), וַיַּכִּרֵם (recognized them), and its cognate, ויתנכר (treated them like strangers, unknown to him). The verb הכיר ('to recognize') belongs to the SF in the broad sense, and in this scene we meet cognitive perception as well as visual perception. The same verb occurs twice more in the following verse (ויכר, הכרהו, 42.8). Although Joseph has recognized his brothers, he talks to them harshly, accusing them of being spies coming to *see* the *nakedness* of the land (ערות הארץ, 42.9). The Hebrew term ערוה ('nakedness') is a derivative of the root ערה which carries the meaning of exposing (e.g. Isa. 3.17).[65] It is this meaning of the root that connects the lexeme ערוה ('nakedness') to the SF.

Then, Joseph commands that they leave one brother behind while the rest return to Canaan and bring the young Benjamin. After that, he promises, he will believe their claims. The brothers talk among themselves about this proposition, a discussion that is crucial to understanding the theme of the story: 'They *said* (ויאמרו) to one another, "Alas, we are paying the penalty for what we did to our brother; we *saw* (ראינו) his anguish when he *pleaded* (בהתחננו) with us, but we *would not listen* (ולא שמענו)"' (Gen. 42.21). The main problem of the narrative is explicitly presented right here, and it is related to Sight and Oral communication; in this rare confession, the relationship between the two fields becomes evident as regards the brothers: they admit that they *saw* his distress but *would not listen* to him.

64. See also Frisch, 'שמע and ראה as a Pair of *Leitwörter*', pp. 89-98 (Hebrew).
65. *HALOT*, pp. 881-82.

Seeing and hearing are dominant in the following passage as well. Reuben, whose name represents the sense of sight, speaks: 'Did I *not tell* (הלוא אמרתי) you not to wrong the boy? But you *would not listen* (ולא שמעתם). So now there comes a reckoning for his blood' (42.22).

At this point, Joseph turns away from them and weeps (ויבך, 42.24); the sounds of weeping are connected to the field of Oral Communication. But Joseph does not want his brothers to hear these sounds, at least not yet. Instead, he returns and *speaks* to them, picking Simeon and binding him before their *eyes* (42.24). The name Simeon stems from the root שמע, 'to hear', which is fundamental in the field of Oral Communication. The 'eyes' mentioned in this verse are connected to the SF. Joseph's selection of Simeon is a symbolic act, as he is trying to punish all the brothers for not hearing his voice so long ago.

Genesis 43.29 reports that Joseph sees Benjamin, stressing it by the use of the long formulaic expression[66]: 'Then he *looked up and saw* (וישא עיניו וירא) his brother Benjamin, his mother's son'. As to Oral Communication, it is told that Joseph still did not want his crying to be heard by his brothers, which means that the brothers are not ready yet, from Joseph's point of view, to recognize their sin of not hearing him: 'With that, Joseph hurried out, because he was overcome with affection for his brother, and he was about *to weep*. So he went into a private room and *wept* there' (Gen. 43.30). The text continues stressing Joseph's calculated restraint: 'Then he washed his face and came out; and controlling himself he said, "Serve the meal"' (v. 31). The 'face' (פניו) is a peripheral constituent in the SF, since the eyes are in the face and by part–whole relations the face can represent the eyes, as for instance in Isa. 5.21 (§2.7).

Genesis 43 and 44 continue and develop the theme of sight through the repetition of the phrase 'to see the face', as I have discussed in §4.7. Genesis 43 is also distinguished by the repetition of the verb ירא ('fear', 43.18, 23), which is a constituent in the SF. Joseph's brothers fear him, and the fact that they are brought to his house alarms them. The brothers' fear is not the fear of God; they are still at a low level of sight.

In Judah's last speech in front of Joseph, in which he asks him first, 'let your servant please *speak a word* in my lord's *ears*...' (44.18), Judah is willing, for the first time, to see and feel empathy for his father's distress. This is expressed with a term from the SF: 'For how can I go back to my father if the boy is not with me? I fear *to see* (פן אראה) the suffering that would come upon my father' (44.34). At this point Joseph is willing to cry in front of the brothers: 'And *he wept so loudly* that the Egyptians *heard* it, and

66. On formulaic expressions in the Hebrew Bible, see Polak, 'Linguistic and Stylistic Aspects of Epic Formulae'.

the household of Pharaoh *heard* it' (45.2). In Hebrew a long formula of crying is used, ויתן את־קלו בבכי, which stresses the special event. His loud, emotional reaction contrasts with the brothers' speechlessness when they hear about his identity: 'But his brothers *could not answer* him, so dismayed were they at his presence' (45.3). In 45.12 Visual Perception and Oral Communication are mentioned together by way of eyes and mouth, and apart from the verbs of these fields: 'And now your *eyes* and the *eyes* of my brother Benjamin *see* that it is my own *mouth* that *speaks* to you'. Sounds of crying, the crying of Joseph and Benjamin, are soon heard in 45.14. Verse 15 mentions more crying of Joseph, on his brothers' shoulders, and there is a reference to the brothers' talk this time. The dialogue between Joseph and his brothers begins after a long period of silence. This time, after Judah's confession, the brothers are changed, in that they have come to terms with their responsibility for their father's catastrophe.

Thus the turning point of the entire narrative—the encounter between Joseph and his brothers in Genesis 45, and his confession to them—is formulated in terms of Sight and Oral Communication. Joseph stands face to face before his brothers and reveals his identity now. Terms and expressions from the SF emphasize the difference between Joseph and his brothers on the level of sight, the two sides are not equal in their sight. In this encounter Joseph knows more. Before he confesses the brothers do not know his identity. Joseph is the seeing–knowing party. He is characterized by a higher level of sight, since he reveals to his brothers that God is responsible for the sequence of events as they occurred: 'And now, do not be distressed, or angry with yourselves (ואל־יחר בעיניכם), because you sold me here; for God sent me before you to preserve life' (45.5), 'And God sent me before you to preserve for you a remnant on earth' (45.7); also 'So it was not you who sent me here, but God' (45.8), and similarly, 'God has made me lord of all Egypt' (45.9).[67]

He who had not been heard is now heard crying. The brothers who in ch. 37 refuse to talk peaceably to Joseph now agree to speak to him. The lack of insight and communication at the human level has almost been resolved. Still, the father mentions his need to see the face of his son Joseph before he dies (45.28). This request is very important for fixing the borders of the unit. Westermann, for instance, ends the Joseph Narrative at ch. 45, and according to him ch. 46 onwards mainly belongs to a different cycle, the Jacob

67. Polliack treats the throwing of Joseph into the pit as clinical trauma and the encounter between him and the brothers in ch. 45 as a recovery from the trauma. Apparently, Joseph telling the story from his point of view (45.5-9) is a crucial part of the recovery process, and his crying signals the stage of giving a voice to what has happened (Polliack, 'Joseph's Trauma', pp. 89-91).

cycle.[68] But the matter of sight arises, links up the end of ch. 45 with the next part of the book, and binds the two parts together. Genesis 46.29-30 describes the meeting of Jacob and Joseph, in the course of which the phrase ראה פנים ('to see the face') appears. The seeing of the face at the time of the renewed encounter between the father and his son is a very significant factor in the life of Jacob, as I have shown in the previous paragraphs, and it is reminiscent of the encounter between Jacob and the angel (Gen. 32.30), and the meeting of reconciliation between Jacob and Esau (Gen. 33.10), two other encounters which were turning-points in Jacob's history.

In Genesis 48, in which Jacob blesses Joseph's sons, matters of sight are again emphasized. Jacob blesses Joseph's sons, relying on God's *appearance* to him at Luz in the land of Canaan (48.3). The beginning of the episode of the blessing is marked by an act of sight: 'When Israel *saw* (וירא) Joseph's sons, he said, "Who are these?"' (48.8). After this it becomes clear that Jacob is quite unable to see clearly: 'Now the *eyes* of Israel were dim (ועיני ישׂראל כבדו) with age, so that *he could not see* (לא יוכל לראות). So Joseph brought them near him…' (48.10). The importance of Jacob's seeing Joseph's face is again mentioned in 48.11. When Joseph *sees* that his father puts his right hand on the head of Ephraim, his younger son, instead of that of Manasseh, his firstborn, he tries to remove his hand and put it on Manasseh's head. Jacob refuses, and says: 'I *know*, my son, I *know* (ידעתי בני ידעתי). He also shall become a people, and he also shall be great; nevertheless his younger brother shall be greater than he, and his descendants shall become a multitude of nations' (48.19). That is to say, in his old age Jacob has no great powers of sensory-visual perception, but he is well endowed with cognitive sight. In this incident, Jacob blesses Joseph's sons, and thereby expresses sight at its highest level, for he is passing on the word of God.

Genesis concludes with ch. 50, which describes Joseph's brothers' apprehension that he will take revenge on them after their father's death. But Joseph affirms his trust in God, and reminds them of God's part in the unfolding history of the family. He pacifies his brothers using the verb ירא ('fear'), from the SF: '*Fear* not (אל־תיראו), for am I in the place of God?' (Gen. 50.19). Joseph explains to them that they should not be afraid of him, and, indirectly, that only God should be dreaded and feared. Lexemes of the CPF, which is close to the SF, are used: 'As for you, you *meant* (חשׁבתם) evil against me; but God *meant* (חשׁבה) it for good… So do not *fear* (אל־תיראו)' (50.20, 21).

68. Westermann, *Genesis 37–50*, pp. 22-25.

Oral Communication also plays an important part in Genesis 50. It opens with the weeping and mourning of Joseph and the Egyptians over the death of Jacob (50.1-3). Joseph weeps when his brothers speak to him (Gen. 50.17). He *comforts* them and *speaks* kindly to them (50.21).

To conclude, the Joseph Narrative is dominated by the fields of Sight and Oral Communication intertwining at critical turning points, and frequently highlighted by special semantic and rhetorical effects. This consistent and unique constellation of occurrences has a thematic value in the human and divine spheres. In the Joseph Narrative God ceases to play a visible central role, and withdraws to behind the scenes. He never again appears to Joseph, the main character in the section, face to face, as he has appeared in the patriarchal narratives; God pulls strings, and functions indirectly. This is also the reason why the field of Oral Communication comes to the front of the stage, and emphasizes this theme in addition to the SF. Speech takes place only on the human level, and God chooses to pass on his blessing through Jacob (Gen. 48 and 49).

Indirect divine activity is emphasized in the recognition that it is God who is responsible for the interpretation of Joseph's dreams. Similarly, it is he who is responsible, as I have pointed out, for Joseph's success in the house of Potiphar, and Potiphar *sees* this (39.3), as does the warder of the prison (39.23). The clearest expression of the change in God's appearance in the world—from an open partner to a hidden supervisor—is that after the encounter between the brothers in Genesis 45 he speaks to Jacob for the last time 'in the *visions of the night*' (במראת הלילה), and no longer through a face-to-face appearance (46.2). Joseph does not experience a direct vision of God, and he has no dreams of such a vision, as had Jacob.

As to the human sphere, the intertwining of the dominant semantic fields of Sight and Oral Communication calls our attention to the development of the characters of Joseph and his brothers. As the story begins, both Joseph and his brothers are cast in a negative light with regard to sight and speech. Joseph dreams of being in a position of superiority over his family and tells his brothers about his dreams. The brothers hate him because of his dreams and his talk. They do not hear his pleading when he is thrown into the pit. The symbol of the sheaves in his dream, which stems from the root אלם and carries an additional meaning of 'dumbness', may allude to the period in which there was no oral communication between Joseph and his brothers. Only Reuben, whose very name is interrelated with sight, has behaved positively in his attempt to save Joseph. Reuben might have served as a role model for his brothers, but they chose not to follow. Other character names also play a symbolic role: Judah, whose name is connected to the field of Oral Communication, contrives to kill his brother, and the Midianites and Ishmaelites, who are also connected by name to this field, stress the negative communication path toward which Joseph and his brothers are heading. As to the divine plane, God is absent from this scene and from the participants' cognition, at least in the explicit sense.

The appearance of lexemes of Sight and Oral Communication at turning points is regular and consistent in every one of the episodes, including Genesis 38 and 39. As the story progresses, we witness the development of Joseph's personality, through his growing recognition of, and faith in, God. The hidden presence of God is illustrated by dreams which are related to the SF. Simeon, whose name contains the verb 'to hear', is taken as a prisoner by Joseph also as a symbolic indication that the brothers should have listened to his plea. Genesis 45 presents a critical turning point in the story, when Joseph stands before his brothers and reveals his identity. This is an episode which is all about Sight and Talk. Suddenly Joseph, whom the brothers have not heard, is crying loudly. In ch. 37, the brothers refused to talk to Joseph in a peaceable manner, but now they speak to him, in addition to seeing him face to face. In accordance with the theme of sight and communication, there is now a more positive relationship between Joseph and his brothers: for the first time they see him for what he is, and carry on a peaceful dialogue with him.

Nevertheless, the issue of sight and speech between the brothers and God has not yet found its full resolution. At the end of Genesis Joseph is conscious of divine providence acting behind the scenes, but it seems that his brothers, who are also the ancestors of ancient Israel, do not yet recognize the hidden supremacy of God. Therefore Joseph has to explain to them that God will *remember* (פקד יפקד) them and bring them up from the land of Egypt to the land of Canaan (Gen. 50.24-25). In Genesis, Jacob's sons, who will in the future become the tribes of Israel, do not experience the sight and fear of God. Hence, we may conclude that for them, the process of seeing is not yet complete. The intense experiences of Sight and Oral Communication continue to evolve in the first part of the book of Exodus, whose climax is the revelation on Mount Sinai, as the descendants of Joseph and his brothers—now the people of Israel—see and hear sounds of the Divine: 'Now when all the people *perceived* (רֹאִים) the *thunderings* (הַקּוֹלֹת) and the *lightnings* (הַלַּפִּידִם) and the *sound* (קוֹל) of the *trumpet* (שֹׁפָר) and the mountain smoking, the people were *afraid* (וַיַּרְא) and trembled; and they stood afar off' (Exod. 20.18).

Chapter 5

Conclusions: Divine Sight Gives Way to Human Sight in Genesis

I have argued above that lexemes from the SF appear at strategic points in various plots, and thus contribute to the cohesion of the individual narratives. The findings have shown that words from the SF were consistently found in openings, at turning-points, in events triggering the central occurrence in the text, and as background details in place-names and personal names. Following this, I went on to examine the occurrence of the field in individual stories, and the implications for the interpretation of the stories' theme. Since the analyses of the individual narratives were centred on small units, they enabled us to examine the clauses and their components more closely. They showed that both sound patterns and semantic resemblances contribute to the prominence of lexemes from the field.

After establishing the role of the semantic field in the individual stories, it was possible to proceed to an overview of the four main sections of Genesis. It was shown how the theme of Sight recurs constantly throughout them, and contributes to an overall coherence of the book. We saw how it shapes the history of major and secondary characters, traits of characters, and outward appearance. Thus, the words of the SF serve to create cohesion between the clauses of the text, and they also sustain the unifying theme of Genesis by virtue of their prominence at strategic points in the individual plots and macro-plot.

From a literary point of view, this investigation into the SF in Genesis has revealed a line of development moving between spheres that eventually meet: seeing on the human sphere and seeing on the divine sphere.

From the primeval times and the beginning of humankind God himself undergoes processes of sight and insight, that is, visual and cognitive perception, and is explicitly presented as an active participant in his world. As the sections of Genesis progress, God gradually becomes a hidden director of human behaviour; his active and explicit presence is felt less and less, and in the story of Joseph his implicit actions are expressed mainly by means of declarations by Joseph himself (Gen. 45.7). The first section of Genesis tells of divine and human sight. God focuses on seeing the beings he has created, in an attempt to learn about them and their behaviour in order to know how to act towards them. At the end of the Flood story he understands that the inclination of the humans is evil from their youth, and at the end of the section, in the story of the Tower of Babel, God sees the behaviour of humans and decides to confuse their languages.

Human sight in Genesis 1–11 is seeing at its lowest levels. Humans engage in the visual perception of the world around them, and their insights are also connected with sensory sight, and not with more exalted views of the world connected with belief in God. For example, Adam and Eve see that they are naked (3.7), at the end of the Flood Noah perceives that the surface of the ground is dry (8.13), and Noah's son sees his father's nakedness (9.22). As the book progresses, we recognize an increase in the number of utterances of sight which show growing awareness on the part of human beings. Furthermore, visual perception becomes more and more abstract and related to God by some of the characters. As we have seen, the theme of sight also appears in the narratives concerning secondary characters, and they are thereby included in the thematic development of Genesis.

In the section of the Abraham narratives God is engaged in the observation of Abraham, the one he has chosen, in such a way that the history of Abraham is characterized by a series of trials imposed by God. From the point of view of visual perception, Abraham is passive, and it is usually God who demonstrates and recognizes Abraham's faith. In two of the climaxes of this section, Genesis 15 (God's Promise and Covenant) and Genesis 22 (the sacrifice of Isaac), God sees that Abraham believes in him. Yet the narrator does not attribute to Abraham an explicit declaration of his fear of God;[1] there is, therefore, a certain degree of lack of clarity in relation to Abraham's level of sight. In other words, Abraham's insight is not represented in an unequivocal expression of faith. An explicit declaration by a character, that he/she recognizes God's presence, takes place in the Abraham section at the time when Hagar calls God *El Roi* ('God of sight', 16.13). According to this text, Hagar experiences sight at a high level.

In the following section, that of the Jacob narrative, in Genesis 28 Jacob experiences sight at a high level, when he awakes from his dream and declares that he knows of God's presence. From the middle of the Jacob narrative (ch. 31) God's explicit intervention in the affairs of humans becomes rare. The spotlight naturally focuses on relations between humans, and the phrase פנים + ראה ('to see the face') often constitutes a bridge between key episodes. Throughout this section Jacob experiences no more direct revelations. Nevertheless, God is revealed in a dream (ch. 31), in the form of a camp (32.1-3), in the form of an unidentified man (the struggle in Penuel, 32.22-32), and in nocturnal visions (46.2). The Jacob stories are

1. See the discussion concerning 'And he *believed* in Yhwh' (Gen. 15.6) in §4.5.

designed in such a way that the combination of different senses carries special weight, and emphasizes the depiction of Isaac as a sensual character in comparison with Jacob. As we have seen, in the story of the theft of the blessing (ch. 27), the sense of hearing (and speech), the sense of touch, and the senses of taste and smell are all active in Isaac. Rebekah's actions are dominated by the field of Oral Communication. Nonetheless, the other senses serve to emphasize the dominant role of Visual Perception in Jacob's life. Seeing attests to Jacob's belief in God, after God is revealed to him (ch. 28). After that Jacob is changed, and his developing ability to perceive others leads him to turn into a better man.

In the story of Joseph God does not reveal himself to humans. The relations between God and the hero, Joseph, are no longer established by God's appearance face to face in front of the main character. In the episode concerning Joseph's confession to his brothers, he admits several times that God was responsible for his ascent to greatness, and the saving of his family, and repeats this at the end of the narrative: 45.7-8; 50.20. Thus Joseph reaches the highest level of sight, since, although God's activity is hidden from sight, Joseph fears him. Divine activity is expressed in indirect communication, by means of symbolic dreams which are not dreams of revelation. Divine activity is also expressed at the level of speech, and in Jacob's blessing of Joseph's sons when his eyes are dim and his sight impaired. Joseph's level of sight is exalted, since he has seen and understood that God has adopted concealed activity; in this respect he differs from his brothers, who do not declare openly that they fear God until the end of Genesis. As I remarked at the end of my analysis of the Joseph narrative, the climax of the processes of sight which Jacob's sons—who later on develop into the Israelite nation—undergo is at the revelation of Mount Sinai in Exodus 20 (§4.8). In this episode the fields of Sight and Oral Communication function in concert, when Israel *sees* the divine *sounds* and draws away from the mountain because of its holiness (Exod. 20.18). Only there do they accept God and acknowledge their faith in him. At this point the fields of Sight and Oral Communication appear together in harmony, celebrating an event in which God is simultaneously seen and hidden, and Israel sees and hears, but takes care to keep physical distance. In the course of this event Israel is given God's Law, and here the process which we have traced from the beginning of Genesis reaches its conclusion.

Through all this, the theme of sight peculiar in Genesis is manifested. In the prophetic writings the concealment of God's face is conceived of as punishment for man's behaviour.[2] This is not so in Genesis. The theme of sight as seen in Genesis reveals a gradual process, in which God is interested in finding a chosen character with whom he can make a covenant, and

2. Balentine, *The Hidden God*, p. 164.

spread the notion of faith in God among humans. From the days of the Flood God adopts concealed activity of his own will, not as a rebuke for human beings, but rather as a consequence of God's close observation of their natural tendencies, and with an intention to allow more Sight between them. The above consideration of the phrase ראה + פנים, which begins to appear in the Jacob narrative, supports this conclusion. Apart from enhancing the cohesiveness of the narratives, it is shown that 'seeing the face' is confined to humans. The subject seeing belongs to a lower status than the one whose face is seen, and it is always an interaction occurring between humans, never with God. We may find justification for this explanation at Exod. 33.20. In this verse God acknowledges to Moses that 'You cannot see my face; for man shall not see me and live', and in 33.23 that 'Then I will take away my hand, and you shall see my back; but my face shall not be seen'. Beginning from the final section of Genesis, God retreats behind the scenes of his own will, in order to leave the arena to human beings rather than because of a desire to punish them.

Another significant feature established through the SF is connected with the construction of the characters of the Matriarchs. Sarah, Rebekah and Rachel are linked to the SF because of their beauty: Sarah is described as 'a woman beautiful to behold' (יפת־מראה, Gen. 12.11), Rebekah as 'fair to look upon' (טובת מראה, 26.7), and Rachel as 'beautiful and lovely' (יפת־תאר ויפת מראה, 29.17). These three matriarchs do not play an active role regarding divine sight. Hagar's case is unlike that of the other matriarchs, since no mention is made of her external appearance. But in fact, as we have seen, she attains a high-level sight. God is revealed to her (through an angel), and she speaks of the visual encounter between them.

In addition to these women, Leah is also described in 29.17 by terms of sight. She is not described as beautiful to behold, rather as having 'tender' eyes (KJV; the RSV has 'weak' eyes; the Hebrew reads ועיני לאה רכות). Her ability to see is hinted at here, but it is unclear whether the text signifies the external appearance of her eyes, or whether a trait of character is meant. Be that as it may, God sees that she is hated and opens her womb, and she bears *Reuben*, 'for she said, "because Yhwh has *looked upon* my affliction"' (29.32). Leah's relationship with God is expressed through her naming of her sons. This is also true of Rachel.

The question of Joseph's beauty also merits discussion, since he is described, like his mother, as 'handsome and good-looking' (39.6; cf. 29.17). Although Joseph is a male, his outward characteristics are described in terms similar to those of the matriarchs. But, unlike Sarah, Rebekah and Rachel, Joseph experiences sight at its highest level, when he explicitly recognizes God's hidden activity in the world. When Flavius Josephus tells the story of Joseph and Potiphar's wife he speaks of Joseph's 'blind faith' in God:

> Now Joseph, commending all his affairs to God, did not betake himself to make his defence, nor to give an account of the exact circumstances of the fact, but silently underwent the bonds and the distress he was in, firmly believing that God, who knew the cause of his affliction, and the truth of the fact, would be more powerful than those that inflicted the punishments upon him.[3]

Thus, among the matriarchs whoever was described as beautiful did not experience the revelation of God, whereas Hagar, whose beauty is not mentioned, experiences the highest level of sight. She who is described as 'soft-eyed' bears a son in whose name divine sight is hinted at (Reuben). Joseph, the male, is granted external beauty, but reaches the highest level of sight.[4]

This complex investigation shows that the SF indeed consistently occurs at key points in the individual stories of Genesis, and throughout its broader sections as well. It connects texts that are by many interpreters considered secondary in Genesis (e.g. Gen. 38), and it runs through distant texts sharing similar motifs, such as the beauty of the matriarchs. In addition, from the point of view of the Documentary Hypothesis, it appears in all of the sources. In the view of all that has been said I wish to conclude that the use of the SF is part of the redactor's scheme, and not merely a device limited to a reader's interpretation.

But the investigation of semantic fields in Genesis does not end here. The present study has focussed on the SF, which contributes to the coherence of Genesis in that it is prominent in the book and emphasizes its theme. This analysis will be completed, however, only when it reveals of which other semantic fields the book is constituted, and how meaningful they are in relation to the SF. Thus, for instance, the dialogue between the SF and the occurrence of lexemes from the fields of the other senses, of hearing, touch, taste and smell, is extremely interesting.[5] I have already shown an example of a dialogue between the SF and the field of Oral Communication in the Joseph narrative and in the analysis of the story of the Tower of Babel. This dialogue is expressed as early as the opening of Genesis, when God creates the world by his pronouncements. Preambles such as 'After these *things* (דברים: "things" or "words") the *word of* Yhwh came to Abram in a *vision*' (Gen. 15.1) are connected with this. We have seen an example of the

3. Josephus, *Ant.* 2.60 (in Josephus, *Complete Works* [trans. William Whiston; Grand Rapids: Kregel Publications, 1978]).

4. The biblical narrator says nothing about the external appearance of Potiphar's wife. This gap is filled in post-biblical literature by a description of her looks: 'For when I was in her house she was wont to bare her arms, and breasts, and legs, that I might lie with her; for she was very beautiful, splendidly adorned in order to beguile me. And the Lord guarded me from her devices' (*Testament of Joseph* 9.5, in Charles [ed.], *The Apocrypha and Pseudepigrapha of the Old Testament*, II).

5. On the senses in the Old Testament see Avrahami, *The Senses of Scripture*.

intertwining of other senses in Genesis 27. It should, therefore, be further considered in what context each of the senses is emphasized. These findings should be compared with those relating to the SF, and thereby a more complete picture of the contribution of the SF to the unity of Genesis will be attained. Nevertheless, this work is an example of a kind of a reading that is attentive to the semantic fields of literary texts. It shows that uncovering a dominant semantic field can illuminate the way to a better understanding of its inner structure and overarching theme.

Bibliography

Abou-Assaf, A., P. Bordreuil and A.R. Millard, *La statue de Tell Fekheriye et son inscription bilingue assyro-araméenne* (Etudes assyriologiques, 7; Paris: Editions recherches sur la civilisation, 1982).

Ahuvia, Abraham, 'סנורים = The Covering of the Eyes' (Hebrew), *Tarbiṣ* 39 (1970), pp. 90-92.

Alter, R., *The Art of Biblical Narrative* (New York: Basic Books, 1981).

—*Genesis: Translation and Commentary* (New York: W.W. Norton, 1996).

Amit, Yairah, *The Book of Judges: The Art of Editing* (trans. Jonathan Chipman; Leiden: Brill, 1999).

—'The Function of Topographical Indications in the Biblical Story' (Hebrew), *Shnaton: An Annual for Biblical and Ancient Near Eastern Studies* 9 (1985), pp. 15-30.

—'The Multi-purpose "Leading Word" and the Problems of its Usage', *Prooftexts* 9 (1989), pp. 99-114.

—*Reading Biblical Stories* (Jerusalem: Ministry of Defence, 2000 [Hebrew]).

—'The Repeated Situation: A Poetic Principle in the Modeling of the Joseph', in *In Praise of Editing in the Hebrew Bible: Collected Essays in Retrospect* (trans. Betty Sigler Rozen; Sheffield: Sheffield Phoenix Press, 2012), pp. 70-83.

Aristotle, *Aristotle's Poetics* (trans. Gerald F. Else; Cambridge, MA: Harvard University Press, 1957).

Auerbach, Erich, *Mimesis: The Representation of Reality in Western Literature* (trans. W.R. Trask; Princeton, NJ; Princeton University Press, 2003).

Avrahami, Yael, 'Name Giving to the Newborn in the Hebrew Bible', *These Are the Names: Studies in Jewish Onomastics* 5 (2011), pp. 15-53.

—*The Senses of Scripture: Sensory Perception in the Hebrew Bible* (New York: T. & T. Clark, 2012).

Baden, Joel S., *The Composition of the Pentateuch: Renewing the Documentary Hypothesis* (New Haven: Yale University Press, 2012).

Bal, Mieke, 'Dealing/with/Women: Daughters in the Book of Judges', in Regina M. Schwartz (ed.), *The Book and the Text: The Bible and Literary Theory* (Oxford: Basil Blackwell, 1990), pp. 16-39.

—*Death and Dissymmetry: The Politics of Coherence in the Book of Judges* (Chicago: University of Chicago Press, 1988).

—*Narratology: Introduction to the Theory of Narrative* (Toronto: University of Toronto Press, 1997).

Balentine, Samuel E., *The Hidden God: The Hiding of the Face of God in the Old Testament* (Oxford: Oxford University Press, 1983).

Bar-Efrat, Shimon, *Narrative Art in the Bible* (trans. Dorothea Shefer-Vanson in conjunction with the author; Sheffield: Almond Press, 1989).

Basset, F.W., 'Noah's Nakedness and the Curse of Canaan: A Case of Incest?', *VT* 21 (1971), pp. 232-37.

Bednarek, Monika A., 'Frames Revisited: The Coherence-Inducing Function of Frames', *Journal of Pragmatics* 37 (2005), pp. 685-705.

Ben Yehuda, Eliezer, *A Complete Dictionary of Ancient and Modern Hebrew* (Ben-Yehuda Hozaa-La'Or: Jerusalem, 1948–59 [Hebrew]).

Bergsma, John, and Scott Hahn, 'Noah's Nakedness and the Curse on Canaan', *JBL* 124 (2005), pp. 25-40.

Berlin, Adele, 'Lexical Cohesion and Biblical Interpretation', *Hebrew Studies* 30 (1989), pp. 29-40.

—*Poetics and Interpretation of Biblical Narrative* (Sheffield: Almond Press, 1983).

Berlin, Brent, and Paul Kay, *Basic Color Terms: Their Universality and Evolution* (Berkeley: University of California Press, 1969).

Bertil, Alberktson, 'A Disputed Sense in a Covenant Context: On the Interpretation of Genesis 15:6', in *Covenant as Context: Essays in Honour of E.W. Nicholson* (New York: Oxford University Press, 2003), pp. 1-9.

Beuken, Willem A.M., 'Job's Imprecation as the Cradle of a New Religious Discourse: The Perplexing Impact of the Semantic Correspondences between Job 3, Job 4–5 and Job 6–7', in W.A.M. Beuken (ed.), *The Book of Job* (Leuven: Leuven University Press, 1994), pp. 41-78.

Blenkinsopp, Joseph, 'The Pentateuch', in John Barton (ed.), *The Cambridge Companion to Biblical Interpretation* (Cambridge: Cambridge University Press, 1998), pp. 181-97.

—*The Pentateuch: An Introduction to the First Five Books of the Bible* (New York: Doubleday, 1992).

Blois, Reinier de, with the assistance of Enio R. Mueller, *Semantic Dictionary of Biblical Hebrew* (United Bible Societies 2000–2009), <http://www.sdbh.org/home-en.html>.

Brenner, Athalya, *Colour Terms in the Old Testament* (JSOTSup, 21; Sheffield: JSOT Press, 1982).

—*The Intercourse of Knowledge: On Gendering Desire and 'Sexuality' in the Hebrew Bible* (Leiden: E.J. Brill, 1997).

—'On the Semantic Field of Humour, Laughter and the Comic in the Old Testament', in Y.T. Radday and A. Brenner (eds.), *On Humour and the Comic in the Hebrew Bible* (Sheffield: Almond Press, 1990), pp. 39-58.

Brenner, Athalya, and Frank Polak (eds.), *Performing Memory in Biblical Narrative and Beyond* (The Bible in the Modern World, 25; Sheffield: Sheffield Phoenix Press, 2009).

Buber, Martin, 'Abraham the Seer (Genesis 12–25)', in N.N. Glatzer (ed.), *On the Bible: Eighteen Studies by Martin Buber* (trans. S. Meyer; New York: Schocken Books, 1968 [first published 1939]), pp. 22-43.

—'Leitwort Style in Pentateuch Narrative', in Buber and Rosenzweig (eds.), *Scripture and Translation*, pp. 114-28.

Buber, Martin, and F. Rosenzweig (eds.), *Scripture and Translation* (trans. L. Rosenwald and E. Fox; Bloomington: Indiana University Press, 1994 [first published 1936]).

Bublitz, Wolfram, Uta Lenk and Eija Ventola (eds.), *Coherence in Spoken and Written Discourse: How to Create It and How to Describe It* (Pragmatics and Beyond, 63; Amsterdam: John Benjamins, 1999).

Buckley, Jerome Hamilton, *Season of Youth: The Bildungsroman from Dickens to Golding* (Cambridge, MA: Harvard University Press, 1974).

Burrows, M. (ed.), *The Dead Sea Scrolls of St. Mark's Monastery*. I. *The Isaiah Manuscript and the Habakkuk Commentary* (New Haven: The American Schools of Oriental Research, 1950).

Canale, M., 'From Communicative Competence to Communicative Language Pedagogy', in J.C. Richards and R.W. Schmidt (eds.), *Language and Communication* (London: Longman, 1983), pp. 2-26.

Carr, David McLain, *The Formation of the Hebrew Bible: A New Reconstruction* (New York: Oxford University Press, 2011).

Cassuto, U., *A Commentary on the Book of Genesis* (trans. Israel Abrahams; Jerusalem: Magnes Press, 1965).

—'The Story of Tamar and Judah', in U. Cassuto, *Biblical and Oriental Studies*. I. *Bible* (trans. I. Abrahams; Jerusalem: Magnes Press, 1973 [first published in Hebrew in 1929), pp. 29-40.

Cassuto, U. *et al.*, 'אלון, אלה' (Hebrew), *Encyclopedia Biblica*, I, cols. 294-95.

Charles, R.H. (ed.), *The Apocrypha and Pseudepigrapha of the Old Testament* (Berkeley, CA: Apocryphile Press, 2004).

Chatman, S., *Story and Discourse: Narrative Structure in Fiction and Film* (Ithaca, NY: Cornell University Press, 1978).

Clifford, R.J., 'Genesis 38: Its Contribution to the Jacob Story', *CBQ* 66 (2004), pp. 519-32.

Clines, David J.A., 'The Image of God in Man', *TynBul* 19 (1968), pp. 62-69.

—*Job 1–20* (WBC, 17; Dallas, TX: Word Books, 1989).

—*The Theme of the Pentateuch* (JSOTSup, 10; Sheffield: JSOT Press, 1997).

Croft, W., and D.A. Cruse, *Cognitive Linguistics* (Cambridge: Cambridge University Press, 2004).

Cun, Antonia, 'Coherence in Discourse', *The Scientific Journal of Humanistic Studies* 1 (2009), pp. 62-67.

Dahood, Mitchell, *Psalms: Introduction, Translation, and Notes* (AB, 16-17A; 3 vols.; Garden City, NY: Doubleday, 1966–70).

Dalley, Stephanie, *Myths from Mesopotamia: Creation, the Flood, Gilgamesh, and Others* (Oxford: Oxford University Press, 1989).

Daube, D., *Studies in Biblical Law* (New York: KTAV; Cambridge: Cambridge University Press, 1969 [reprint of 1947]).

Donald, T., 'The Semantic Field of "Folly" in Proverbs, Job, Psalms, and Ecclesiastes', *VT* 13 (1963), pp. 285-92.

Dozeman, Thomas B., Thomas Römer and Konrad Schmid (eds.), *Pentateuch, Hexateuch, or Enneateuch: Identifying Literary Works in Genesis through Kings* (Atlanta, GA: Society of Biblical Literature, 2011).

Dozeman, Thomas B., and Konrad Schmid (eds.), *A Farewell to the Yahwist? The Composition of the Pentateuch in Recent European Interpretation* (Atlanta: Society of Biblical Literature, 2006).

Dozeman, Thomas B., Konrad Schmid and Baruch J. Schwartz, *The Pentateuch: International Perspectives on Current Research* (Tübingen: Mohr Siebeck, 2011).

Driver, S.R., *A Treatise on the Use of the Tenses in Hebrew and Some Other Syntactical Questions* (Oxford: Clarendon Press, 3rd edn, 1969 [first published 1882]).

Dundes, A., *The Morphology of North American Indian Folk Tales* (Helsinki: Suomalainen Tiedeakatemia, 1980).

Embry, Brad, 'The "Naked Narrative" from Noah to Leviticus: Reassessing Voyeurism in the Account of Noah's Nakedness in Genesis 9.22-24', *JSOT* 35 (2011), pp. 417-33.

Ewen, J., *Milon LeMunachei HaSiporet* (Jerusalem: Academon, 1978 [Hebrew]).

Faber, Pamela, and Celia Wallhead, 'The Lexical Field of Visual Perception in *The French Lieutenant's Woman* by John Fowles', *Language and Literature* 4 (1995), pp. 127-44.

Fabry, H.J., 'נחש', in *TDOT*, IX, pp. 356-69.

Fidler, Ruth, *'Dreams Speak Falsely?' Dream Theophanies in the Bible* (Jerusalem: Magnes Press, 2005 [Hebrew]).

Fields, Weston W., *Sodom and Gomorrah: History and Motif in Biblical Narrative* (JSOTSup, 231; Sheffield: Sheffield Academic Press, 1997).

Fokkelman, J.P., 'Genesis', in R. Alter and F. Kermode (eds.), *The Literary Guide to the Bible* (Cambridge, MA: Belknap Press, 1987), pp. 36-55.

—'Genesis 37 and 38 at the Interface of Structural Analysis and Hermeneutic', in L.J. de Regt *et al.* (eds.), *Literary Structure and Rhetorical Strategies in the Hebrew Bible* (Assen: Van Gorcum, 1996), pp. 152-87.

—*Narrative Art in Genesis: Specimens of Structural and Stylistic Analysis* (Assen: Van Gorcum, 1975).

Foster, Benjamin R. (trans. and ed.), *The Epic of Gilgamesh: A New Translation, Analogues, Criticism* (New York: W.W. Norton, 2001).

Freedman, H., and Maurice Simon (trans. and ed.), *Midrash Rabbah* (London: Soncino Press, 1939).

Freytag, Gustav, *Freytag's Technique of the Drama* (trans. Elias J. MacEwan; New York: Johnson Reprint Corp, 1968).

Frisch, Amos, 'שמע and ראה as a Pair of *Leitwörter*' (Hebrew), *Proceedings of the Twelfth World Congress of Jewish Studies: Jerusalem, July 29–August 5 1997* (Jerusalem: World Union of Jewish Studies, 1999), pp. 89-98.

—'The Conveyance of the *Leitwort* in English Translations of the Bible (KJV, JPS, RSV, JB, NAB, NEB, NJPS, NRSV)' (Hebrew), *Studies in Bible and Exegesis* 6 (2002), pp. 235-51.

Galinier, Jacques *et al.*, 'Anthropology of the Night: Cross-Disciplinary Investigations', *Current Anthropology* 51 (2010), pp. 819-47.

Galpaz-Feller, Pnina, *Va' Yoled: Relations between Parents and Children in Biblical Stories and Laws* (Jerusalem: Carmel, 2006 [Hebrew]).

Garsiel, Moshe, *Biblical Names: A Literary Study of Midrashic Derivations and Puns* (trans. Phyllis Hackett; Ramath Gan: Bar-Ilan University Press, 1991).

Geertz, C., *The Interpretation of Cultures* (New York: Basic Books, 1973).

Giora, R., 'Notes Towards a Theory of Text Coherence', *Poetics Today* 6 (1985), pp. 699-715.

Goldingay, J., 'The Patriarchs in Scripture and History', in Millard and Wiseman (eds.), *Essays on the Patriarchal Narratives*, pp. 1-34.

Grandy, Richard E., 'In Defense of Semantic Fields', in E. LePore (ed.), *New Directions in Semantics* (London: Academic Press, 1987), pp. 259-80.

Gunkel, Hermann, *Genesis: übersetzt und erklärt* (Göttingen: Vandenhoeck & Ruprecht, 1966).

—*The Legends of Genesis: The Biblical Saga and History* (intro. by William F. Albright; trans. W.H. Carruth; New York: Schocken Books, 1964 [from the 1901 German edn]).

Guralnik, David B., and Joseph H. Friend (eds.), *Webster's New World Dictionary of the American Language: Encyclopedia Edition* (Cleveland, OH: World Company, 1964).

Habermas, T., and S. Bluck, 'Getting a Life: The Emergence of the Life Story in Adolescence', *Psychological Bulletin* 126 (2000), pp. 748-69.

Halliday, M.A.K., and R. Hasan, *Cohesion in English* (London: Longman, 1976).

—*Language, Context, and Text: Aspects of Language in a Social-Semiotic Perspective* (Oxford: Oxford University Press, 1989).

Hamilton, Victor P., *The Book of Genesis: Chapters 1–17* (Grand Rapids: Eerdmans, 1990).

Harman, A.M., 'עַיִן', in W.A. VanGemeren (general ed.), *New International Dictionary of Old Testament Theology and Exegesis* (Grand Rapids, MI: Zondervan, 1997), III, pp. 385-90.

Hasan, Ruqaiya, *Linguistics, Language, and Verbal Art* (Oxford: Oxford University Press, 1989).

—'Rime and Reason in Literature', in Seymour Chatman (ed.), *Literacy Style: A Symposium* (New York: Oxford University Press, 1971), pp. 299-326.

Hasel, G., 'The Meaning of "Let Us" in Gn 1:26', *AUSS* 13 (1975), pp. 58-66.

Heard, Christopher R., *Dynamics of Diselection: Ambiguity in Genesis 12–36 and Ethnic Boundaries in Post-Exilic Judah* (Atlanta: Society of Biblical Literature, 2001).

Huddlestun, J.R., 'Divestiture, Deception, and Demotion: The Garment Motif in Genesis 37–39', *JSOT* 98 (2002), pp. 47-62.

Hunter, Jannie, *Faces of a Lamenting City: The Development and Coherence of the Book of Lamentations* (Frankfurt am Main: P. Lang, 1996).

Ibn Ezra, *Rabbi Abraham Ibn Ezra's Commentary on Genesis*, in Menahem Cohen (ed.), *Mikra'ot Gedolot 'HaKeter'* (Ramath Gan: Bar-Ilan University Press, 1997 [Hebrew]).

Ipsen, G., 'Der alte Orient und die Indogermanen', in J. Friedrich *et al.* (eds.), *Stand und Aufgaben der Sprachwissenschaft: Festschrift für W. Streitberg* (Heidelberg: C. Winter, 1924), pp. 200-37.

Jacobs, Jonathan, 'Willing Obedience with Doubts: Abraham at the Binding of Isaac', *VT* 60 (2010), pp. 546-59.

Joines, Karen Randolph, 'The Bronze Serpent in the Israelite Cult', *JBL* 87 (1968), pp. 245-56.

—'The Serpent in Gen 3', *ZAW* 87 (1975), pp. 1-11.

Jones, T.J., *Quelle, Brunnen und Zisterne im Alten Testament* (Leipzig: E. Pfriffer, 1928).

Josephus, *Complete Works* (trans. William Whiston; Grand Rapids: Kregel Publications, 1978).

Joüon, P., and T. Muraoka, *A Grammar of Biblical Hebrew* (Subsidia Biblica, 27; Rome: Editrice Pontificio Istituto biblico, 2006).

Kaddari, Menahem Z., *A Dictionary of Biblical Hebrew* (Ramath Gan: Bar-Ilan University Press, 2006 [Hebrew]).

—'Semantic Fields in the Language of the Dead Sea Scrolls' (Hebrew), *Leshonenu* 29 (1965), pp. 226-37.

—*Semantic Fields in the Language of the Dead Sea Scrolls* (Jerusalem: Kiryath Sepher, 1968 [Hebrew]).

Kapelrud, Arvid S., 'Genesis xlix 12', *VT* 4 (1954), pp. 426-28.

Kasher, Hannah *et al.* (eds.), *Abraham, Father of Believers* (Ramath Gan: Bar-Ilan University Press, 2002 [Hebrew]).

Kessler, Martin (ed.), *Reading the Book of Jeremiah: A Search for Coherence* (Winona Lake, IN: Eisenbrauns, 2004).

Kim, Seenam, *The Coherence of the Collections in the Book of Proverbs* (Eugene, OR: Pickwick Publications, 2007).

Klein, Daniel, 'Who Counted Righteousness to Whom? Two Clashing Views by Shadal on Genesis 15:6', *Jewish Bible Quarterly* 36 (2008), pp. 28-32.

Kleparski, Grzegorz A., and Angelina Rusinek, 'The Tradition of Field Theory and the Study of Lexical Semantic Change', *Zeszytynaukowe Uniwersytetu Rzeszowskiego* 47 (2007), pp. 188-205.

Kress, Gunther, 'Cohesion', in Paul Cobley (ed.), *The Routledge Companion to Semiotics and Linguistics* (London: Routledge, 2001), pp. 173-74.

Krispijn, Th.J.H., 'The Sumerain Lexeme URUM, a Lexico-Etymological Approach', in W.H. van Soldt *et al.* (eds.), *Veenhof Anniversary Volume: Studies Presented to Klaas R. Veenhof on the Occasion of his Sixty-fifth Birthday* (Leiden: Nederlands Instituut voor het Nabije Oosten, 2001), pp. 251-61.

Lakoff, G., *Women, Fire and Dangerous Things: What Categories Reveal about the Mind* (Chicago: University of Chicago Press, 1987).

Lambrecht, Knud, *Information Structure and Sentence Form: Topic, Focus and the Mental Representations of Discourse Referents* (Cambridge: Cambridge University Press, 1994).

Lane, E.W., *An Arabic–English Lexicon* (Beirut: Librairie du Liban, 1968).

Leder, Arie C., 'The Coherence of Exodus: Narrative Unity and Meaning', *CTJ* 36 (2001), pp. 251-69.

Licht, Jacob, *Testing: In the Hebrew Scriptures and in Post-Biblical Judaism* (Jerusalem: Magnes Press, 1973 [Hebrew]).

Loewenstamm, Samuel Ephraim, 'The Death of Moses' (Hebrew), *Tarbiẓ* 27 (1958), pp. 142-57.

—'Reuben and Judah in the Cycle of Joseph-Stories', in *From Babylon to Canaan* (Jerusalem: Magnes Press, Hebrew University, 1992), pp. 35-41.

Loewenstamm, Samuel Ephraim, and J. Blau (eds.), *Otzar Leshon haMikra* (Jerusalem: The Bible Concordance Press, 1957–68).

Long, V. Philips, *The Reign and Rejection of King Saul: A Case for Literary and Theological Coherence* (Atlanta, GA: Scholars Press, 1989).

Longacre, Robert E., *The Grammar of Discourse* (New York: Plenum Press, 1996).

—'Interpreting Biblical Stories', in T. van Dijk (ed.), *Discourse and Literature: New Approaches to the Analysis of Literary Genres* (Philadelphia: John Benjamins, 1985), pp. 169-85.

—*Joseph: A Story of Divine Providence: A Text Theoretical and Textlinguistic Analysis of Genesis 37 and 39–48* (Winona Lake, IN: Eisenbrauns, 1989).

Lyons, J., *Semantics* (Cambridge: Cambridge University Press, 1977).

—*Structural Semantics* (Oxford: Blackwell, 1963).

Malul, M., *Knowledge, Control and Sex: Studies in Biblical Thought, Culture and Worldview* (Tel Aviv: Archaeological Center Publication, 2002).

—'Law in the Narratives: A Study of the Expressions הכירו and וייטב בעיניהם in 2 Sam 3:36', *JNSL* 17 (1991), pp. 23-36.

Matthews, Victor H., 'The Anthropology of Clothing in the Joseph Narrative', *JSOT* 65 (1995), pp. 25-36.

McAlpine, Thomas, *Sleep, Divine and Human, in the Old Testament* (JSOTSup, 38; Sheffield: JSOT Press, 1987).

Mckeown, James, *Genesis* (Two Horizons Old Testament Commentary; Grand Rapids: Eerdmans, 2008).

Merwe, C.H.J. van der, 'A Cognitive Linguistic Perspective on הִנֵּה in the Pentateuch, Joshua, Judges, and Ruth', *Hebrew Studies* 48 (2007), pp. 101-40.

—'Lexical Meaning in Biblical Hebrew and Cognitive Semantics: A Case Study', *Biblica* 87 (2006), pp. 85-95.

Mettinger, Tryggve N.D., *The Eden Narrative: A Literary and Religio-Historical Study of Genesis 2–3* (Winona Lake, IN: Eisenbrauns, 2007).

Millard, A.R., and D.J. Wiseman (eds.), *Essays on the Patriarchal Narratives* (Winona Lake, IN: Eisenbrauns, 1983).

Moberly, R.W.L., 'The Earliest Commentary on the Akedah', *VT* 38 (1988), pp. 302-23.

Morag, Shelomo, '"ומתערה כאזרח רענן" (Psalms XXXVI, 35)', in *Studies on Biblical Hebrew* (Jerusalem: Magnes Press, 1995 [Hebrew]), pp. 194-217 (first published 1972).

Mukarovsky, J.R., 'Standard Language and Poetic Language', in P.L. Garvin (ed.), *A Prague School Reader on Esthetics, Literary Structure, and Style* (Washington, DC: Georgetown University Press, 1964), pp. 17-30.

Murphy, M. Lynne, *Semantic Relations and the Lexicon* (Cambridge: Cambridge University Press, 2003).

Nerlich, Brigitte, and David D. Clarke, 'Semantic Fields and Frames: Historical Explorations of the Interface between Language, Action, and Cognition', *Journal of Pragmatics* 32 (2000), pp. 125-50.

Nicolopoulou, Ageliki, 'The Elementary Forms of Narrative Coherence in Young Children's Storytelling', *Narrative Inquiry* 18 (2008), pp. 299-325.

Oberhuber, Karl, *Innsbrucker sumerisches Lexicon* (Innsbruck: Institut für Sprachwissenschaft der Universität Innsbruck, 1990).

Okoye, James C., 'Sarah and Hagar: Genesis 16 and 21', *JSOT* 32 (2007), pp. 163-75.

Olshtein, E., and M. Celce-Murcia, 'Discourse Analysis and Language Teaching', in Schiffrin, Tannen and Hamilton (eds.), *The Handbook of Discourse Analysis*, pp. 707-24.

Onega, S., and J.A. Garcia Landa, *Narratology: An Introduction* (London: Longman, 1996).

Otto, E., *Gott und Mensch nach den ägyptischen Tempelinschriften der griechisch-romischen Zeit* (Heidelberg: C. Winter, 1964).

Ottoson, M., 'חלום', in *TDOT*, IV, pp. 423-25.

Palache, J.L., *Semantic Notes on the Hebrew Lexicon* (trans. R.J. Werblowsky; Leiden: E.J. Brill, 1959).

Pirson, R., *The Lord of the Dreams: A Semantic and Literary Analysis of Genesis 37–50* (JSOTSup, 355; London: Sheffield Academic Press, 2002).

Polak, Frank, 'לא בקורא תגר: A Structural and Thematic Analysis of the Covenant among the Divided Parts (Genesis 15.1-21)' (Hebrew), in Y. Avishur and J. Blau (eds.), *Mehqarim Bamikrah Uvamizrah Haqadum* (Jerusalem: Rubinstein, 1978), pp. 319-27.

—*Biblical Narrative: Aspects of Art and Design* (Jerusalem: Mosad Bialik, 1999 [Hebrew]).

—'Epic Formulae in Biblical Narrative and the Origins of Ancient Hebrew Prose' (Hebrew), *Te'uda* 7 (1991), pp. 9-54.

—'Linguistic and Stylistic Aspects of Epic Formulae in Ancient Semitic Poetry and Biblical Narrative', in S. Fassberg and A. Hurvitz (eds.), *Biblical Hebrew in its Northwest Semitic Setting* (Winona Lake, IN: Eisenbrauns, 2006), pp. 285-304.

Polliack, Meira, 'Joseph's Trauma: Memory and Resolution', in Brenner and Polak (eds.), *Performing Memory*, pp. 72-105.

Porzig, W., 'Wesenhafte Bedeutungsbeziehungen', *Beiträge zur deutchen Sprache und Literature* 58 (1934), pp. 70-97.

Prince, Gerald, *A Dictionary of Narratology* (Lincoln: University of Nebraska Press, 1987).

Rabbi David Kimhi, *Rabbi David Kimhi's Commentary on Genesis*, in Menahem Cohen (ed.), *Mikra'ot Gedolot 'HaKeter'* (Ramath Gan: Bar-Ilan University Press, 1997 [Hebrew]).

Rabin, Chaim, 'Comments on: "סנורים = The Covering of the Eyes"' (Hebrew), *Tarbiẓ* 39 (1970), pp. 214-15.

Rad, G. von, *Genesis: A Commentary* (trans. J.H. Marks; Old Testament Library; London: SCM Press, 1963).

—*Old Testament Theology*. I. *The Theology of Israel's Historical Traditions* (trans. D.M.G. Stalker; Edinburgh: Oliver & Boyd, 1962).

Rashbam, *Rabbi Shmuel Ben Meir's Commentary on Genesis*, in Menahem Cohen (ed.), *Mikra'ot Gedolot 'HaKeter'* (Ramath Gan: Bar-Ilan University Press, 1997 [Hebrew]).

Redford, D.B., *A Study of the Biblical Story of Joseph (Genesis 37–50)* (VTSup, 20; Leiden: E.J. Brill, 1970).

Reinhart, Tanya, 'Conditions for Text Coherence', *Poetics Today* 1 (1980), pp. 161-80.

Rendtorff, Rolf, *The Problem of the Process of Transmission in the Pentateuch* (JSOTSup, 89; trans. J.J. Scullion; Sheffield: JSOT Press, 1990).

Rosch, Eleanor, 'Principles of Categorization', in E. Rosch and B.B. Lloyd (eds.), *Cognition and Categorization* (Hillsdale, NJ: Erlbaum, 1978), pp. 27-48.

Rosenzweig, F., 'The Secret of Biblical Narrative Form', in Buber and Rosenzweig (eds.), *Scripture and Translation*, pp. 129-42.

Rubinstein, Eliezer, 'The Hidden Perceiver' (Hebrew), *Hebrew Computational Linguistics* 19 (1982), pp. 63-68.

Sanders, Ted, and Henk Pander Maat, 'Cohesion and Coherence: Linguistic Approaches', in K. Brown *et al.* (eds.), *Encyclopedia of Language and Linguistics* (London: Elsevier, 2006), pp. 591-95.

Sarna, Nahum, *The JPS Torah Commentary: Genesis* (Philadelphia: Jewish Publication Society, 1989).

Saussure, Ferdinand de, *Course in General Linguistics* (ed. Charles Bally and Albert Sechehaye with the collaboration of Albert Reidlinger; trans. Wade Baskin; New York: Philosophical Library, 1959 [based on de Saussure's lectures given between 1906 and 1911, first published 1916]).

Sawyer, J.F.A., *Semantics in Biblical Research: New Methods of Defining Hebrew Words for Salvation* (London: SCM Press, 1972).
Schank, Roger C., and Robert P. Abelson, *Scripts, Plans, Goals, and Understanding* (Hillsdale, NJ: Erlbaum, 1977).
Schatz, Rabbi Morris, *Ethics of the Father in the Light of Jewish History* (New York: Bloch, 1970).
Schiffrin, D., D. Tannen and H.E. Hamilton (eds.), *The Handbook of Discourse Analysis* (Malden, MA: Blackwell, 2001).
Schneider, J., and A.B. Weiner (eds.), *Cloth and Human Experience* (Washington, DC: Smithsonian Institution Press, 1989).
Schwarzenbach, A., *Die geographische Terminologie im Hebräischen des Alten Testamentes* (Leiden: E.J. Brill, 1954).
Skinner, J., *A Critical and Exegetical Commentary on Genesis* (ICC; Edinburgh: T. & T. Clark, 1930).
Soden, von W., *Akkadisches Handwörterbuch* (3 vols.; Wiesbaden: Harrassowitz, 1959–81).
Sommer, Benjamin D., *The Bodies of God and the World of Ancient Israel* (New York: Cambridge University Press, 2009).
Sovran, Tamar, 'Exploring the Semantic Field of the Positive' (Hebrew), in Shimon Sharvit (ed.), *Studies in Ancient and Modern Hebrew: In Honour of M.Z. Kaddari* (Ramath Gan: Bar-Ilan University Press, 1999), pp. 375-81.
—*Semantic Fields: A Linguistic-Philosophical Study of Meaning Relations* (Jerusalem: Hebrew University/Magnes Press, 2000 [Hebrew]).
Speiser, E.A., 'The "Elative" in West-Semitic and Akkadian', *JCS* 6 (1952), pp. 81-92.
—*Genesis* (AB, 1; Garden City, NY: Doubleday, 1964).
Spooren, W., and T. Sanders, 'The Acquisition Order of Coherence Relations: On Cognitive Complexity in Discourse', *Journal of Pragmatics* 40 (2008), pp. 2003-26.
Stadler-Sutskover, Talia, 'The Leading Word and its Roles in Judges 19–21', in Johann Cook (ed.), *Bible and Computer: The Stellenbosch AIBI-6 Conference. Proceedings of the Association Internationale Bible et Informatique 'From Alpha to Byte' University of Stellenbosch 17–21 July, 2000* (Leiden: E.J. Brill, 2002), pp. 295-307.
Stendebach, F.J., 'עין', in *TDOT*, XI, pp. 28-44.
Sternberg, M., 'What Is Exposition? An Essay in Temporal Delimitation', in J. Halperin (ed.), *The Theory of the Novel: New Essays* (New York: Oxford University Press, 1974), pp. 25-70.
Stol, Marten, 'Blindness and Night-Blindness in Akkadian', *JNES* 45 (1986), pp. 295-99.
Sutskover, Talia, 'Lexical Fields and Coherence in the Jacob Narrative', in Brenner and Polak (eds.), *Performing Memory*, pp. 126-39.
—'Lot and his Daughters (Gen 19:30-38): Further Literary and Stylistic Examinations', *JHS* 11 (2011), pp. 2-11.
—'The Semantic Fields of Seeing and Oral Communication in the Joseph Narrative', *JNSL* 33.2 (2007), pp. 33-50.
Sweetser, Eva, *From Etymology to Pragmatics: Metaphorical and Cultural Aspects of Semantic Structure* (Cambridge: Cambridge University Press, 1990).
Talmon, Shemaryahu, 'Synonymous Readings in the Textual Traditions of the Old Testament', *Scripta Hierosolymitana* 8 (1961), pp. 335-83.

Talmud Bavli: The Gemara: The Classic Vilna Edition, with an Annotated, Interpretive Elucidation, as an Aid to Talmud Study (elucidated by Gedaliah Zlotowitz; Brooklyn, NY: Mesorah Publications, 2000).

Tomashevski, Boris, 'Thematics', in L.T. Lemon and M.J. Reis (eds. and trans.), *Russian Formalist Criticism: Four Essays* (Lexington: University of Nebraska Press, 1965 [first published in 1925]), pp. 61-98.

Trier, Jost, 'Das sprachliche Feld: eine Auseinandersetzung', *Neue Jahrbücher für Wissenschaft und Jugenbildung* 10 (1934), pp. 428-49.

—'Sprachliche Felder', in Jost Trier, A. van der Lee and O. Rechmann, *Aufsätze und Vorträge zur Wortfeldtheorie* (The Hague: Mouton, 1973), pp. 93-109.

Turner, Laurence A., *Announcements of Plot in Genesis* (JSOTSup, 96; Sheffield: JSOT Press, 1990).

—'The Rainbow as the Sign of the Covenant in Genesis ix 11-13', *VT* 43 (1993), pp. 119-24.

Ungerer, F., and Hans-Jörg Schmid, *An Introduction to Cognitive Linguistics* (London: Longman, 2006).

Van Seters, John, *Abraham in History and Tradition* (New Haven: Yale University Press, 1975).

—*The Pentateuch: A Social-Science Commentary* (Sheffield: Sheffield Academic Press, 1999).

Vaux, Roland de, *Ancient Israel* (trans. John McHugh; London: Darton, Longman & Todd, 1965).

Viberg, Ake, *Symbols of Law: A Contextual Analysis of Legal Symbolic Acts in the Old Testament* (Stockholm: Almqvist & Wiksell International, 1992).

Vriezen, T.C., and A.S. van der Woude, *Ancient Israelite and Early Jewish Literature* (trans. Brian Doyle; Leiden: Brill, 2005).

Waltke, B.K., and M. O'Connor, *An Introduction to Biblical Hebrew Syntax* (Winona Lake, IN: Eisenbrauns, 1990).

Walzel, O., *Das Wortkunstwerk* (Darmstadt: Wissenschaftliche Buchgesellschaft, 1968 [1st edn 1926]).

Wellhausen, J., *Die Composition des Hexateuchs und der historischen Bücher des Alten Testaments* (Berlin: W. de Gruyter, 1963 [repr. 3rd edn 1899]).

—*Prolegomena zur Geschichte Israels* (Berlin: G. Reimer, 1905).

Wenham, G.J., *Genesis 1–15* (WBC, 1; Waco, TX: Word Books, 1987).

—*Genesis 16–50* (WBC, 2; Dallas, TX: Word Books, 1995).

Westermann, Claus, *Genesis 1–11: A Commentary* (trans. J.J. Scullion; Minneapolis: Augsburg, 1984).

—*Genesis 12–36: A Commentary* (trans. J.J. Scullion; London: SPCK, 1985).

—*Genesis 37–50: A Commentary* (trans. J.J. Scullion; London: SPCK, 1987).

White, H.C., 'Reuben and Judah: Duplicates or Complements?', in J.T. Butler, E.W. Conrad and B.C. Ollenburger (eds.), *Understanding the Word: Essays in Honor of Bernhard W. Anderson* (JSOTSup, 37; Sheffield: JSOT Press, 1985), pp. 73-97.

Widdowson, H.G., *Discourse Analysis* (Oxford: Oxford University Press, 2007).

Wilson, Leslie S., *The Serpent Symbol in the Ancient Near East* (Lanham, MD: University Press of America, 2001).

Wittgenstein, L., *Philosophical Investigations* (trans. G.E.M. Anscombe; Oxford: Basil Blackwell, 1958).

Wolde, E.J. van, *Reframing Biblical Studies: When Language and Text Meet Culture, Cognition, and Context* (Winona Lake, IN: Eisenbrauns, 2009).

—*Words Become Worlds: Semantic Studies of Genesis 1–11* (Leiden: E.J. Brill, 1994).

Wyatt, Nick, 'Circumcision and Circumstance: Male Genital Mutilation in Ancient Israel and Ugarit', *JSOT* 33 (2009), pp. 405-31.

Zadka, Y., '"Noah found grace in the eyes of the Lord": A Semantic and Syntactic Analysis' (Hebrew), *Criticism and Interpretation* 24 (1988), pp. 113-40.

Zakovitch, Yair, '"The voice of the LORD... upon many waters"—The God Who Leads his World and People in the Water' (Hebrew), in Yair Zakovitch and Avigdor Shinan (eds.), '*... Like Watercourses in the Negeb': Water in the Bible and Rabbinic Literature* (Jerusalem: The Presidential Residence, 1998), pp. 13-23.

Zohori, Menahem, '"Light"—Its Meanings in the Hebrew Bible' (Hebrew), in *Bamiqra Uvolamo: Studies and Essays on Biblical and Oriental Subjects* (Jerusalem: Carmel, 1998), pp. 7-18.

Zucker, David Jeremy, and Aurora Colorado, 'Seeing and Hearing: The Interrelated Lives of Sarah and Hagar', *Women in Judaism* 7 (2010), <http://wjudaism.library.utoronto.ca/index.php/wjudaism/article/view/14663>.

Indexes

Index of References

Hebrew Bible/
Old Testament

Genesis

1–11 3, 92, 138, 140, 141, 179
1–4 141
1–3 149
1 61, 90, 94, 95, 145, 147
1.1–2.3 92, 135
1.1 145
1.2 61
1.3-4 1
1.3 61
1.4 1, 61, 92, 143, 145
1.5 21, 61, 89, 92
1.8 89
1.10 1, 92, 143
1.12 1, 92
1.13 89
1.14 90, 93
1.15 61, 90, 93
1.16 90, 91
1.17 61, 93
1.18 1, 61, 92
1.21 1, 92
1.25 1, 92
1.26 54, 55, 93
1.27 55, 93
1.31 1, 41, 81, 92, 93, 147
2–4 94
2 94, 95
2.3 94
2.4–3.24 94, 135
2.4 94, 95
2.7 95
2.9 52, 76, 95, 97
2.10 79
2.17 76, 95, 96
2.19 96
2.20 96
2.21-22 96
2.21 80, 81, 96
2.22-24 98
2.22 98
2.23 111
2.24 98
2.25–3.1 2
2.25 63, 96-98
3 68, 95, 145
3.1 38, 68, 77, 96, 97
3.2-3 97
3.4-5 97
3.4 68
3.5 97
3.6 96, 97
3.7 1, 39, 63, 68, 94, 96, 97, 145, 179
3.8 63, 89, 98
3.9 98
3.10 63, 96, 98
3.11 63, 98
3.12 98
3.13 98
3.16 97
3.20 98
3.21 72, 98
3.22 95, 97
3.24 95
4 66
4.1 146
4.4-5 49, 146
4.5 59
4.6 59
4.9 146
4.12 66
4.14 64, 66
4.15 146
4.17 146
4.25 146
5 35
5.1-5 147
5.1 54, 94, 146
5.3 54, 55, 146
6–9 141
6 1
6.1-4 147
6.2 1, 147
6.5 147
6.8 57, 147
6.9 94
6.12 147
7.1 147
7.11 60, 70, 147
7.16 22
7.19 63, 147
7.20 63, 147
8.1 75, 148
8.2 60, 70, 147
8.5 3, 147
8.8 148
8.11 148

Genesis (cont.)
8.13 64, 148, 179
8.21 150
9 66
9.2 148
9.6 55
9.9 148
9.12 28, 66, 148
9.13 148
9.14-16 66, 148
9.14 148
9.15 75, 148
9.16 75, 148
9.18-29 40
9.21 40, 62
9.22 40, 62, 149, 179
9.23 62, 63
9.24 40, 80, 81, 148
9.25 149
11 92, 100, 145
11.1-9 29, 99, 149
11.1 99
11.3 99
11.4 99
11.5 45, 99, 149
11.6 99
11.7 99
11.9 99
11.27 86, 94, 100
11.28 82, 100
11.31 82, 86, 100
12–50 140
12–25 140, 150
12 62, 100, 136
12.1–25.18 3
12.1-9 100
12.1-3 100, 138
12.1 100, 150, 151, 156, 158
12.2-3 100
12.4-5 100
12.4 86, 100, 101
12.5 86, 101
12.6 62, 78, 83, 84, 100, 101
12.7 62, 83, 86, 100, 101, 151
12.8-9 101
12.8 35, 101
12.10-20 100, 112, 156
12.10 112
12.11-12 112
12.11 52, 113, 181
12.12 62, 113
12.13 113
12.14 113
12.15 113, 143
12.17 113
12.18 113
12.19 81, 113
12.20 113
13 156
13.1-4 86
13.10-13 50
13.10 57, 143
13.14 57
13.15 151, 156
13.18 83, 84
14 84
14.7 70, 87
14.12-13 37
14.12 86
14.13 83
14.16 86
14.24 86, 87
15 61, 100, 101, 151, 152, 179
15.1-5 89
15.1 52, 101, 182
15.2 101
15.4-5 153
15.5 48, 91, 101, 114
15.6 74, 76, 101, 102, 153, 179
15.7 82, 101, 102
15.8 102, 153
15.12 61, 81, 88, 91, 102
15.13-16 102
15.16 102
15.17 62, 79, 89, 91, 102
15.18 151
16 69, 82, 100, 107, 111
16.1-6 107
16.1 107
16.2 107
16.3 107
16.4 58, 107-109
16.5 58, 108, 109
16.6 58, 85, 108, 109
16.7-14 107
16.7 37, 45, 69, 70, 85, 108
16.9 108, 109
16.10 108
16.11 108, 109
16.12 108
16.13 82, 85, 109, 116, 156, 179
16.14 37, 81, 83, 85, 109
16.15-16 107, 109
17 67, 154
17.1 86, 154

17.6-7 154
17.11 67, 110, 154
18 154
18.1-15 154
18.1 1, 39, 83, 86, 89, 114, 154
18.2 1, 39, 57, 104, 155
18.3 57, 155
18.4 155
18.5 155
18.8 155
18.9 155
18.10 155
18.12 144, 154
18.15 154, 157
18.16 1, 50, 155
18.17 64, 154
18.19 76, 155
18.21 155
18.28 154
18.29 154
18.30 59, 154
18.31 154
18.32 154
19 37, 46, 100, 113, 114, 155, 156
19.1-29 113
19.1 1, 86, 113-15, 155
19.2 80, 86
19.5 39, 86, 114, 115, 155
19.6-8 39
19.6 86
19.8 58, 114, 115
19.9 39, 46, 86
19.10 86
19.11 13, 40, 46, 114, 115, 156
19.12 86
19.14 59, 86, 115
19.15 86, 90, 115
19.17 48, 156
19.18 86
19.19 57, 115
19.21 115
19.23 86, 91, 115
19.24 79, 115
19.26 48, 114, 155, 156
19.27 113, 115
19.28 1, 50, 113, 114, 155
19.29 75, 86, 114, 155
19.30-38 87
19.30 86
19.33-36 87
19.33-35 36
19.33 40, 88, 155
19.35 40, 88, 155
19.36 86
20 112
20.1 85
20.13 93
20.15 58
20.16 59
21 30, 69, 100, 109, 111, 115
21.1-21 110
21.1-8 110
21.1-7 110
21.1-2 110
21.1 77
21.3 110, 111
21.4 67, 110
21.7 111
21.8-21 110
21.8 110, 111
21.9 1, 39, 110, 111
21.10 111
21.11 58, 111
21.12-13 109
21.12 58, 111
21.13 111
21.14 36, 109-11
21.15-16 112
21.15 111
21.16 110, 112
21.17 110, 112
21.19 69, 110, 112
21.21 110
22 30, 84, 100, 103, 105, 107, 109, 179
22.1 103
22.2 7, 37, 78, 84, 86, 109
22.3 36, 103, 110
22.4-8 110
22.4 57, 90, 104
22.5 104
22.6 79, 104
22.7 79, 104
22.8 45, 104
22.9 105
22.10 105, 110
22.11-12 105
22.12 106, 110, 112, 156
22.13 57, 105, 110
22.14 37, 84, 86, 105, 110
22.15-18 106
22.16-17 106
22.17 91, 106
22.19 106

Genesis (cont.)
22.24 41
23.17 86
23.19 86
24 65
24.13 70
24.15-16 36
24.16 52, 70
24.21 48, 49
24.23 80
24.25 80
24.29 70
24.30 70
24.42 70
24.43 70
24.45 70
24.54 80
24.62 85
24.63-64 85
24.63 89, 104
24.65 64, 65, 85
25–36 140
25 121
25.8-10 157
25.9 86, 121, 157
25.11 85, 121, 157
25.12-18 157
25.12 94
25.18 41, 85, 109, 121, 157
25.19-36 3
25.19-26 157
25.21 158
25.22 158
25.23 158
25.25 111, 158
25.26 111
25.30 158
26 112, 158, 159
26.2 158
26.3-4 158
26.4 91
26.5 78
26.7 52, 159
26.8 50, 143, 159
26.12-22 159
26.12 159
26.19 159
26.24 77, 159
26.25 159
26.28 159
26.32 159
27 38, 71, 116, 118, 120, 159, 180, 183
27.1 13, 38, 47, 56, 116, 159
27.2 116, 118
27.4 116
27.7 116
27.8 117
27.9 116
27.10 118
27.11 117
27.12 59, 117
27.13 117
27.14 116, 117
27.17 116
27.21 117
27.22-25 117
27.22 117, 118
27.23 71, 118
27.26-27 118
27.27 117, 118
27.42-43 118
27.45 77
28–32 163
28 160, 168, 179, 180
28.6 160
28.8 58, 160
28.10-22 118
28.11-12 89
28.11 79, 80, 91, 118, 119
28.12-15 119
28.12 53, 119
28.13 160
28.16-17 4, 144
28.16 80, 119, 160
28.17 2, 119, 160
28.18-20 119
28.18 79, 119
28.19 119
29 36, 118, 161
29.1-2 161
29.10 161
29.17 52, 55, 56, 161, 181
29.20 59
29.23 36, 88
29.25 36, 88
29.31 161
29.32 37, 41, 88, 161, 181
30 39
30.1 3, 39, 143, 161
30.8 161
30.9 161
30.14 88, 161
30.22 75
30.25-26 162
30.27 57
30.32 162
30.37 21, 63, 67, 162
30.40 162
30.41 162
31 169, 179
31.1 120
31.2 78, 162, 165, 168
31.3 162, 165
31.5 162, 165
31.10 53, 57, 81
31.12 57, 162
31.15 76
31.19 163
31.24 163
31.27 63

31.29	163, 168	33.15	57	37.18-30	124
31.32	71, 163	34	67, 164	37.19	124
31.33	163	34.1-2	1, 38	37.20	54, 124
31.34	163	34.1	164	37.21-22	125
31.35	59, 70, 163	34.2	164	37.21	88
		34.7	59	37.22	88
31.36-42	163	34.11	57	37.23	72, 73, 124
31.37	163	34.18	58		
31.39	70	35–36	164	37.24	124
31.40	59, 80	35	164	37.25	57, 124
31.42	163	35.1	164	37.26	64, 126
31.43	163, 168	35.7	62, 93, 164	37.27	126
31.49	48, 64, 87, 165			37.28	126
		35.9	39, 164	37.29	74, 88
31.51	78	35.22	88	37.31-35	126
31.54	80	35.23	88	37.31-33	127
31.55	120	35.27	86	37.32-33	127, 171
32	161, 163, 168	36	35, 164	37.32	71, 73, 126, 129
		36.9	164		
32.1-3	179	36.13	86	37.33	71, 129
32.1	80	36.17	86	37.34	74, 126
32.2-3	120, 168	36.21	164	37.35	126
32.6	57	36.31	164	37.36	126
32.10	168	36.33	86	38	28, 65, 121, 127, 129-32, 171, 177, 182
32.14	80	37–50	3, 140, 170		
32.20-21	165				
32.22-32	120, 179	37	71, 73, 121, 122, 126, 129-32, 170, 177		
32.22-23	120				
32.22	80			38.1	127
32.24	120			38.2	128
32.25	90, 120			38.3	87
32.26	120	37.2	94, 122	38.6	87, 128
32.27	90	37.3	72, 73, 122	38.7	58, 87
32.30	37, 120, 165, 175			38.10	58, 128
		37.4	122, 170	38.12	128
32.31	62, 88, 121, 163	37.5	53, 123	38.14	28, 37, 64, 65, 73, 87, 128, 129
		37.6	53, 123		
32.32	88, 91	37.7	81		
32.34	114	37.8	123	38.15	15, 64, 76, 127, 129, 166
33.1	57, 104, 164	37.9-10	168		
		37.9	53, 91, 123, 124		
33.5	57, 104, 164			38.16	128, 129
		37.10	53, 124	38.19	65, 73
33.8	57	37.12-17	124	38.21	87
33.10	40, 57, 164, 165, 175	37.14	124	38.25-26	73, 127
		37.15	70, 124	38.25	71, 87, 129
		37.16	70, 124		

Genesis (cont.)
38.26 71, 129
38.28 73
38.29 111
38.30 73, 86
39 121, 130-32, 171, 177
39.1–41.23 72
39.1 127
39.3 131, 171, 176
39.4 57, 77, 131, 171
39.5 77
39.6 52, 55, 131, 171, 181
39.7 57, 131, 171
39.10 131
39.11 72
39.12-13 131
39.12 72
39.14 131
39.15 72
39.16 72
39.18 72, 131
39.19 131
39.21 57
39.23 45, 131, 176
40 171
40.4 77
40.5 53
40.8 53, 171
40.14 75
40.23 40, 75, 77
40.28 78
40.33 75
40.38 75
41 80, 171
41.1 53
41.2 52
41.3 52
41.4 52, 80
41.5 53, 80
41.7 80
41.9 75
41.11 53
41.14 74
41.15 53
41.16 171
41.18 55
41.19 55
41.21 52, 80
41.22 54
41.25 171
41.28 171
41.30 77
41.33 45
41.34 77
41.37 58
41.42 72
42 171
42.1 2, 172
42.2 172
42.4 172
42.7 28, 71, 172
42.8 71, 172
42.9 53, 62, 63, 75, 166, 172
42.12 62, 63
42.20 74
42.21 172
42.22 88, 173
42.24 173
42.27 80
42.35 77
42.37 88
43 173
43.3 166
43.5 166
43.9 70
43.18 173
43.21 80
43.23 173
43.29 57, 104, 173
43.30 70, 173
43.31 173
44 173
44.3 61, 89
44.12 70
44.18 173
44.23-24 168
44.23 166
44.26 166
44.34 173
45 121, 132, 174, 175, 177
45.1 40, 132
45.2 174
45.3 40, 174
45.5-9 174
45.5 59, 132, 174
45.7-8 180
45.7 132, 174, 178
45.8 132, 174
45.9 132, 174
45.12 40, 132, 174
45.13 132
45.14 174
45.15 174
45.16 58
45.20 59
45.22 72
45.26 74
45.27 132
45.28 132, 174
46 174
46.2 54, 176, 179
46.4 59
46.8 88
46.9 88
46.12 86, 87
46.16 88
46.28 78
46.29-30 175
46.30 120, 166, 168

47.25 57
47.29 57
48 175, 176
48.3 175
48.5 88
48.8 175
48.10 38, 56, 175
48.11 120, 167, 168, 175
48.17 58
48.18-19 38
48.18 38
48.19 175
48.28 78
48.29 78
49 176
49.1 140
49.3 88
49.8-9 60
49.8 125
49.10 60
49.11 60
49.12 60, 80
49.22 70, 85
49.30 86
50 77, 175, 176
50.1-3 176
50.4 57
50.13 86
50.17 176
50.19 175
50.20 4, 76, 175, 180
50.21 175, 176
50.24-25 177
50.24 77
50.25 77

Exodus
1–2 23
2.25 76
3.1-6 118
3.1-2 86
3.3 51
4.11 45
4.24 114
5.9 50
10.22-23 61
10.28 167
10.29 167
14.31 77
18.21 45
20 180
20.18 177, 180
22.9-12 126
23.15 167
24.11 45
26 64
26.20 96
33 168
33.20 167, 181
33.23 167, 181
35 64
36 64
39 64
40 64

Leviticus
13 42
21.20 56
22.22 47

Numbers
3 64
4 64
12.6 54
15.39-40 148
16–17 29
21.4-9 68
21.5 68
21.6 68
21.9 68
24.4 45, 52
24.16 45, 52
26.16 88

Deuteronomy
2.9 86
3.28 150
11.2 76
11.30 83
28.10 77
28.28 45, 47
28.65 56
30.1-10 30
34.1-5 100, 150
34.7 48, 56

Joshua
2 114
24.31 76

Judges
2.7 76
16.6-21 34
19–21 114

1 Samuel
3.2 48
3.15 54
5.2-15 89
6.11 55
11 69
11.1-2 69
13.18 51
18.23 58
21.10 86
23.22 76
24.12 76
25.17 76
28.5 77
28.13 77

2 Samuel
3.13 167
3.36 58, 71
6.16 50
6.22 58
13.18 72
19.5 86
24.20 51

1 Kings
3.5 54
19.6 81

2 Kings
3.18 58
6 47
6.17 46
6.18 46, 114
6.20 46
14.8 172
14.11 172

1 Chronicles
21.21 51

2 Chronicles
3.1 84
25.17 172
25.21 172

Ezra
4.14 45

Nehemiah
8.3 90

Esther
6.1 59

Job
3.9 91
6.21 77
6.30 75
7.14 54
7.19 50
9.17 98
9.30 118
14.6 50
20.8 54
33.15 54

Psalms
40.4 77
51.9 118
58.10 75
65.13 65
83.9 86
139.11 98
144.3 15, 76
147.4-5 31
148.3 91

Proverbs
2.4 70
4.18 90
7.7 75
23.29 60
29.10 75

Ecclesiastes
12.3 60

Song of Songs
2.14 51
5.14 65
7.4 69

Isaiah
1.18 118
3.17 172
5.21 6, 78, 173
13.10 91
17.7 49
17.8 49
22.4 50
25.7 86
29.10 79
41.5 77
41.10 49
41.23 49
47.8 76
51.20 65
53.7 123
57.5 84

Jeremiah
2.23 76
8.23 79
9.1 79
15.10 126
52.25 167

Ezekiel
1.22-23 66
1.26 66
1.28 66
3.26 123
13.7 52

Joel
2.10 91

Amos
5.18 90
5.26 55
8.13 65

Habakkuk
1.3 126

Zechariah
9.5 77
11.17 56

PSEUDEPIGRAPHA
Jubilees
12.16-19 151
18.14 84

Testament of Joseph
9.5 182

MISHNAH
'Abot 5.4 150

BABYLONIAN TALMUD
Baba Batra
16b 152

TOSEFTA
Berakot
81 84

MIDRASH
Genesis Rabbah
3.8 145
3.9 150
44.12 152
55.2 153
65.15 117

Pirqe deRabbi Eliezer
26 103

Qohelet Rabbah
10 164

Sifre Deuteronomy
352 84

Tanḥuma
19 164

Tehillim
76 84

ARISTOTLE
Poetics
52a.12-21 105
52a.22 34
55b.26-27 34
55b.28-29 34

JOSEPHUS
Antiquities
1.224 84
4.8 152
4.48 152

ANCIENT NEAR EASTERN TEXTS
Enuma Elish
VI.83-94 66

Index of Authors

Abelson, R.P. 5
Abou-Assaf, A. 55
Ahuvia, A. 47
Alter, R. 96, 128, 140
Amit, Y. 29-31, 33, 34, 84, 94, 95, 100, 103, 106, 108, 109, 123, 124, 127, 130, 131
Auerbach, E. 104
Avrahami, Y. 8, 11, 111, 182

Baden, J.S. 135
Bal, M. 24, 34, 75, 142
Balentine, S.E. 7, 12, 45, 63-65, 128, 165, 167, 180
Bar-Efrat, S. 36, 107
Basset, F.W. 149
Bednarek, M.A. 1, 5, 7, 20
Ben Yehuda, E. 51, 55, 67, 74, 79, 90
Bergsma, J. 149
Berlin, A. 9, 20, 31, 81, 113
Bertil, A. 153
Beuken, W.A.M. 8
Blau, J. 53, 81
Blenkinsopp, J. 135
Blois, R. de 43
Bluck, S. 21
Bordreuil, P. 55
Brenner, A. 8, 9, 16, 42, 60, 61, 75, 81, 158, 159, 162
Buber, M. 29, 32, 103, 107, 130, 137
Bublitz, W. 20
Buckley, J.H. 39
Burrows, M. 76

Canale, M. 21
Carr, D.M. 135
Cassuto, U. 84, 94
Celce-Murcia, M. 23
Charles, R.H. 151, 182
Chatman, S. 33
Clarke, D.D. 4
Clifford, R.J. 127-29
Clines, D.J.A. 50, 60, 93, 139
Colorado, A. 108
Croft, W. 11
Cruse, D.A. 11
Cun, A. 21

Dahood, M. 98
Dalley, S. 66
Daube, D. 71, 100, 150
Donald, T. 7, 9
Dozeman, T.B. 24, 135
Driver, S.R. 151
Dundes, A. 106

Embry, B. 149
Ewen, J. 34

Faber, P. 3, 10, 127, 142
Fabry, H.J. 68
Fidler, R. 53, 54
Fields, W.W. 114
Fokkelman, J.P. 119, 125, 141, 142, 160
Foster, B.R. 57
Freedman, H. 117, 145, 150, 153
Freytag, G. 33
Friend, J.H. 44
Frisch, A. 30, 31, 69, 77, 84, 172

Galinier, J. 90
Galpaz-Feller, P. 109
Garcia Landa, J.A. 33
Garsiel, M. 37, 83, 85, 86
Geertz, C. 67
Giora, R. 20, 24
Goldingay, J. 139
Grandy, R.E. 7
Gunkel, H. 105, 106, 109, 135, 161
Guralnik, D.B. 44, 53

Habermas, T. 21
Hahn, S. 149
Halliday, M.A.K. 6, 21-23
Hamilton, V.P. 93, 98
Harman, A.M. 57
Hasan, R. 2, 6, 21-28, 30, 32, 35

Hasel, G. 93
Heard, C.R. 118, 136
Huddleston, J.R. 170
Hunter, J. 24

Ipsen, G. 4

Jacobs, J. 107
Joines, K.R. 68
Jones, T.J. 69
Joüon, P. 52

Kaddari, M.Z. 8, 9, 43
Kapelrud, A.S. 60
Kasher, H. 152
Kay, P. 9
Kessler, M. 24
Kim, S. 23, 24
Klein, D. 153
Kleparski, G.A. 7
Kress, G. 20
Krispijn, Th.J.H. 82

Lakoff, G. 6, 13, 51
Lambrecht, K. 89
Lane, E.W. 50, 55
Leder, A.C. 23
Lenk, U. 20
Licht, J. 145
Loewenstamm, S.E. 53, 81, 125, 127, 153
Long, V.P. 23
Longacre, R.E. 20, 35, 98, 146
Lyons, J. 5

Maat, H.P. 20
Malinowitz, C. 152
Malul, M. 8, 58, 71, 126
Matthews, V.H. 14, 71, 72, 122, 170
McAlpine, T. 8
Mckeown, J. 135
Merwe, C.H.J. van der 11, 81
Mettinger, T.N.D. 95
Millard, A.R. 55
Moberly, R.W.L. 105
Morag, S. 48, 62
Mueller, E.R. 43
Mukarovsky, J.R. 30, 35
Muraoka, T. 52
Murphy, M.L. 6

Nerlich, B. 4
Nicolopoulou, A. 21

O'Connor, M. 81, 113
Oberhuber, K. 82
Okoye, J.C. 107
Olshtein, E. 23
Onega, S. 33
Otto, E. 56
Ottoson, M. 53

Palache, J.L. 62, 72, 89
Pirson, R. 125, 129
Polak, F. 8, 30, 32-34, 36, 57, 75, 84, 89, 93, 97, 103, 106, 118, 146, 153, 161, 163, 173
Polliack, M. 166, 174
Porzig, W. 4, 5
Prince, G. 30

Rabin, C. 47
Rad, G. von 101, 106, 118, 127, 136, 138, 155
Redford, D.B. 121, 125
Reinhart, T. 20, 24
Rendtorff, R. 136, 139
Römer, T. 24
Rosch, E. 11, 12, 44
Rosenzweig, F. 31, 32
Rubinstein, E. 58, 65, 66, 73
Rusinek, A. 7

Sanders, T. 20
Sarna, N. 96
Saussure, F. de 77
Sawyer, J.F.A. 8
Schank, R.C. 5
Schatz, M. 150
Schmid, H.-J. 1
Schmid, K. 24, 135
Schneider, J. 72
Schorr, Y.S. 152
Schwartz, B.J. 135
Schwarzenbach, A. 69
Simon, M. 117, 145, 150, 153
Skinner, J. 50, 56, 58, 64, 66, 83, 93, 107, 112, 118, 125, 127, 135, 155
Sommer, B.D. 155
Sovran, T. 7, 9, 11, 74

Speiser, E.A. 46, 47, 49, 57, 59, 60, 86, 93, 94, 127
Spooren, W. 20
Stadler-Sutskover, T. 31
Stendebach, F.J. 56, 57, 69, 128
Sternberg, M. 33
Stol, M. 46, 47
Sutskover, T. 40, 116, 122, 158
Sweetser, E. 6, 11, 44

Talmon, S. 15, 76
Tomashevski, B. 33
Trier, J. 4
Turner, L.A. 66, 137

Ungerer, F. 1

Van Seters, J. 136, 138
Vaux, R. de 83
Ventola, E. 20
Viberg, A. 67
Vriezen, T.C. 135

Wallhead, C. 3, 10, 127, 142
Waltke, B.K. 81, 113
Walzel, O. 30
Weiner, A.B. 72
Wellhausen, J. 83, 135
Wenham, G.J. 86, 94, 96, 103, 104, 107, 110, 118, 125, 128, 135, 137
Westermann, C. 47, 49, 56-59, 64, 76, 83, 85, 95, 98, 103-107, 111, 112, 122, 136, 140, 175
White, H.C. 122, 125
Widdowson, H.G. 21
Wilson, L.S. 68
Wittgenstein, L. 11
Wolde, E.J. van 8, 95
Woude, A.S. van der 135
Wyatt, N. 67

Zadka, Y. 56
Zakovitch, Y. 69
Zohori, M. 61
Zucker, D.J. 108

www.ingramcontent.com/pod-product-compliance
Ingram Content Group UK Ltd.
Pitfield, Milton Keynes, MK11 3LW, UK
UKHW020843290926
15470UKWH00004B/1531

9 781907 534942